W9-DFP-128

TAILORING HEART FAILURE THERAPY

Edited by

Ronnie Willenheimer, MD, PhD
Associate Professor of Cardiology
Lund University
Head, Heart Failure Unit
Head, Echocardiography Unit
Head, Out-Patient Unit
Assistant Director, Department of Cardiology
University Hospital
Malmö
Sweden

Karl Swedberg, MD, PhD
Professor of Medicine
Göteborg University
Department of Medicine
Sahlgrenska University Hospital/Östra
Göteborg
Sweden

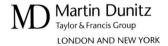
Martin Dunitz
Taylor & Francis Group
LONDON AND NEW YORK

© 2003 Martin Dunitz, an imprint of the Taylor & Francis Group plc

First published in the United Kingdom in 2003
by Martin Dunitz, an imprint of the Taylor and Francis Group plc,
11 New Fetter Lane, London EC4P 4EE

Tel.:   +44 (0) 20 7583 9855
Fax.:   +44 (0) 20 7842 2298
E-mail: info@dunitz.co.uk
Website: http://www.dunitz.co.uk

Although every effort has been made to ensure that all owners of copyright material
have been acknowledged in this publication, we would be glad to acknowledge in
subsequent reprints or editions any omissions brought to our attention.

A CIP record for this book is available from the British Library.

ISBN 1 84184 148 X

Distributed in the USA by
Fulfilment Center
Taylor & Francis
10650 Tobben Drive
Independence, KY 41051, USA
Toll Free Tel.: +1 800 634 7064
E-mail: taylorandfrancis@thomsonlearning.com

Distributed in Canada by
Taylor & Francis
74 Rolark Drive
Scarborough, Ontario M1R 4G2, Canada
Toll Free Tel.: +1 877 226 2237
E-mail: tal_fran@istar.ca

Distributed in the rest of the world by
Thomson Publishing Services
Cheriton House
North Way
Andover, Hampshire SP10 5BE, UK
Tel.: +44 (0)1264 332424
E-mail: salesorder.tandf@thomsonpublishingservices.co.uk

Composition by EXPO Holdings, Malaysia
Printed and bound in Great Britain by Biddles, Guildford and King's Lynn

Contents

Contributors

Wendy M Book MD
Assistant Professor
Emory University School of Medicine
Department of Medicine
Division of Cardiology
Atlanta GA, USA

A John Camm MD
Professor of Clinical Cardiology
Department of Cardiological Sciences
St George's Hospital Medical School
London, UK

Charles Cline MD PhD
Department of Cardiology
Malmö University Hospital
Malmö, Sweden

Kenneth Dickstein MD
Cardiology Department
Central Hospital in Rogaland
Stavanger, Norway

Barry H Greenberg MD
Professor of Medicine
Director, Heart Failure/Cardiac
Transplant Program
University of California San Diego
University of California San Diego
Medical Center
San Diego CA, USA

Anjan Gupta
Professor of Medicine
University of Bergen
Norway

Alborz Hassankhani MD PhD
Department of Medicine
Division of Cardiology
University of California San Diego
School of Medicine
San Diego CA, USA

Karen Hogg BN BSc MBChB
Clinical Research Initiative in Heart Failure
University of Glasgow
Glasgow, UK

Jeffrey D Hosenpud MD, FACC
Cardiovasular Associates LPD
Milwaukee WI, USA

Brenda J Hott MD
Emory University School of Medicine
Department of Medicine
Division of Cardiology
Atlanta GA, USA

Wei Jiang MD
Assistant Professor of Medicine
Assistant Professor of Psychiatry and
Behavioral Sciences
Duke University Medical Center
Durham NC, USA

Cord Manhenke MD
Cardiology Department
Central Hospital in Rogaland
Stavanger, Norway

John McMurray MD FRCP
Professor of Medical Cardiology
Honorary Consultant Cardiologist
Western Infirmary
Glasgow, UK

Christopher M O'Connor MD
Department of Medicine
Duke University Medical Center
Durham NC, USA

Jan Östergren MD PhD
Associate Professor
Department of Medicine
Karolinska Hospital
Stockholm, Sweden

Helen Oxenham MD
Research Fellow
Cardiovascular Research Department
University of Auckland
Auckland, New Zealand

Patrizia Presbitero MD
Chief Consultant in Interventional
Cardiology
Istituto Clinico Humanitas
Rozzano-Milano
Italy

Irina Savelieva MD
Department of Cardiological Sciences
St George's Hospital Medical School
London, UK

Neilander Sawhney MD
Department of Medicine
Division of Cardiology
University of California San Diego
School of Medicine
San Diego CA, USA

Norman Sharpe MD FRACP
Professor, Department of Medicine
University of Auckland
Auckland, New Zealand

Allan D Struthers MD
Professor of Cardiovascular Medicine and
Therapeutics
Department of Clinical Pharmacology and
Therapeutics
Ninewells Hospital and Medical School
Dundee, UK

Tullia Todros MD
Associate Professor of Obstetrics and
Gynecology
Maternal-Fetal Medicine Unit
University of Turin
Italy

Viola Vaccarino MD
Emory University School of Medicine
Department of Medicine
Division of Cardiology
Atlanta GA, USA

Clyde W Yancy MD
Associate Professor of Internal
Medicine/Cardiology
Medical Director, Heart Failure/
Cardiac Transplantation
University of Texas Southwestern Medical
Center
Director, Cardiovascular Institute
St Paul Medical Center
Dallas TX, USA

Preface

Chronic heart failure is a common and steadily increasing syndrome, afflicting around 2-3 % of the adult population in the industrialized world. The majority of patients with heart failure are elderly and their prognosis is poor. Adequate diagnostic measures, always including echocardiography, are a prerequisite for adequate treatment, which is imperative to improve morbidity and survival, as well as quality of life and physical function among these patients. The treatment of heart failure comprises non-pharmacological and pharmacological therapy and the latter, in particular, has developed dramatically over the last few years. Today, several classes of drugs have been convincingly shown to improve morbidity and survival in patients with chronic heart failure with left ventricular systolic dysfunction. Most of these drugs also improve quality of life and physical performance.

The aim of this book is to guide the treating physician in the daily choice of therapy to a wide range of categories of patients with chronic heart failure. Many of these categories are less well studied and the book focuses on how the treatment of chronic heart failure in these patients compares with the general treatment rule in chronic heart failure. The first chapter briefly outlines the general rule of treatment of chronic heart failure. The following chapters focus on the treatment of special categories of patients with chronic heart failure and heart failure patients with various concomitant diseases.

Ronnie Willenheimer, Malmö, Sweden
Karl Swedberg, Göteborg, Sweden

1

Modern treatment of chronic heart failure: the general rule

Ronnie Willenheimer and Karl Swedberg

Introduction

This chapter deals predominantly with the treatment of the 'general' patient with chronic heart failure. The present information on treatment is based almost exclusively on trials investigating patients with left ventricular systolic dysfunction, and the knowledge about the treatment of patients with heart failure with preserved left ventricular systolic function is very limited.

General measures

The chance of therapeutic success in chronic heart failure increases if the patient and the family are educated about the disease. This includes explaining the disease and its symptoms, the probable cause of heart failure, signs and symptoms that indicate worsening heart failure, therapeutic strategies, and the benefit of therapy. It is essential to inform the patient to avoid drugs that may worsen heart failure symptoms, such as nonsteroidal anti-inflammatory drugs (NSAIDs). The patient's active participation in the care is also important, including frequent body weight monitoring, smoking cessation, and modest alcohol use. The underlying disease(s) – such as coronary artery disease, hypertension, and diabetes – should always be adequately treated, and risk factors for atherosclerosis must obviously be carefully

modified. It is also important that the patient is properly immunized against influenza and pneumococcal disease.

Several randomized, controlled studies have shown that regular exercise training at a level suitable for the patients is valuable with regard to symptoms, physical function, and quality of life. There is some indication that exercise training might improve survival and decrease the need for heart failure hospitalization. The European Society of Cardiology recently published guidelines for exercise training in chronic heart failure.[1]

Pharmacological therapy

Diuretics (except spironolactone)

Diuretics have been shown to reduce symptoms and improve exercise capacity in patients with fluid overload. Also, in patients without clinical evidence of edema, but with excessively increased left ventricular filling pressures, diuretics may reduce symptoms. No clinical trials have been performed showing that diuretics improve prognosis in chronic heart failure, but a lifesaving effect in patients with severe fluid retention seems obvious. The consensus today is that diuretics should be used when the patient has fluid retention. However, it is debated whether diuretics can be avoided when the heart failure patient is stable without signs of fluid retention or overly increased filling pressures. It is recommended that the dose should be kept as low as possible. Diuretics increase neurohormonal activation, e.g. of the renin–angiotensin–aldosterone system, which is potentially harmful to the patient. Furthermore, electrolyte imbalance and a negative metabolic effect can be induced.

Thiazide diuretics are rarely used for the treatment of chronic heart failure, but may suffice in mild heart failure. Usually, loop diuretics such as furosemide are recommended. In patients with severe fluid retention not responding adequately to loop diuretics, metolazone is often more effective. However, particular caution should be exercised, since metolazone can induce severe disturbances in electrolyte and acid–base balance. If the patient responds insufficiently to a diuretic, it is usually more effective to use slow-release preparations, administer the total daily dosage on two or three occasions instead of one, or give the drug intravenously. The combination of a loop diuretic and a thiazide has a synergistic effect and is another way to increase the efficacy of diuretics. Sometimes the reason for a poor diuretic response is a low urine pH value with a clear increase in blood base excess, in which case a carbanhydrase inhibitor usually works well.

Since loop diuretics, thiazides, and metolazone generally cause a loss of electrolytes such as potassium and magnesium, they should never be used without proper protection against such losses. Potassium tablets alone are not adequate, since they do not protect against magnesium loss. Patients with chronic heart failure usually receive an angiotensin-converting enzyme (ACE) inhibitor, which often offers sufficient protection against electrolyte deficiency.

Angiotensin-converting enzyme inhibitors

Treatment with an ACE inhibitor constitutes first-line treatment in chronic heart failure. Several clinical trials in patients with chronic heart failure with left ventricular systolic dysfunction have shown that these agents improve survival and decrease the need for hospitalization due to worsening of heart failure.[2] Most clinical trials in this patient category have also shown that ACE inhibitors improve symptoms of heart failure[2,3] and exercise capacity,[3] whereas effects on quality of life have been less well-documented.[4] The clinical effects of ACE inhibitors develop after several weeks of treatment.

ACE inhibitors have also been shown to improve survival and morbidity in patients with asymptomatic left ventricular systolic dysfunction,[5,6] as well as in patients with established atherosclerotic disease without heart failure and with preserved left ventricular systolic function.[7] ACE inhibitors have not been investigated with regard to mortality and morbidity in patients with chronic heart failure with preserved left ventricular systolic function. However, in the light of all available information, the findings of the HOPE trial[7] can be translated to a recommendation to use ACE inhibitors in patients with chronic heart failure and preserved left ventricular systolic function who need treatment with diuretics.

ACE inhibitors should be initiated when the patient is clinically stable. However, they can be started even if the patient has some fluid retention and should then be combined with a diuretic. The initial dose should be low, and doubling of the dose by 1- or 2-week intervals, or more, is recommended. One should aim to titrate the ACE inhibitor to a target dose, as documented in the trials (Table 1.1). If the patient cannot tolerate the target dose, a low dose is most likely better than no ACE inhibitor at all. Electrolytes and creatinine should be monitored during titration. Symptoms of hypotension may limit the dose titration. A pronounced increase in serum creatinine (50% or more), especially if it is rapid, may be indicative of bilateral renal artery stenosis. In such cases the ACE inhibitor should be discontinued, the patient examined with regard to renal artery stenosis, and any stenosis properly treated to allow for ACE inhibitor treatment.

Caution should be exercised when initiating an ACE inhibitor in patients with renal dysfunction, hypotension, electrolyte imbalance, and in severely atherosclerotic patients. Significant aortic and mitral valve stenosis are considered contraindications to ACE inhibitor therapy, although this is based on theory rather than evidence.

Beta-blockers

Treatment with a beta-blocker is first-line treatment of patients with chronic heart failure with left ventricular systolic dysfunction. This therapy should be added to a background therapy with an ACE inhibitor unless there are any contraindications. Bisoprolol, metoprolol, and carvedilol have been documented to have beneficial effects in chronic heart failure.[8–10] Beta-blockade may be the most important principle for the treatment of chronic heart failure with left ventricular systolic dysfunction. This therapy, in addition to an ACE inhibitor, reduces mortality by a further 34–35%.[8–10] The effects on morbidity are equally impressive, and beta-blockers either have neutral or beneficial effects on exercise capacity and quality of life. The clinical benefit of a beta-blocker might not be evident until several weeks or months after initiation of therapy. Also, patients with left ventricular systolic dysfunction following an acute myocardial infarction have been shown to have a prognostic benefit from beta-blockade with carvedilol.[11]

Similar to ACE inhibitors, beta-blockers should be initiated when the patient is clinically stable. Although there is a long-term positive inotropic effect of beta-blockers, they have an initial negative inotropic effect. Due to this initial negative inotropic effect, they are not recommended for patients with clear fluid retention. The initial dose should be low, around 10–20% of the target dose, and may be doubled every 2–4 weeks. One should aim to titrate the beta-blocker to the target dose documented in clinical trials. Symptoms of hypotension and bradycardia

Drug	Initiating dose[†]	Target dose[†]
Captopril	6.25 mg t.i.d.	50 mg t.i.d.
Enalapril	2.5 mg b.i.d.	10 mg b.i.d.
Ramipril	1.25–2.5 mg b.i.d.	5 mg b.i.d.
Trandolapril	1 mg daily	4 mg daily

* Manufacturers' or regulatory recommendations.
† b.i.d. = twice a day; t.i.d. = three times a day.

Table 1.1 Recommended initiating* and target doses for ACE inhibitors with documented beneficial effects on survival and morbidity in patients with left ventricular systolic dysfunction with or without symptoms of heart failure

may limit the titration. Patients with chronic obstructive pulmonary disease often tolerate the highly beta$_1$-selective blockers bisoprolol and metoprolol.

Spironolactone

Despite adequate treatment with an ACE inhibitor, circulating aldosterone levels are often increased.[12] This observation could explain why the RALES (Randomized ALdactone Evaluation Study) trial demonstrated that the addition of a small dose of the aldosterone receptor antagonist spironolactone (mean dose 27 mg/day) to standard heart failure treatment, including an ACE inhibitor, substantially improved survival and decreased morbidity.[13] Patients in the RALES trial had a reduced left ventricular ejection fraction and pronounced symptoms of heart failure; 80% were in New York Heart Association (NYHA) class IV. Thus, this effect has not been shown in patients with modest symptoms and/or more preserved left ventricular systolic function. The 11% of the patients in RALES who received both a beta-blocker and an ACE inhibitor had just as much benefit from the addition of spironolactone as patients with only an ACE inhibitor. The average baseline dose of the ACE inhibitors used was less than the recommended target doses, which might have affected the result.

In the RALES trial, problems with hyperkalemia and gynecomastia were quite rare. However, these problems should not be underestimated in clinical practice. Hyperkalemia can sometimes arise after several weeks of spironolactone treatment. Painful gynecomastia may limit the use of spironolactone. The more specific aldosterone receptor antagonist eplerenone may be better tolerated in this respect, and its efficacy is currently being evaluated.

Angiotensin receptor blockers

Angiotensin receptor blockers (specific angiotensin type 1 receptor blockers, ARB), sometimes called angiotensin II antagonists, should be considered in patients who are intolerant to ACE inhibitors, usually due to cough. Trials conducted so far suggest that ARBs have an efficacy similar to ACE inhibitors on symptoms, whereas the effect on survival is yet uncertain.[14] In Val-HeFT (Valsartan Heart Failure Trial), the addition of the ARB valsartan to standard therapy for chronic systolic heart failure, including an ACE inhibitor, substantially reduced heart failure hospitalization but did not affect survival.[15] In patients on both an ACE inhibitor and a beta-blocker there was no benefit of valsartan and harm of this triple combination is presently not precluded. Therefore, ARBs may be recommended to patients with chronic heart failure who either cannot tolerate ACE inhibitors, beta-blockers, or both. An ongoing large trial (CHARM, Candesartan in Heart Failure – Assessment of Reduction in Mortality and Morbidity) will probably provide insight in this context.

ARBs should be titrated in a manner similar to ACE inhibitors, and the same precautions with regard to hypotension, hyperkalemia, and renal dysfunction should be taken.

Digitalis

Digitalis is considered indicated in patients with heart failure and atrial fibrillation to control heart rate and improve symptoms. The effect on survival is neutral, based on the findings of the DIG (Digitalis Investigation Group) trial.[16] In this trial, digoxin was compared with placebo on top of standard heart failure therapy, including an ACE inhibitor, in patients with chronic heart failure and sinus rhythm.[16] Digoxin had no effect on survival but reduced the need for heart failure hospitalization. However, the narrow therapeutic interval of digoxin leads to some problems, including additional hospitalizations due to digitalis intoxication. Largely based on this trial, digoxin is recommended to heart failure patients with left ventricular systolic dysfunction and sinus rhythm who have clear heart failure symptoms despite therapy with an ACE inhibitor, a beta-blocker, and spironolactone.

Antiarrhythmic agents (except beta-blockers)

There is no indication for prophylactic treatment with an antiarrhythmic agent in chronic heart failure. Amiodarone is the only antiarrhythmic drug that has been convincingly shown to be safe for antiarrhythmic use in patients with chronic heart failure. Dofetilide, another class III antiarrhythmic agent, has also been reported to have a neutral effect on mortality and a beneficial effect on heart failure hospitalization in patients with chronic heart failure and left ventricular systolic dysfunction.[17] The safety of class I antiarrhythmic agents is questionable in patients with heart failure and left ventricular systolic dysfunction.

Positive inotropic agents

In patients with severely symptomatic heart failure, positive inotropic agents may improve symptoms of heart failure, exercise capacity, and left ventricular systolic function. However, the prognostic effects of phosphodiesterase inhibitors (e.g. milrinone, amrinone) and beta$_1$-agonists (e.g. dobutamine) given as intermittent intravenous support is largely unknown and appears to be negative. By oral administration, these agents have convincingly been shown to decrease survival and are therefore not recommended for long-term treatment. According to preliminary data, the calcium sensitizer levosimendan is safe when administered as a single intravenous infusion for 24 hours to patients with acute worsening of heart failure,[18] or acute heart failure after acute myocardial infarction.[19] The infusion was associated with a clear reduction in symptoms of heart failure and the effect on survival appears to be better than that of dobutamine.

Calcium channel blockers

Calcium channel blockers are not to be considered for treatment of chronic heart failure. Sometimes it is necessary to give a calcium channel blocker to a patient with chronic heart failure due to angina pectoris or hypertension. Among calcium channel blockers, only amlodipine has been convincingly shown to be safe for use in patients with heart failure with left ventricular systolic dysfunction,[20,21] although other highly vascular-selective agents such as felodipine are probably safe.

Antithrombotic agents

Guidelines generally recommend the use of warfarin in patients with chronic heart failure and atrial fibrillation due to beneficial effects on thromboembolic complications. There is no evidence from prospective trials that any antithrombotic or anticoagulant agents are beneficial in patients with chronic heart failure without atrial fibrillation. The effects of anticoagulants on survival in patients with chronic heart failure are largely unknown, although there are some retrospective analyses that indicate the benefit of warfarin. It has been argued that acetyl salicylic acid may interact with diuretics and ACE inhibitors in patients with chronic heart failure, but retrospective analysis shows no such interaction with regard to survival and morbidity.[22]

Surgical therapy

Implantable cardioverter–defibrillator therapy

The role of implantable cardioverter–defibrillator (ICD) devices in patients with chronic heart failure is not clear, although promising.[23] Although trials in high-risk patients with coronary artery disease and left ventricular systolic dysfunction have shown a survival benefit of an ICD, the role of ICD in chronic heart failure is not yet defined.

Revascularization therapy

There is no evidence that revascularization therapy improves prognosis in chronic heart failure in general. However, a systematic overview shows that coronary bypass surgery improves survival in patients with chronic heart failure and limiting angina.[24] In patients with chronic heart failure who have hibernating myocardium, i.e. myocardium that is viable but non-contracting, revascularization may improve left ventricular systolic function.[25] Unless revascularization therapy is considered on the grounds of ischemic symptoms, demonstration of myocardial contractile reserve seems essential for a beneficial outcome of revascularization therapy.

Valvular surgery

Correction of significant primary valvular disease may improve symptoms in selected patients. Observational studies have shown that surgical correction of mitral regurgitation secondary to left ventricular dilatation is beneficial with regard to symptoms and physical function.[26]

Cardiac resynchronization therapy

Cardiac resynchronization therapy using biventricular pacing has been tested in a subset of patients with chronic heart failure who have intraventricular conduction delays with asynchronous contraction of the ventricles. Recent short-term studies have shown beneficial effects on symptoms and submaximal exercise capacity. The prognostic effect of this treatment is currently being investigated.

Ventricular assist devices and artificial hearts

Ventricular assist devices and artificial hearts are used as a bridge to heart transplantation and during recovery of cardiac function in patients with acute myocarditis. The long-term prognostic benefit of such therapy is unclear at present. In one randomized trial in patients with advanced heart failure not considered for heart transplantation, the one-year survival was significantly improved compared to optimal medical therapy, from 25% to 52%.[27] The two-year survival was not significantly better with a left ventricular assist device. More complications, mainly infections, were associated with the device. The treatment is associated with considerable costs and its place in the treatment of advanced heart failure is not clear.

Heart transplantation

No controlled trials have examined the value of heart transplantation; however, it is considered to improve survival, morbidity, exercise capacity, and quality of life in patients with end-stage heart failure. The 5-year survival after heart transplant is approximately 70%.[28] The shortage of donor hearts, the consequences of the immunosuppressive therapy, and the intense follow-up have dictated the many contraindications.

Prevention of heart failure

Despite the best-available treatment, the prognosis of chronic heart failure is dismal; therefore, there is reason to prevent the development of symptomatic heart failure. It has been shown that treatment of asymptomatic left ventricular systolic dysfunction by ACE inhibition[5,6] and beta-blockade[11] can delay the onset of heart failure and improve survival. Also, ACE inhibition given to patients with atherosclerotic disease without left ventricular systolic dysfunction or heart failure symptoms was shown to delay the onset of heart failure and to improve survival.[7] In general, intervention trials in hypertension show that effective antihypertensive therapy has a greater impact on the development of heart failure than on any other clinical endpoint. Recently, RENAAL (Losartan Renal Protection Study) showed that therapy with the ARB losartan compared with placebo in patients with type 2 diabetes and renal insufficiency, almost all of whom had hypertension, substantially decreased a first hospitalization for heart failure, on top of standard therapy.[29] ACE inhibition given to patients with diabetes seems to have a preventive effect similar to that shown in patients with atherosclerotic disease.[7] Simvastatin has been shown to delay the onset of heart failure in patients with coronary artery disease and increased plasma cholesterol levels.[30]

Thus, by adequately treating the main precursors of chronic heart failure – coronary artery disease, hypertension, and diabetes – prevention of heart failure may be achieved. Modern treatment of chronic heart failure is prevention of heart failure.

References

1. Working Group on Cardiac Rehabilitation & Exercice Physiology and Working Group on Heart Failure of the European Society of Cardiology. Recommendations for exercise training in chronic heart failure patients. Eur Heart J 2001; 22:125–35.
2. Garg R, Yusuf S. Overview of randomized trials of angiotensin-converting enzyme inhibitors on mortality and morbidity in patients with heart failure. Collaborative Group on ACE Inhibitor Trials. JAMA 1995; 273:1450–6.
3. Narang R, Swedberg K, Cleland JG. What is the ideal study design for evaluation of treatment for heart failure? Insights from trials assessing the effect of ACE inhibitors on exercise capacity. Eur Heart J 1996; 17:120–34.
4. Wolfel EE. Effects of ACE inhibitor therapy on quality of life in patients with heart failure. Pharmacotherapy 1998; 18:1323–34.
5. The SOLVD investigators. Effect of enalapril on mortality and the development of heart failure in asymptomatic patients with reduced left ventricular ejection fractions. N Engl J Med 1992; 327:685–91.
6. Pfeffer MA, Braunwald E, Moyé LA, et al. Effect of captopril on mortality and morbidity in patients with left ventricular dysfunction after myocardial infarction. Results of the survival and ventricular enlargement trial. N Engl J Med 1992; 327:669–77.
7. Yusuf S, Sleight P, Pogue J, et al. Effects of an angiotensin-converting-enzyme inhibitor, ramipril, on

cardiovascular events in high-risk patients. The Heart Outcomes Prevention Evaluation Study Investigators. N Engl J Med 2000; 342:145–53.

8. CIBIS-II Investigators and Committees. The Cardiac Insufficiency Bisoprolol Study II (CIBIS-II): a randomised trial. Lancet 1999; 353:9–13.

9. MERIT-HF Study Group. Effect of metoprolol CR/XL in chronic heart failure: Metoprolol CR/XL Randomised Intervention Trial in Congestive Heart Failure (MERIT-HF). Lancet 1999; 353:2001–7.

10. Packer M, Coats AJ, Fowler MB, et al. Effect of carvedilol on survival in severe chronic heart failure. N Engl J Med 2001; 344:1651–8.

11. Dargie HJ. Effect of carvedilol on outcome after myocardial infarction in patients with left-ventricular dysfunction: the CAPRICORN randomised trial. Lancet 2001; 357:1385–90.

12. MacFadyen RJ, Lee AF, Morton JJ, et al. How often are angiotensin II and aldosterone concentrations raised during chronic ACE inhibitor treatment in cardiac failure? Heart 1999; 82:57–61.

13. Pitt B, Zannad F, Remme WJ, et al. The effect of spironolactone on morbidity and mortality in patients with severe heart failure. Randomized Aldactone Evaluation Study Investigators. N Engl J Med 1999; 341:709–17.

14. Pitt B, Poole-Wilson PA, Segal R, et al. Effect of losartan compared with captopril on mortality in patients with symptomatic heart failure: randomized trial – the Losartan Heart Failure Survival Study ELITE II. Lancet 2000; 355:1582–7.

15. Cohn JN, Tognoni G, for the Valsartan Heart Failure Trial Investigators. A randomized trial of the angiotensin-receptor blocker valsartan in chronic heart failure. N Engl J Med 2001; 345:1667–75.

16. The Digitalis Investigation Group. The effect of digoxin on mortality and morbidity in patients with heart failure. N Engl J Med 1997; 336:525–33.

17. Torp-Pedersen C, Møller M, Bloch-Thomsen PE, et al. Dofetilide in patients with congestive heart failure and left ventricular dysfunction. Danish Investigations of Arrhythmia and Mortality on Dofetilide Study Group. N Engl J Med 1999; 341:857–65.

18. Jones CG, Cleland JG. Meeting report – the LIDO, HOPE, MOXCON and WASH studies. Heart Outcomes Prevention Evaluation. The Warfarin/Aspirin Study of Heart Failure. Eur J Heart Fail 1999; 1:425–31.

19. Gomes UC, Cleland JG. Heart failure update. Eur J Heart Fail 1999; 1:301–2.

20. Packer M, O'Connor CM, Ghali JK, et al. Effect of amlodipine on morbidity and mortality in severe chronic heart failure. Prospective Randomized Amlodipine Survival Evaluation Study Group. N Engl J Med 1996; 335:1107–14.

21. Thackray S, Witte K, Clark AL, et al. Clinical trials update: OPTIME-CHF, PRAISE-2, ALLHAT. Eur J Heart Fail 2000; 2:209–12.

22. Flather MD, Yusuf S, Køber L, et al. Long-term ACE-inhibitor therapy in patients with heart failure of left-ventricular dysfunction: a systematic overview of data from individual patients. Lancet 2000; 355:1575–81.

23. Hsia HH, Jessup ML, Marchlinski FE. Debate: Do all patients with heart failure require implantable defibrillators to prevent sudden death? Curr Control Trials Cardiovasc Med 2000; 1:98–101.

24. Baker DW, Jones R, Hodges J, et al. Management of heart failure. III. The role of revascularization in the treatment of patients with moderate or severe left ventricular systolic dysfunction. JAMA 1994; 272:1528–34.

25. La Canna G, Alfieri O, Giubbini R, et al. Echocardiography during infusion of dobutamine for identification of reversible dysfunction in patients with chronic coronary artery disease. J Am Coll Cardiol 1994; 23:617–26.

26. Bolling SF, Pagani FD, Deeb GM, et al. Intermediate-term outcome of mitral reconstruction in cardiomyopathy. J Thorac Cardiovasc Surg 1998; 115:381–6.

27. Rose EA, Gelijns AC, Moskowitz AJ, et al. Randomized Evaluation of Mechanical Assistance for the Treatment of Congestive Heart Failure (REMATCH) Study Group. N Engl J Med 2001; 345:1435–43.

28. Bennett LE, Keck BM, Daily OP, et al. Worldwide thoracic organ transplantation: a report from the UNOS/ISHLT International Registry for Thoracic Organ Transplantation. Clin Transpl 2000:31–44.

29. Brenner BM, Cooper ME, de Zeeuw D, et al. RENAAL Study Investigators. Effects of losartan on renal and cardiovascular outcomes in patients with type 2 diabetes and nephropathy. N Engl J Med 2001; 345:910–2.

30. Kjekshus J, Pedersen TR, Olsson AG, et al. The effects of simvastatin on the incidence of heart failure in patients with coronary heart disease. J Card Fail 1997; 3:249–54.

2

Tailoring of neurohormonal modulating therapy in chronic heart failure

Allan D Struthers

Neurohormonal modulation in chronic heart failure

The strategy which has so far proved to be the most successful in the treatment of patients with chronic heart failure is neurohormonal modulation.

Angiotensin-converting enzyme inhibition

This era began with the CONSENSUS I trial showing the enormous benefits of giving enalapril to grade IV patients.[1] Innumerable multicenter trials confirmed this idea. The Studies of Left Ventricular Dysfunction (SOLVD)[2] and the Survival and Ventricular Enlargement (SAVE)[3] trials were the next to show the benefits of angiotensin-converting enzyme (ACE) inhibition. These were followed by the Acute Infarction Ramipril Efficacy (AIRE) study,[4] the Trandolapril Cardiac Eval-uation (TRACE)[5] study and the Survival of Myocardial Infarction Long Term Evaluation (SMILE)[6] study. A recent meta-analysis showed that ACE inhibitors improve total mortality by 20% in patients with left ventricular systolic dysfunction.[7]

Beta-blockade

The next therapy to be shown to yield unequiv-ocal benefit in chronic heart failure was beta-

blocker therapy. This was first found in the US Carvedilol Trials[8] and was confirmed by the Cardiac Insufficiency Bisoprolol Study II (CIBIS II),[9] the Metoprolol Intervention Trials (MERIT)[10] and more recently by COPERNI-CUS[11] and CAPRICORN.[12] Only one such trial, the Beta Blocker Evaluation of Survival Trial (BEST) did not seem to confirm this effect.[13] The additional survival benefit due to beta-blockers added to an ACE inhibitor seems to be larger than that of ACE inhibitors com-pared with placebo, i.e. approximately 35% mortality reduction for beta-blockers.[9,10]

Aldosterone receptor blockade

The third neurohormonal strategy which was found to produce benefit was aldosterone block-ade, i.e. spironolactone. In the Randomised Aldactone Evaluation Study (RALES), spirono-lactone on top of ACE inhibition reduced mor-tality by 30%.[14] Although there is only one trial showing this, the RALES results are definitive and backed up by a lot of mechanistic data showing that aldosterone escape is common and that aldosterone is a major cardiovascular culprit in itself. However, it is worth mentioning that at baseline the doses of the ACE inhibitors used in RALES were somewhat suboptimal.

Angiotensin receptor blockade

The fourth neuroendocrine strategy involves the angiotensin type 1-receptor blockers

(ARBs). Here, for once, the data for neuroendocrine blockade are not as promising. In the Evaluation of Losartan in the Elderly 2 (ELITE 2) trial,[15] losartan and captopril were probably equivalent as monotherapy. In the Randomized Evaluation of Strategies of LV Dysfunction (RESOLVD), adding candesartan to enalapril produced further neurohormonal blockade but no benefit with regard to mortality or morbidity, although it was not designed to assess the latter.[16] In the Valsartan Heart Failure Trial (Val-HeFT),[17] valsartan added to an ACE inhibitor certainly reduced hospitalizations but had no effect whatsoever on mortality. In Val-HeFT, subgroup analysis suggests that chronic heart failure patients who are already on beta-blockade at randomization may do better if they remain on the ACE inhibitor and beta-blocker rather than have an ARB added to this combination. This could be the first sign that endless sequential neuroendocrine blockade may not be the correct way to go. Perhaps there is a limit to the amount of neuroendocrine blockade that should be employed.

Current guideline recommendations

How have guidelines reacted to the above information? Guidelines suggest that all chronic heart failure patients should be tried on ACE inhibitors and beta-blockers unless there are any contraindications.[18] Guidelines also suggest spironolactone should be initiated in moderate-to-severe chronic heart failure.

With regard to ARBs, it is suggested that they be used in patients who are intolerant to ACE inhibitors, especially if the intolerance is due to cough. ARBs are also recommended in chronic heart failure patients on ACE inhibitor therapy who are intolerant of beta-blocker therapy. In general, therefore, guidelines suggest that ACE inhibitors and beta-blockers are used in nearly all chronic heart failure patients, with spironolactone being added in all moderate-to-severe chronic heart failure cases. ARBs are recommended in both ACE-inhibitor-intolerant patients and beta-blocker-intolerant patients.

Tailoring heart failure therapy
What do trial results mean to the individual?

The above response is perfectly legitimate with regard to what was found in the large multicenter trials. However, one must always bear in mind that the result of any trial reflects the mean effect of the intervention in the respective study population and that the response in an individual may range from exceptional efficacy to neutral effects or even to harm. Subgroup analysis is often undertaken to try to identify patient subgroups who either benefited particularly or who had no benefit, or were even harmed. Although such subgroup analysis can be helpful, the subgroups often become too small for the subgroup result to be definitive. Furthermore, statisticians are often uneasy about trawling through datasets too much as, inevitably, chance can lead to spurious positive findings. Therefore, it can be hard to identify responders versus nonresponders within the results of a multicenter trial. Another way to express the same feeling is that, once completed, the entry criteria for each trial unfortunately become a bit of a straitjacket for future clinical practice. That is, those patients who fulfil the entry criteria are given the new therapy even if a subgroup of them actually comes to harm, whereas all patients who just missed the entry criteria are denied the therapy even if they may well benefit. For example, the SAVE trial used an entry criterion of a left ventricular ejection fraction 40% or less. This meant that patients with left ventricular ejection fractions of 42% would be denied ACE inhibitor therapy, even although it is now recognized that formal left ventricular ejection fraction measurement is not the ideal way to choose patients in routine practice.

Problems with polypharmacy

Side effects

Another problem arising from these trials is that each new neuroendocrine inhibiting therapy further reduces the already low blood pressure of chronic heart failure patients. It is already the case that a low blood pressure is a limiting factor in being able to give full neuroendocrine inhibition therapy to all patients. This problem is likely to get even worse in the future as many of the new therapeutic advances on the horizon also reduce the blood pressure further, e.g. endothelin antagonists, neutral endopeptidase inhibitors. Yet another problem with all this neuroendocrine-inhibiting polypharmacy is that compliance/adherence with medication generally becomes worse as more and more drugs are employed. This is likely to be the case even more in chronic heart failure where patients are elderly and where they are probably already taking many non-neuroendocrine modulating therapies such as furosemide, aspirin and statins as well as therapy for their many comorbid conditions such as arthritis and chronic obstructive pulmonary disease.

Possible interactions

A further key problem is that some of these neuroendocrine blocking therapies may not actually go well together. The best example is the idea of combining an ACE inhibitor, a beta-blocker, and an ARB, as subgroup analysis of Val-HeFT raises the possibility that such a combination may produce more harm than good. The reason

for such an adverse interaction (if there is one) is unknown. It may even simply be chance, especially, as in RALES, patients on beta-blockers did particularly well with spironolactone therapy and it is hard to envisage why ARBs and spironolactone should have diametrically oppos- ite effects in beta-blocked patients.

Possible benefits of tailored therapy

The above problems have led to the new idea that neuroendocrine inhibiting therapy ought to be targeted better to those who are known to benefit most, so that one is able to avoid unnecessary hypotension, unnecessary nonadherence, and unnecessary adverse drug interactions. In addition, such targeting might well reduce total drug costs if some drugs are truly superfluous.

In theory, better targeting or tailoring of therapy is obviously always desirable. The real question is whether there are means available or not to perform this better targeting. It is also worth saying that targeting does not simply mean whether the drug is prescribed or not. It also applies to the height of the dose of the drug used in an individual patient. Some patients may need larger doses to achieve the same target effect as in other patients.

Means to tailor neuroendocrine inhibiting therapy

Three possibilities arise (Table 2.1).

| 1. Specific plasma hormone levels |
| 2. Specific gene polymorphisms |
| 3. Plasma brain natriuretic peptide (BNP) as general guide |

Table 2.1 Ways of targeting neuroendocrine inhibiting therapy

Assess neurohormonal activation

The first, obvious, method of targeting neuroendocrine inhibiting therapy would be to measure plasma neurohormone levels and to target neuroendocrine inhibition in those patients with high hormone levels. This strategy is backed up with a limited amount of data. Lim et al.[19] showed that only those with high plasma renin levels appeared to retain sodium if their ACE inhibitor therapy was stopped. Data from the CONSENSUS I trial similarly suggest that ACE inhibitors improve mortality mainly in those with neuroendocrine activation.[1] A similar picture was seen in V-HeFT 2 for high versus low renin.[20]

One potential problem with such a strategy is that it may really be tissue hormone levels that matter rather than plasma hormone levels. Plasma and tissue levels may be dissociated and it would be very difficult if not impossible to sample tissues in routine clinical practice.

A second problem with this strategy is that, although patients with high hormone levels may be the ones who benefit the most, they are very likely to also be the ones who get the most side effects, especially hypotension. Hence one of the main rationales for targeting neuroendocrine therapy (i.e. avoidance of side effects) may not work in practice. Of course this does raise a wider issue for all of clinical medicine, which is that trying to target a drug's benefits at the same time as avoiding its side effects may be a forlorn hope, as benefits and side effects may well usually track together. One example of this is that in RALES, patients on digoxin get more benefit from spironolactone in terms of mortality reduction than those not on digoxin, yet patients on digoxin and spironolactone also get more gynecomastia than those on spironolactone but not on digoxin.[14]

Assess gene polymorphisms

The second possible means of targeting such therapy would be to tailor therapy by assessing an individual's relevant gene polymorphisms. As yet, there are no data exploring this concept. Its advantage might be that it could represent an indirect way of assessing tissue hormonal activation without having to biopsy inaccessible tissues. Its disadvantage is that it would not circumvent the problem that drug benefits and drug side effects might track together.

The role of brain natriuretic peptide

A third possibility is to use plasma brain natriuretic peptide (BNP) levels in the same way as a diabetologist uses HbAlc levels to decide if diabetic control is adequate or not. In chronic heart failure, BNP could be used to guide how intense the neuroendocrine inhibition should be in each individual patient. The value of such an approach has recently been demonstrated by Troughton et al.,[21] who found that treatment guided by BNP resulted in fewer cardiovascular events than did treatment guided by standard clinical assessment. However, it must be emphasized that Troughton et al. had already initiated standard neuroendocrine inhibitory therapy in all patients and, therefore, although the study supports the overall principle of using BNP to guide therapy, it cannot be taken as evidence to withhold ACE inhibitors or beta-blockers in certain individuals.

Tailoring therapy: the ethical dilemma

The main problem facing the idea of tailoring therapy is that it is now ethically difficult to withhold ACE inhibitors or beta-blockers from any chronic heart failure patient. This makes it difficult to conduct the clinical research that would be needed to advance the idea that some patients do not need ACE inhibitors or beta-blockers. This illustrates a further 'problem' with multicenter randomized controlled trial results, which is that they make a permanent irreversible imprint on what research can ethically be done in the future. However, the problem of polypharmacy and hypotension is becoming so great that all future therapies should be investigated with regard to their better targeting.

In that regard, one could say that our hand was only now being forced to address this issue but address this issue we must, as we have clearly reached the limit of 'all drugs for all patients' in chronic heart failure. There is a particular opportunity now to address the question of which patients should get ARB therapy (on top of ACE inhibitor therapy), because Val-HeFT raises the possibility that not all patients with chronic heart failure necessarily benefit from ARB therapy. Studies should now be undertaken to see if ARB therapy should be given on the basis of plasma angiotensin II levels, angiotensin gene polymorphisms, plasma BNP levels, or even simple clinical criteria.

Tailoring therapy today

In the meantime, is there any tailoring of therapy that we should do now? My own opinion is that all chronic heart failure patients should be given a trial of ACE inhibitor and beta-blocker (plus spironolactone if their disease is severe). The doses of the ACE inhibitor and the beta-blocker should be those used in the main trials. If side effects (hypotension) prevent the ACE inhibitor and/or the beta-blocker being used at the full trial doses, my view is that the patient is better off on multiple therapy at less than full dose rather than being on full dose of one drug and none of the other. There is little evidence to back up this view except that in ATLAS,[22] the benefit of increasing the lisinopril dose to a high dose was substantially less than the benefit seen when a beta-blocker was added in CIBIS 2 and MERIT.

If patients are able to tolerate the full trial doses of ACE inhibitor, beta-blocker, and spironolactone, I would predict that we will in the future use plasma BNP to decide which patients should receive even more therapy. Those with a remaining high BNP level despite apparently optimum therapy may well in the future be given either higher doses of diuretics, or higher than trial doses of ACE inhibitors, beta-blockers, or spironolactone, or alternatively, have an ARB added. Research will need to be undertaken to explore these various possibilities.

References

1. Swedberg K, Eneroth P Kjekshus J, Snapinn S. Effects of enalapril and neuroendocrine activation on prognosis in severe congestive heart failure (follow-up of the CONSENSUS trial). CONSENSUS Trial Study Group. Am J Cardiol 1990; 66:40–4D.
2. Effect of enalapril on mortality and the development of heart failure in asymptomatic patients with reduced left ventricular ejection fractions. The SOLVD Investigators. N Engl J Med 1992; 327:685–91.
3. Pfeffer MA, Braunwald E, Moyé LA, et al. Effect of captopril on mortality and morbidity in patients with left ventricular dysfunction after myocardial infarction. Results of the survival and ventricular enlargement trial. N Engl J Med 1992; 327:669–77.
4. The Acute Infarction Ramipril Efficacy (AIRE) Study Investigators. Effect of ramipril on mortality and morbidity of survivors of acute myocardial infarction with clinical evidence of heart failure. Lancet 1993; 342:821–8.

5. Køber L, Torp-Pedersen C, Carlsen JE, et al. A clinical trial of the angiotensin-converting-enzyme inhibitor trandolapril in patients after myocardial infarction. Trandolapril cardiac evaluation (TRACE) study group. N Engl J Med 1995; 333:1670–6.

6. Ambrosioni E, Borghi C, Magnani B. The effect of the ACE inhibitor, zofenopril on mortality and morbidity after anterior myocardial infarction. The Survival of Myocardial Infarction Long Term Evaluation (SMILE) Study investigators. N Engl J Med 1995; 332:80–5.

7. Flather MD, Yusuf S, Køber L, et al. Long-term ACE-inhibitor therapy in patients with heart failure or left-ventricular dysfunction: a systematic overview of data from individual patients. Lancet 2000; 355:1575–81.

8. Packer M, Bristow MR, Cohn JN, for the US Carvedilol Heart Failure Study Group. The effect of carvedilol on morbidity and mortality in patients with chronic heart failure. N Engl J Med 1996; 334:1349–55.

9. The Cardiac Insufficiency Bisoprolol Study II (CIBIS-II): a randomised trial. Lancet 1999; 353:9–13.

10. Effect of Metoprolol CR/XL in chronic heart failure: Metoprolol CR/XL Randomised Intervention Trials in Congestive Heart Failure (MERIT-HF). Lancet 1999; 353:2001–7.

11. Packer M, Coats AJS, Fowler MB, et al. Effect of carvedilol on survival in severe chronic heart failure. N Engl J Med 2001; 344:1651–8.

12. Dargie HJ. Effect of carvedilol on outcome after myocardial infarction in patients with left ventricular dysfunction: the CAPRICORN randomised trial. Lancet 2001; 357:1385–90.

13. The BEST Investigators. A trial of the beta blocker bucindolol in patients with advanced chronic heart failure. N Engl J Med 2001; 344:1659–67.

14. Pitt B, Zannad F, Remme WJ, et al. The effect of spironolactone on morbidity and mortality in patients with severe heart failure. Randomized Aldactone Evaluation Study Investigators. N Engl J Med 1999; 341:709–17.

15. Pitt B, Poole-Wilson PA, Segal R, et al. Effect of losartan compared with captopril on mortality in patients with symptomatic heart failure: randomized trial – the Losartan Heart Failure Survival Study ELITE II. Lancet 2000; 355:1582–7.

16. McKelvie RS, Yusuf S, Pericak D, et al. Comparison of candesartan, enalapril, and their combination in congestive heart failure: randomized evaluation of strategies for left ventricular dysfunction (RESOLVD) pilot study. The RESOLVD Pilot Study Investigators. Circulation 1999; 100:1056–64.

17. Val-HeFT

18. Task Force for Diagnosis and Treatment of Chronic Heart Failure. Guidelines for the diagnosis and treatment of chronic heart failure. Eur Heart J 2001; 22:1527–60.

19. Lim PO, MacFadyen RJ, Struthers AD. Is there a role for renin profiling in selecting chronic heart failure patients for ACE inhibitor treatment? Heart 2000; 83:257–61.

20. Francis GS, Cohn JN, Johnson G, et al. Plasma norepinephrine, plasma renin activity, and congestive heart failure. Relations to survival and the effects of therapy in V-HeFT II. The V-HeFT VA Cooperative Studies Group. Circulation 1993; 87:VI,40–8.

21. Troughton RW, Frampton CM, Yandle TG, et al. Treatment of heart failure guided by plasma aminoterminal brain natriuretic peptide (N-BNP) concentrations. Lancet 2000; 355:1126–30.

22. Packer M, Poole-Wilson PA, Armstrong PW, et al. Comparative effects of low and high doses of the angiotensin-converting enzyme inhibitor, lisinopril, on morbidity and mortality in chronic heart failure. ATLAS Study Group. Circulation 1999; 100:2312–8.

3

Heart failure in the elderly
Charles Cline

Introduction

The prevalence of chronic heart failure has increased dramatically over the past two decades, an increase that has been described as epidemic.[1] A major contributor to this increase is the growing proportion of elderly in the population, heart failure being to a large extent a disease of old age. The prevalence of heart failure approximately doubles with each decade from the age of 50 years.[2] United Nations statistics show that in developed countries 22% of the population were older than 60 years in the year 2000.[3] This number is projected to increase 30% by the year 2020. Worldwide, approximately 10% of the population are currently 60 years or more. This proportion is expected to double during the next 50 years and in the next 150 years time it will have increased even further to one in three.[4] At the same time the elderly population is itself aging.

Heart failure is associated with significantly reduced quality of life and a high level of morbidity and mortality.[5–7] It has been shown to be the most common cause of hospitalization in the elderly, and hospitalization is the primary determinant of costs for the management of heart failure.[8] Heart failure accounts for 2–3% of the total health care budget in developed countries and, as such, is one of the major sources of health care expenditure. Thus, heart failure in the elderly emerges as an area in need of acute attention from a humanitarian and also from an economic perspective.

Epidemiology

The incidence and prevalence of chronic heart failure in relation to age varies in epidemiologic studies. This is due to a number of factors, such as selection of the study population, criteria for heart failure diagnosis, methods used to establish diagnosis, and possible true differences between geographic or ethnic populations.

The Framingham Study reported that the annual incidence of heart failure was 11 per 1000 in men and 9 per 1000 in women aged 65–94 years.[9] This incidence was approximately four times that found in persons under the age of 65 years.[10] A Swedish study recently reported that the incidence of heart failure was 11.5 per 1000 in the age group 75–79 years.[11] This was more than fivefold higher than in those aged 55–54 years. A study of the incidence of heart failure in Olmsted Country, Minnesota showed that 88% of incident cases were 65 years or older and nearly half (49%) were 80 years or older.[12]

Analysis of 34 years of follow-up of the Framingham Study cohort found the prevalence of heart failure to be approximately 10% among persons in their eighties, a 10-fold increase compared with persons in their fifties.[13] In Sweden, Eriksson and et al. found a sixfold increase to 13% in a cohort of men aged 67 years compared with men aged 50 years.[14] In Scotland, McDonagh et al. studied a relatively young population aged 25–74. Nonetheless, they noted that the prevalence of heart failure in combination with left ventricular systolic dysfunction was 3.2% in men aged 65–74 years and 3.6% in women aged 65–74 years, more than double the prevalence in the age group 45–54 years.[15] A study in Rotterdam found that the prevalence of heart failure increased from about 1% in the age group 55–64 years to 13% in 75–84 year olds.[16] Similarly, it has been reported from the Heart of England study that the prevalence of definite heart failure was 2.3% among subjects 45–54 years of age but increased to 3.1% in those 85 years or older.[17]

Etiology

Although the etiology of heart failure varies somewhat between different studies, with regard to relative proportions, coronary heart disease and hypertension have been found to be the two most common conditions predating the onset of heart failure.[18,19] Some investigators state that coronary heart disease and hypertension are responsible for more than half of all cases of heart failure. Cowie et al. reported that coronary artery disease was the cause of more than half of incident cases of heart failure.[20] They concluded that clinical assessment without coronary angiography underestimated the proportion of patients with coronary artery disease, which may in part explain some of the variation seen in different studies. Further, the risk of developing heart failure following myocardial infarction increases with age and appears double in those aged 75–80 years compared with younger patients.[21,22] Age, itself, is an independent predictor of the development of heart failure after myocardial infarction. Diabetes also predisposes for the development of heart failure in the elderly and was, in one study, associated with a 30% increased risk of developing heart failure over a 3–4-year period.

Therapy

Angiotensin-converting enzyme inhibitors

Angiotensin-converting enzyme (ACE) inhibitors are recommended as first-line therapy for heart failure in patients with impaired left ventricular systolic function expressed as reduced ejection fraction, i.e. <40–45%.[23,24] In general, ACE inhibitors should be uptitrated to the dosages shown to be effective in large controlled trials in heart failure and not titrated based on symptomatic improvement alone.[25] ACE inhibitors have been shown to significantly reduce morbidity and mortality, as well as hospitalization, in patients with moderate-to-severe heart failure due to left ventricular systolic dysfunction.[25–28] ACE inhibitors should be given first but in patients with volume overload or signs of fluid retention, together with diuretics.[23,24]

The mean age of patients in heart failure mortality trials, as shown in Table 3.1, has tended to be lower than in clinical practice, in which as many as 78% have been reported to be 65 years or older.[29] The Co-operative North Scandinavian Enalapril Survival Study (CONSENSUS) was the first to show that an ACE inhibitor, enalapril, reduced mortality compared with placebo in patients with severe heart failure.[26] The mean age of patients was relatively high, 70–71 years. In comparison, the mean age of patients in other major trials of ACE inhibitors in heart failure was 60–64 years.[25,27,28]

Is there then data to support the use of ACE inhibition in the elderly and are ACE inhibitors tolerated in elderly patients? Reliable information on the risk–benefit ratio can be derived by use of data from individuals in each trial compared using a meta-analysis based on published data. Recently, a collaborative overview was published which sought to estimate the overall effect (on deaths, admissions for heart failure, and reinfarction) and risks of ACE inhibitors in clinically important subgroups, including elderly heart failure patients.[30] The overview included patients with heart failure or left ventricular systolic dysfunction following myocardial infarction,[31–33] as well as patients in the Study of Left Ventricular Dysfunction (SOLVD) prevention trial.[34]

Trial	Drug	Mean age (years)
CONSENSUS[26]	Enalapril	71
V-HeFT II[27]	Enalapril	61
SOLVD treatment[28]	Enalapril	61
AIRE[53]	Ramipril	65
SAVE[31]	Captopril	59
TRACE[32]	Trandolapril	67
ATLAS[25]	Lisinopril	64
ELITE[40]	Losartan	73
ELITE II[49]	Losartan	71
Val-HeFT[50]	Valsartan	63
RALES[68]	Spirorolactone	61
CIBIS II[55]	Bisoprolol	61
MERIT-HF[53]	Metoprolol	64
COPERNICUS[54]	Carvedilol	63
DIG[82]	Digoxin	63

Table 3.1 Mean age of patients included in major clinical trials on the treatment of heart failure

With stratification for age (<55 years, 55–64 years, 65–74 years, >75 years) there was no heterogeneity in the benefits of treatment for the combined outcomes of death or myocardial infarction and death or readmission for heart failure. The meta-analysis demonstrated a clear and graded relation between the baseline ejection fraction and the effects of ACE inhibition.

Greater benefits on mortality and hospital admission for heart failure were observed in patients with lower ejection fractions. Although there was a less clear interaction on the composite outcome of death, myocardial infarction, or admission for heart failure, there seemed to be a greater benefit of the ACE inhibitor among patients with the lowest ejection fractions. However, it is clear that even among patients with relatively preserved ejection fractions, there is a clinically important benefit. These data support the prescription of ACE inhibitors to elderly heart failure patients even if there is only a moderate impairment of left ventricular ejection fractions.

Aging is not only associated with extensive changes in cardiovascular structure and function but also with changes in other organ systems. Glomerular filtration rate (GFR) declines with increasing age.[35] A major concern when treating elderly heart failure patients with ACE inhibitors is the side effect of renal impairment.[36] Significant renal artery disease, defined as renal artery stenosis of more than 50%, is present in one-third of elderly patients.[37] It has even been suggested that high-risk elderly heart failure patients should be screened for renal artery stenosis to identify the need for further examination with renal angiography. There is, however, no knowledge to support that there are any positive effects of screening for renal impairment that would improve outcomes with regard to serious episodes of renal dysfunction in conjunction with ACE inhibitor treatment. Although a large proportion of elderly heart failure patients have renal artery disease, only a few have bilateral disease. Elderly patients with unilateral disease tolerate ACE inhibitors well. Therefore, at the present time, there is no justification for screening for renal artery disease before prescribing ACE inhibitor therapy for elderly patients with heart failure.[38]

Acute renal failure is usually preceded by a rise in serum creatinine concentrations. Renal function can deteriorate acutely when ACE inhibitor therapy is initiated as well as in patients receiving chronic ACE inhibitor therapy, particularly in elderly patients with chronic heart failure.[39] It is important to keep in mind that acute renal failure can occur even if ACE inhibitor doses and creatinine levels have been stable for months or years. The frequency with which renal function changes in patients with heart failure has been evaluated and reported in several studies.[26,28,40] In SOLVD, decreased renal function was defined as a rise in serum creatinine of ≥ 0.5 mg/dl (44 μmol/l) from baseline. Sixteen percent of patients randomly assigned to enalapril had a decrease in renal function compared with 12% in the placebo controls. By multivariate analysis, in both the placebo and enalapril groups, old age, diuretic therapy, and diabetes were associated with decreased renal function, whereas beta-blocker therapy and a higher ejection fraction were renoprotective.[28,36]

A number of factors leading to renal hypoperfusion may result in the development of acute renal failure in elderly heart failure patients receiving ACE inhibitor treatment. These factors include systemic hypotension, which is not uncommon in heart failure as many patients are treated with combinations of diuretics, ACE inhibitors, beta-blockers, and possibly vasodilators, either for heart failure or concomitant conditions such as angina. Introduction of an ACE inhibitor leads to a fall in angiotensin II levels and hence vasodilatation. Other mechanisms may also be involved.

A number of heart failure patients may be volume-depleted due to intense diuretic therapy. Diuretics have been reported to increase the risk of acute renal failure more than 10-fold when ACE inhibitors are administered.[39] Other risk factors are bilateral renal artery stenosis, stenosis of a dominant or single kidney, atherosclerotic disease in smaller preglomerular vessels, and afferent arteriolar narrowing due to hypertension.[37]

If elderly patients are carefully monitored, the development of acute renal failure due to ACE inhibitors can be identified early. Serum creatinine and electrolyte levels should be evaluated before and at least 1 week after therapy with ACE inhibitors is started in heart failure patients. If sustained oliguria or hypotension develop, creatinine should be monitored earlier. A rise in creatinine of more than 30% from a serum creatinine value of less than 200 μmol/l should lead to dose adjustment. If the creatinine level continues to increase, the medication should be stopped while additional renal evaluation is undertaken. Renal failure complicating ACE inhibitor therapy is almost always reversible.[41] Withdrawal of the ACE inhibitor therapy, or at least a reduction in dose, is appropriate in the light of clinical experience.

In addition, withdrawal of interacting drugs, supportive management of fluid and electrolytes, and temporary dialysis where indicated are the mainstay of therapy. The underlying causes of volume depletion and renal hypoperfusion should be identified and corrected. If this can be performed satisfactorily, the ACE inhibitor can usually be reintroduced after the improvement of systemic hemodynamics and renal function. When chronic renal insufficiency is present, it could be advantageous to select an ACE inhibitor that is eliminated in part by hepatic clearance rather than by renal excretion and therefore is less likely to accumulate in the presence of renal dysfunction. Fosinopril and trandolapril, for example, are ACE inhibitors that have dual (renal and hepatic) elimination pathways.

Guidelines recommend that ACE inhibitors should be prescribed in doses used in clinical trials. ACE inhibitors are often not prescribed to elderly heart failure patients and, when prescribed, are not used in doses proven effective in major randomized clinical.[42–45] The ATLAS study addressed the issue of comparative effects of low and high doses of the ACE inhibitor lisinopril on morbidity and mortality in heart failure.[25] The combined risk of morbidity and mortality was significantly lower in the high-dose group than in the low-dose group. The results of the ATLAS study suggest that patients with heart failure should not be maintained on very low doses of an ACE inhibitor unless these are the only doses that can be tolerated.

The pre-randomization titration and stabilization period of the ATLAS trial provides information about the tolerability of low- to medium-dose lisinopril in previously ACE-naive subjects as well as in patients who had previously received ACE inhibitor treatment.[46] For the patients who had not received an ACE inhibitor before entry, these adverse reactions were subdivided into whether they occurred at the first or second open-label dose. It was found that 4.4% of patients who had not previously received an ACE inhibitor, and 3.0% of patients who had, withdrew because of such events. The reasons were divided approximately equally between effects possibly related to hypotension or dizziness and renal dysfunction or hyperkalemia. These figures

provide a maximum estimate of drug-related discontinuations in these categories, as there was no concomitant placebo-treated group to provide an indication of the frequency of discontinuations for reasons unrelated to ACE inhibitor therapy.

Post-randomization data on the occurrence of hypotension and dizziness in patients younger than 70 years and patients 70 years or older in the high- and low-dose groups showed that there was a slightly higher frequency in both dose groups among the elderly (Table 3.2). However, there was no major discrepancy between the increase in these symptoms, depending on age, between the high-dose and low-dose groups. There was possibly a greater tendency to withdraw elderly patients from blinded treatment in the high-dose group. The difference was small, in the order of 1%. The occurrence of renal dysfunction or hyperkalemia increased to a greater extent when comparing the high- and low-dose groups. However, these changes rarely led to withdrawal (Table 3.3). Post-randomization data on overall withdrawals showed that high-dose lisinopril was tolerated slightly better than low-dose lisinopril in both young and elderly patients and, although more elderly were withdrawn from study treatment, more were also withdrawn from low-dose treatment (Table 3.3).[47] Further analysis of data from the ATLAS study has shown that for all-cause mortality and all-cause hospitalization, there was no effect of age on outcome, with uniform hazard ratios in the different 5-year age groups. Analysis using age as a continuous covariate showed no interaction between age and treatment.[47]

It can be concluded that ACE inhibitors are indicated in the treatment of heart failure, when systolic function is reduced, even in the elderly. Elderly patients may be at a greater risk of developing renal failure due to ACE inhibitor treatment; however, if creatinine levels

Subgroups	Treatment group, percent of patients					
	Any occurrence		Classified as serious		Leading to withdrawal	
	HD	LD	HD	LD	HD	LD
Hypotension/dizziness:						
Age ≥70 years ($n = 988$)	36.8	24.8	14.6	10.7	2.3	0.8
Age <70 years ($n = 2176$)	30.7	21.9	11.8	8.3	1.5	1.2
Renal dysfunction/hyperkalemia:						
Age ≥70 years	32.2	21.7	12.9	10.3	3.3	3.8
Age <70 years	18.5	15.3	6.3	6.9	1.9	1.7

HD indicates high-dose group; LD, low-dose group.

Table 3.2 Incidence of possible dose-related side effects in elderly patients compared with younger patients in the ATLAS trial[47]

Age at entry (years)	Percentage of patients withdrawn from therapy	
	High-dose lisinopril	Low-dose lisinopril
<70	24.5	28.8
70–74	33.6	34.7
>75	31.2	35.2
Overall	27.1	30.7

Table 3.3 Patient withdrawals by lisinopril dose and age group in the ATLAS study[47]

are checked regularly on the initiation of treatment, serious side effects can be avoided. When treatment is initiated in the elderly, doses should be uptitrated to the doses used in major mortality trials if possible.

Angiotensin type 1 receptor blockers

Angiotensin type 1 receptor blockers (ARBs) are recommended as an alternative treatment in patients in whom an ACE inhibitor is indicated but not tolerated due to ACE inhibitor-specific side effects such as cough.[23,24,48] Whereas ACE inhibitors block the production of angiotensin II, ARBs block the angiotensin

II type 1 receptor. The detrimental effects of angiotensin II in heart failure have been attributed to stimulation of this receptor. The ARB losartan has been compared to an ACE inhibitor, captopril, specifically with regard to efficacy and safety in elderly patients with congestive heart failure and impaired left ventricular systolic dysfunction in the ELITE trial.[40] Patients included had symptomatic heart failure and were 65 years or older (mean age 73–74 years). These patients had not previously been treated with an ACE inhibitor. The primary aim was to study the frequency of persisting increases in serum creatinine apart from the secondary aim, which was to compare the composite measure of death and/or hospital admission for heart failure. The frequency of persisting creatinine increase was the same in the losartan and captopril groups. Fewer losartan patients discontinued therapy for adverse experiences, suggesting that tolerability for ARBs in elderly patients with heart failure is better than for ACE inhibitors. There was also a 32% reduction in death and/or hospital admission for heart failure, which was mainly as a result of a fewer number of deaths in the losartan group. Subsequently, the ELITE II trial attempted to confirm the finding of improved efficacy of losartan in this population.[49] Patients in ELITE II were slightly younger, 60 years or older (mean age 71–72 years), and almost one of four patients had previously been treated with an ACE inhibitor. This trial could not confirm that losartan was superior to captopril in improving survival in heart failure but did confirm that losartan was significantly better tolerated.[49]

Although losartan compared favorably with captopril with regard to tolerability, this did not seem to have had an impact on well-being. In a substudy to ELITE, quality of life significantly improved to a similar degree in both treatment groups. However, there was a trend toward greater improvement in the losartan group. Almost twice as many patients withdrew from captopril due to adverse events. This finding could be the reason for the trend toward greater improvement in quality of life in the losartan-treated patients.

The effects of angiotensin II are not completely blocked despite the use of an ACE inhibitor or an ARB. The hypothesis that more complete blockade of the renin–angiotensin system would result in improved outcomes was addressed in a study in which the angiotensin II receptor antagonist valsartan or placebo was added to conventional therapy that could include an ACE inhibitor, as well

as diuretics, digoxin, and a beta-blocker.[50] The primary outcomes were mortality and the combined endpoint of mortality and morbidity. Approximately half of the patients included were aged 65 years or older. Overall mortality was similar in the two randomized groups. The incidence of the combined endpoint, however, was lower with valsartan than with placebo. The effect was similar in patients younger than 65 years compared to those who were 65 years or older. Treatment with valsartan also resulted in significant improvements in New York Heart Association (NYHA) class, ejection fraction, signs and symptoms of heart failure, and quality of life as compared with placebo. In a posthoc analysis of the combined endpoint and mortality in subgroups, defined according to baseline treatment with ACE inhibitors or beta-blockers, valsartan had a favorable effect in patients receiving neither or one of these types of drugs but an adverse effect in patients receiving both types of drugs. This finding has raised concern about the potential safety of this specific combination, which should generally be avoided pending the results of ongoing clinical trials. In the subgroup of patients not receiving an ACE inhibitor, mortality was significantly reduced.

Several ARBs are currently available for the treatment of heart failure but only losartan and valsartan have been evaluated in heart failure mortality trials. All share a common mechanism of action: antagonism of angiotensin type 1 receptors; however, their receptor-binding kinetics differ, as well as their pharmacokinetics. It remains to be determined whether the observed pharmacologic and pharmacokinetic differences among the members of this class of drugs will have a clinically significant impact on long-term cardiovascular outcomes and mortality.[51] The present recommendation – that ARBs should be prescribed to patients who do not tolerate ACE inhibitors – applies to the elderly. It is important to observe that the prescription of ARBs to elderly patients requires the same considerations with regard to renal impairment as the prescription of ACE inhibitors.

Beta-blockers

Beta-blockers have been extensively studied for the treatment of heart failure in patients with impaired left ventricular systolic function. As early as 1974, Waagstein et al. reported that a beta-1 selective beta-blocker, practolol, was well tolerated by patients who had suffered a myocardial infarction complicated by signs of heart failure.[52] Subsequently, overwhelming evidence of the positive effects of beta-blockers has been published, including data on the effect of treatment in high-risk group such as the elderly. Beta-blockers are recommended, in addition to ACE inhibitors, for all patients with stable heart failure and impaired left ventricular systolic function unless they have contraindications to their use or have been shown to be unable to tolerate treatment with these drugs.[23,24]

Beta-1 selective beta-blockers (bisoprolol, metoprolol) and a nonselective beta-blocker (carvedilol) have been shown to be effective in reducing morbidity and mortality in heart failure.[53–55] The effect of bisoprolol on mortality was reported from the second Cardiac Insufficiency Bisoprolol Study (CIBIS II),[55] in patients in NYHA classes III–IV, aged 22–80 years (mean age 61 years). Treatment had to include a diuretic and an ACE inhibitor, although other vasodilators were allowed if patients were intolerant of ACE inhibitors, and the use of digoxin was optional. Compared with placebo, bisoprolol significantly reduced the primary endpoint all-cause mortality by 34%, and also reduced morbidity significantly.

A post hoc analysis of data from CIBIS II evaluated the effect of bisoprolol on high-risk patient groups randomized in the study, including patients over the age of 70 years.[56] The reduction in mortality was similar in patients over the age of 70 years to those aged 70 years or less.

Secondary endpoints (all-cause hospital admissions, cardiovascular mortality and cardiovascular hospital admissions, a composite endpoint, and permanent premature treatment withdrawals) did not significantly differ in older compared with younger patients, although permanent treatment withdrawals were more common in the bisoprolol-treated elderly patients compared with placebo, in contrast to the case in the younger patients.

The Metoprolol CR/XL Randomized Intervention Trial in Congestive Heart Failure (MERIT-HF) trial included patients with heart failure in NYHA functional classes II–IV with impaired left ventricular systolic function.[53] The primary endpoint, all-cause mortality, was reduced from 11% to 7.2% during 1 year of follow-up by metoprolol compared with placebo. The investigators concluded that metoprolol was effective and well tolerated in the treatment of heart failure. Interestingly, patients were relatively evenly distributed between the age groups <60, 60–69, and ≥70 years. The positive effects of metoprolol were similar in the upper age group compared with the middle and lower age groups.

In contrast to bisoprolol and metoprolol, carvedilol is a nonselective beta-1 and beta-2 receptor blocker as well as an alpha-1 receptor blocker. It also has antioxidant properties. Carvedilol has proven efficacy for the treatment of heart failure with regard to mortality and hospitalization in a broad spectrum of heart failure patients with left ventricular systolic dysfunction.[54,57] The reduction in mortality risk and in the combined risk of death or hospitalization with carvedilol was similar in direction and in magnitude in subgroups defined according to age <65 years or ≥65 years. Smaller studies have shown that carvedilol is well tolerated for the treatment of heart failure, even in elderly patients.[58,59]

Contrary to current belief, it appears that the occurrence of side effects, even in the initial phase of treatment with a beta-blocker, are relatively rare, although the most common side effects of fatigue, hypotension, and bradycardia occur at times.[60] Initiation at low doses and careful monitoring during uptitration is recommended, especially in elderly heart failure patients.

Diuretics

Diuretics, most commonly loop diuretics, are recommended for the treatment of heart failure in the presence of signs of fluid retention or volume overload.[23,24] From a clinical perspective, diuretics appear to be therapeutically superior to other drugs for the treatment of heart failure in their efficacy in relieving symptoms.[61-63] Whether administered intravenously or orally, all diuretics result in a substantial reduction in the raised pulmonary vascular pressures. Diuretics are the only available drugs that can control fluid retention in heart failure. Attempts to circumvent diuretic therapy in favor of an ACE inhibitor have been futile.[64] However, diuretics stimulate release of renin, with subsequent activation of the renin–angiotensin–aldosterone system, which could be detrimental in the long run if unchecked. It is therefore recommended that they be prescribed in combination with ACE inhibitors and beta-blockers if left ventricular systolic dysfunction is present.[23]

It has been reported that, in elderly patients with decompensated heart failure, infusion with a loop diuretic is more efficacious in terms of costs than repeat intravenous bolus doses.[61] Comparisons between furosemide and torasemide suggest that the latter may be more effective in preventing readmission for heart failure, improving symptoms and quality of life, as well as yielding pharmacoeconomic benefits;[65,66] this, however, needs to be confirmed in a large-scale trail. Due to impaired renal function, diuretic resistance may be more likely to occur in elderly patients than in younger patients. It can be circumvented by segmental nephron blockade with a combination of low-dose diuretics that simultaneously block sodium reabsorption in the proximal tubule, the loop of Henle, the distal tubule, and the collecting duct.[67]

There are adverse reactions to chronic diuretic therapy in all patients, including the elderly, and serum electrolytes should be monitored for hypokalemia and hypomagnesemia. Elderly patients may be particularly susceptible to other side effects as well, specifically hypotension and azotemia. The impact of diuretics on prognosis of heart failure patients, both younger and older, is unknown; however, diuretics have been used in all the survival trials with ACE inhibitors and beta-blocking drugs.

Spironolactone is a potassium-sparing diuretic that exerts its effect by blockade of the aldosterone receptor. The rationale for studying the effect of spironolactone was the knowledge that aldosterone has an important role in the pathophysiology of heart failure. It promotes the retention of sodium, the loss of magnesium and potassium, sympathetic activation, parasympathetic inhibition, myocardial and vascular fibrosis, baroreceptor dysfunction, and vascular damage, and impairs arterial compliance. Inhibition of the renin–angiotensin–aldosterone system by ACE inhibitors does not completely suppress the formation of aldosterone. It has been shown that addition of a low-dose spironolactone, in addition to treatment with ACE inhibitors, diuretics, and digoxin, improves survival and reduces hospitalization for worsening heart failure in patients with moderate-to-severe heart failure and left ventricular systolic dysfunction.[68] The median age of patients included was 67 years. Subgroup analysis showed that the effect of spironolactone was similar in those <67 years and those ≥67 years.

Although there were few side effects of treatment with spironolactone in this study, later reports on side effects seen with the clinical implementation of spironolactone treatment for heart failure show the need for caution, especially in the elderly.[69] Hyperkalemia that develops with the combination of ACE inhibitors and spironolactone can be life threatening; however, with the use of low doses and prudent monitoring of electrolytes, this complication can be avoided.

Digoxin

Cardiac glycosides have played a central role in the treatment of heart failure since the 18th century; nevertheless, controversy exists as to the benefits, and also the risks, of treatment in patients with heart failure, particularly the elderly. These drugs are believed to exert their effect by increasing the availability of activator Ca^{2+} in the cardiac myocytes, resulting in positive inotropic effects. Digoxin is the most commonly prescribed cardiac glycoside. Digoxin is excreted exponentially, with an elimination half-life of 36–48 hours in patients with normal renal function, resulting in the loss of about one-third of body stores daily.[70] Renal excretion of digoxin is proportional to the GFR. For patients not previously given digoxin, institution of daily maintenance therapy without a loading dose results in the

development of steady-state plateau concentrations after 4–5 half-lives, or 7–10 days, in subjects with normal renal function. Renal function is often impaired in elderly heart failure patients.[71] In these patients the length of time before steady state is reached on a daily maintenance dose is proportionally prolonged. Furthermore, the steady-state volume of distribution of digoxin is decreased in chronic renal failure and, therefore, loading as well as maintenance doses of digoxin should be decreased.[72] In heart failure there is rarely a need to prescribe a loading dose unless for the treatment of concomitant supraventricular arrhythmias.

An analysis of the consensus based on clinical trial data has led to the recommendation of a therapeutic range between 0.5 and 1.5 ng/ml.[70] As a result of the narrow therapeutic window for digoxin, there is an increased risk for toxicity in the elderly. The incidence of digitalis toxicity is further increased due to interactions with diuretics. The increased risk of digitalis toxicity is due to decreased GFR as a result of volume depletion and electrolyte disturbances. In a study of hospitalized patients treated with digoxin, over 4% had clinical evidence of digoxin toxicity.[73] A study of 56 US academic hospitals showed that 0.07% of all admissions were due to digoxin toxicity, resulting in considerable costs.[74] It was suggested that 53% of the cases could have been prevented. In the case of life-threatening digitalis toxicity, such as serious ventricular arrhythmias, administration of digoxin-specific antibody fragments is the first-line treatment.[75]

Some studies suggest that the decrease in sympathetic nervous system tone and positive inotropic effects of digoxin, as well as negative side effects, appear to occur at different doses or serum concentration levels.[76,77] However, other studies have found that the beneficial effects of digoxin on common clinical endpoints, such as worsening heart failure, are similar, regardless of serum digoxin concentrations.[78] In fact, it has also been suggested that digoxin treatment for heart failure increases mortality.[79–81] These suggestions are not based on prospective data and are therefore not conclusive. The Digitalis Investigation Group (DIG) study, however, was a prospective, randomized, double-blind, placebo-controlled clinical trial designed to evaluate the effects of digoxin on mortality and hospitalizations in patients with chronic heart failure and sinus rhythm.[82] Treatment was administered on a background of diuretic and ACE inhibitor therapy. Patients were included in the main trial if the left ventricular ejection fraction was ≤45% ($n = 7788$), and in the ancillary trial if the left ventricular ejection fraction was >45% ($n = 988$). The mean age of patients in the study was 64 years, and 32% were 70 years of age or older. The primary endpoint was all-cause mortality. The principal finding of the DIG study was that, although digoxin had no discernible effect on total mortality, the composite endpoint of heart failure death or hospitalization was reduced 24% in patients randomized to digoxin.[82] The effect of age on mortality, hospitalizations, and response to digoxin has also been analysed in the DIG study data.[71] Study patients were retrospectively grouped into five age categories: <50 years, 50–59 years, 60–69 years, 70–79 years, and ≥80 years. Increasing age was found to be associated with a progressive increase in the incidence of death, hospitalization, heart failure hospitalization, and heart failure death or hospitalization. Similar to the overall results, digoxin reduced the risk for heart failure hospitalizations within each age. The frequency of drug withdrawal, however, increased progressively with age, offsetting an interaction between age and digoxin toxicity.

It would appear therefore, that digoxin therapy, especially if combined with diuretic and ACE inhibitor treatment, does confer some benefit in the treatment of elderly heart failure patients and digoxin is recommended for the treatment of heart failure in the presence of left ventricular systolic dysfunction.[23,24]

Left ventricular diastolic dysfunction

Heart failure due to left ventricular diastolic dysfunction without impaired systolic function is common in heart failure patients, especially among the elderly.[83–85] It is commonly associated with hypertension and left ventricular hypertrophy. Whereas there are numerous studies on the effects of therapy on heart failure due to left ventricular systolic dysfunction, this is not true for diastolic dysfunction. It has been suggested that the treatment of diastolic heart failure should target symptoms and the causal disease, as well as the mechanism responsible for the development of diastolic dysfunction.[86]

Calcium antagonists lower elevated blood pressure and control tachycardia, both of which may be aims of treatment in diastolic heart failure. Also, theoretically, they may facilitate the energy-dependent transport of calcium ions from the actin–myosin complex into the sarcoplasmic reticulum. Verapamil has been shown to improve exercise capacity and improve indices of diastolic dysfunction in patients with diastolic heart failure, including the elderly.[87,88] ACE inhibitors reverse left ventricular hypertrophy and improve diastolic function.[89,90] ARBs improve exercise tolerance, diastolic filling, and quality of life in hypertensive patients with diastolic dysfunction.[91] Beta-blockers reduce ischemia and can control heart rate. Diuretics decrease pulmonary venous pressure and volume overload due to fluid retention. Long-acting nitrates also can play a role in decreasing central blood volume and reducing ischemia.

Summary

Heart failure is particularly common in the elderly. ACE inhibitors or, if not tolerated, ARBs, should be prescribed in these patients, although impaired renal function in many elderly patients requires special considerations. When signs of fluid retention or volume overload are present, diuretics are indicated, and treatment results in symptomatic improvement and increased exercise capacity. Aldosterone antagonism with spironolactone confers additional benefits beyond diuresis. Beta-blockers have proven efficacy in elderly heart failure patients with left ventricular systolic dysfunction. Digoxin, especially in combination with diuretics and ACE inhibitors, reduces morbidity but requires careful monitoring due to an increased risk of toxicity in the elderly. Heart failure treatment trials have generally included patients with a mean age well below the age of 70 (see Table 3.1). Clinical trials specifically aimed at studying possible age-dependent treatment differences with regard to elderly heart failure patients are lacking. However, available data does not suggest the existence of age-dependent differences if other selection criteria are taken into consideration. Heart failure due to left ventricular diastolic dysfunction – i.e. no or only mild impairment of left ventricular systolic function – is common in elderly heart failure patients, but there is a paucity of clinical trials on which to base treatment recommendations. The drugs used for the treatment of diastolic heart failure are similar to those used for the treatment of systolic heart failure, but the considerations guiding their usage differ.

References

1. Hoes AW, Mosterd A, Grobbee DE. An epidemic of heart failure? Recent evidence from Europe. Eur Heart J 1998; 19(Suppl L):L2–9.
2. Kannel WB. Epidemiological aspects of heart failure. Cardiol Clin 1989; 7:1–9.
3. Anonymous. World population prospects: sex and age. New York: United Nations Publications, 1998.
4. Anonymous. World population projections to 2150. New York: United Nations Publications, 2001.
5. Cline CM, Willenheimer RB, Erhardt LR, et al. Health-related quality of life in elderly patients with heart failure. Scand Cardiovasc J 1999; 33:278–85.
6. Cowie MR, Wood DA, Coats AJ, et al. Survival of patients with a new diagnosis of heart failure: a population based study. Heart 2000; 83:505–10.
7. Cline CM, Broms K, Willenheimer RB, et al. Hospitalization and health care costs due to congestive heart failure in the elderly. Am J Geriatr Cardiol 1996; 5:10–14.
8. Ryden-Bergsten T, Andersson F. The health care costs of heart failure in Sweden. J Intern Med 1999; 246:275–84.

9. McKee PA, Castelli WP, McNamara PM, Kannel WB. The natural history of congestive heart failure: the Framingham study. N Engl J Med 1971; 285:1441–6.

10. Kannel WB, Ho K, Thom T. Changing epidemiological features of cardiac failure. Br Heart J 1994; 72(2 Suppl):S3–9.

11. Wilhelmsen L, Rosengren A, Eriksson H, Lappas G. Heart failure in the general population of men – morbidity, risk factors and prognosis. J Intern Med 2001; 249:253–61.

12. Senni M, Redfield MM. Congestive heart failure in elderly patients. Mayo Clin Proc 1997; 72:453–60.

13. Kannel WB, Belanger AJ. Epidemiology of heart failure. Am Heart J 1991; 121(3 Pt 1):951–7.

14. Eriksson H, Svardsudd K, Larsson B, et al. Risk factors for heart failure in the general population: the study of men born in 1913. Eur Heart J 1989; 10:647–56.

15. McDonagh TA, Morrison CE, Lawrence A, et al. Symptomatic and asymptomatic left-ventricular systolic dysfunction in an urban population. Lancet 1997; 350:829–33.

16. Mosterd A, Hoes AW, de Bruyne MC, et al. Prevalence of heart failure and left ventricular dysfunction in the general population; the Rotterdam Study. Eur Heart J 1999; 20:447–55.

17. Davies M, Hobbs F, Davis R, et al. Prevalence of left-ventricular systolic dysfunction and heart failure in the Echocardiographic Heart of England Screening study: a population based study. Lancet 2001; 358:439–44.

18. Ho KK, Pinsky JL, Kannel WB, Levy D. The epidemiology of heart failure: the Framingham Study. J Am Coll Cardiol 1993; 22(4 Suppl A):3A–6A.

19. Wilhelmsen L, Eriksson H, Svardsudd K, Caidahl K. Improving the detection and diagnosis of congestive heart failure. Eur Heart J 1989; 10(Suppl C):13–18.

20. Cowie MR, Wood DA, Coats AJ, et al. Incidence and aetiology of heart failure; a population-based study. Eur Heart J 1999; 20:421–8.

21. Emanuelsson H, Karlson BW, Herlitz J. Characteristics and prognosis of patients with acute myocardial infarction in relation to occurrence of congestive heart failure. Eur Heart J 1994; 15:761–8.

22. Petrie MC, Berry C, Stewart S, McMurray JJ. Failing ageing hearts. Eur Heart J 2001; 22:1978–90.

23. Hunt SA, Baker DW, Chin MH, et al. ACC/AHA guidelines for the evaluation and management of chronic heart failure in the adult: executive summary. A report of the American College of Cardiology/American Heart Association Task Force on Practice Guidelines (Committee to revise the 1995 Guidelines for the Evaluation and Management of Heart Failure). J Am Coll Cardiol 2001; 38:2101–13.

24. Remme WJ, Swedberg K. Guidelines for the diagnosis and treatment of chronic heart failure. Eur Heart J 2001; 22:1527–60.

25. Packer M, Poole-Wilson PA, Armstrong PW, et al. Comparative effects of low and high doses of the angiotensin-converting enzyme inhibitor, lisinopril, on morbidity and mortality in chronic heart failure. ATLAS Study Group. Circulation 1999; 100:2312–18.

26. The CONSENSUS Trial Study Group. Effects of enalapril on mortality in severe congestive heart failure. Results of the Cooperative North Scandinavian Enalapril Survival Study (CONSENSUS). N Engl J Med 1987; 316:1429–35.

27. Cohn JN, Johnson G, Ziesche S, et al. A comparison of enalapril with hydralazine-isosorbide dinitrate in the treatment of chronic congestive heart failure. N Engl J Med 1991; 325:303–10.

28. The SOLVD Investigators. Effect of enalapril on survival in patients with reduced left ventricular ejection fractions and congestive heart failure. N Engl J Med 1991; 325:293–302.

29. McMurray J, McDonagh T, Morrison CE, Dargie HJ. Trends in hospitalization for heart failure in Scotland 1980–1990. Eur Heart J 1993; 14:1158–62.

30. Flather MD, Yusuf S, Kober L, et al. Long-term ACE-inhibitor therapy in patients with heart failure or left-ventricular dysfunction: a systematic overview of data from individual patients. ACE-Inhibitor Myocardial Infarction Collaborative Group. Lancet 2000; 355:1575–81.

31. Pfeffer MA, Braunwald E, Moye LA, et al. Effect of captopril on mortality and morbidity in patients with left ventricular dysfunction after myocardial infarction. Results of the survival and

ventricular enlargement trial. The SAVE Investigators. N Engl J Med 1992; 327: 669–77.

32. Kober L, Torp-Pedersen C, Carlsen JE, et al. A clinical trial of the angiotensin-converting-enzyme inhibitor trandolapril in patients with left ventricular dysfunction after myocardial infarction. Trandolapril Cardiac Evaluation (TRACE) Study Group. N Engl J Med 1995; 333:1670–6.

33. The Acute Infarction Ramipril Efficacy (AIRE) Study Investigators. Effect of ramipril on mortality and morbidity of survivors of acute myocardial infarction with clinical evidence of heart failure. Lancet 1993; 342:821–8.

34. Effect of enalapril on mortality and the development of heart failure in asymptomatic patients with reduced left ventricular ejection fractions. The SOLVD Investigators. N Engl J Med 1992; 327:685–91.

35. Schoolwerth AC, Sica DA, Ballermann BJ, Wilcox CS. Renal considerations in angiotensin converting enzyme inhibitor therapy: a statement for healthcare professionals from the Council on the Kidney in Cardiovascular Disease and the Council for High Blood Pressure Research of the American Heart Association. Circulation 2001; 104:1985–91.

36. Knight EL, Glynn RJ, McIntyre KM, et al. Predictors of decreased renal function in patients with heart failure during angiotensin-converting enzyme inhibitor therapy: results from the studies of left ventricular dysfunction (SOLVD). Am Heart J 1999; 138(5 Pt 1):849–55.

37. MacDowall P, Kalra PA, O'Donoghue DJ, et al. Risk of morbidity from renovascular disease in elderly patients with congestive cardiac failure. Lancet 1998; 352:13–16.

38. Krumholz HM. Time to focus on the more typical heart-failure patients. Lancet 1998; 352: 3–4.

39. Mandal AK, Markert RJ, Saklayen MG, et al. Diuretics potentiate angiotensin converting enzyme inhibitor-induced acute renal failure. Clin Nephrol 1994; 42:170–4.

40. Pitt B, Segal R, Martinez FA, et al. Randomised trial of losartan versus captopril in patients over 65 with heart failure (Evaluation of Losartan in the Elderly Study, ELITE). Lancet 1997; 349:747–52.

41. Ljungman S, Kjekshus J, Swedberg K. Renal function in severe congestive heart failure during treatment with enalapril (the Cooperative North Scandinavian Enalapril Survival Study [CONSENSUS] Trial). Am J Cardiol 1992; 70:479–87.

42. Andersson F, Cline C, Ryden-Bergsten T, Erhardt L. Angiotensin converting enzyme (ACE) inhibitors and heart failure. The consequences of underprescribing. Pharmacoeconomics 1999; 15:535–50.

43. Philbin EF, Andreaou C, Rocco TA, et al. Patterns of angiotensin-converting enzyme inhibitor use in congestive heart failure in two community hospitals. Am J Cardiol 1996; 77:832–8.

44. Philbin EF. Factors determining angiotensin-converting enzyme inhibitor underutilization in heart failure in a community setting. Clin Cardiol 1998; 21:103–8.

45. Packer M. Do angiotensin-converting enzyme inhibitors prolong life in patients with heart failure treated in clinical practice? J Am Coll Cardiol 1996; 28:1323–7.

46. Massie BM, Armstrong PW, Cleland JG, et al. Toleration of high doses of angiotensin-converting enzyme inhibitors in patients with chronic heart failure: results from the ATLAS trial. The Assessment of Treatment with Lisinopril and Survival. Arch Intern Med 2001; 161:165–71.

47. Ryden L, Armstrong PW, Cleland JG, et al. Efficacy and safety of high-dose lisinopril in chronic heart failure patients at high cardiovascular risk, including those with diabetes mellitus. Results from the ATLAS trial. Eur Heart J 2000; 21:1967–78.

48. Heart Failure Society of America. HFSA guidelines for the management of patients with heart failure due to left ventricular dysfunction. Pharmacological approaches. Congest Heart Fail 2000; 6:11–39.

49. Pitt B, Poole-Wilson PA, Segal R, et al. Effect of losartan compared with captopril on mortality in patients with symptomatic heart failure: randomised trial – the Losartan Heart Failure Survival Study ELITE II. Lancet 2000; 355:1582–7.

50. Cohn JN, Tognoni G. A randomized trial of the angiotensin-receptor blocker valsartan in chronic heart failure. N Engl J Med 2001; 345:1667–75.

51. Oparil S. Newly emerging pharmacologic differences in angiotensin II receptor blockers. Am J Hypertens 2000; 13(1 Pt 2):18S–24S.

53. Waagstein F, Hjalmarson AC, Wasir HS. Apex cardiogram and systolic time intervals in acute

myocardial infarction and effects of practolol. Br Heart J 1974; 36:1109–21.

53. Effect of metoprolol CR/XL in chronic heart failure: Metoprolol CR/XL Randomised Intervention Trial in Congestive Heart Failure (MERIT-HF). Lancet 1999; 353:2001–7.

54. Packer M, Coats AJ, Fowler MB, et al. Effect of carvedilol on survival in severe chronic heart failure. N Engl J Med 2001; 344:1651–8.

55. The Cardiac Insufficiency Bisoprolol Study II (CIBIS-II): a randomised trial. Lancet 1999; 353:9–13.

56. Erdmann E, Lechat P, Verkenne P, Wiemann H. Results from post-hoc analyses of the CIBIS II trial: effect of bisoprolol in high-risk patient groups with chronic heart failure. Eur J Heart Fail 2001; 3:469–79.

57. Packer M, Bristow MR, Cohn JN, et al. The effect of carvedilol on morbidity and mortality in patients with chronic heart failure. U.S. Carvedilol Heart Failure Study Group. N Engl J Med 1996; 334:1349–55.

58. Cioffi G, Stefenelli C. Tolerability and clinical effects of carvedilol in patients over 70 years of age with chronic heart failure due to left ventricular dysfunction. Ital Heart J 2001; 2(12 Suppl):1319–29.

59. Owen A. Experience of commencing carvedilol in elderly patients with heart failure in a routine outpatient clinic. Eur J Heart Fail 2000; 2:287–9.

60. Gottlieb SS, Fisher ML, Kjekshus J, et al. Tolerability of beta-blocker initiation and titration in the Metoprolol CR/XL Randomized Intervention Trial in Congestive Heart Failure (MERIT-HF). Circulation 2002; 105: 1182–8.

61. Howard PA, Dunn MI. Aggressive diuresis for severe heart failure in the elderly. Chest 2001; 119:807–10.

62. Packer M, Medina N, Yushak M, Meller J. Hemodynamic patterns of response during long-term captopril therapy for severe chronic heart failure. Circulation 1983; 68:803–12.

63. Hall SA, Cigarroa CG, Marcoux L, et al. Time course of improvement in left ventricular function, mass and geometry in patients with congestive heart failure treated with beta-adrenergic blockade. J Am Coll Cardiol 1995; 25:1154–61.

64. Anand IS, Kalra GS, Ferrari R, et al. Enalapril as initial and sole treatment in severe chronic heart failure with sodium retention. Int J Cardiol 1990; 28:341–6.

65. Murray MD, Deer MM, Ferguson JA, et al. Open-label randomized trial of torsemide compared with furosemide therapy for patients with heart failure. Am J Med 2001; 111:513–20.

66. Stroupe KT, Forthofer MM, Brater DC, Murray MD. Healthcare costs of patients with heart failure treated with torasemide or furosemide. Pharmacoeconomics 2000; 17:429–40.

67. Sica DA, Gehr TW. Diuretic combinations in refractory oedema states: pharmacokinetic–pharmacodynamic relationships. Clin Pharmacokinet 1996; 30:229–49.

68. Pitt B, Zannad F, Remme WJ, et al. The effect of spironolactone on morbidity and mortality in patients with severe heart failure. Randomized Aldactone Evaluation Study Investigators. N Engl J Med 1999; 341:709–17.

69. Schepkens H, Vanholder R, Billiouw JM, Lameire N. Life-threatening hyperkalemia during combined therapy with angiotensin-converting enzyme inhibitors and spironolactone: an analysis of 25 cases. Am J Med 2001; 110:438–41.

70. Hauptman PJ, Kelly RA. Digitalis. Circulation 1999; 99:1265–70.

71. Rich MW, McSherry F, Williford WO, Yusuf S. Effect of age on mortality, hospitalizations and response to digoxin in patients with heart failure: the DIG study. J Am Coll Cardiol 2001; 38:806–13.

72. Cheng JW, Charland SL, Shaw LM, et al. Is the volume of distribution of digoxin reduced in patients with renal dysfunction? Determining digoxin pharmacokinetics by fluorescence polarization immunoassay. Pharmacotherapy 1997; 17:584–90.

73. Williamson KM, Thrasher KA, Fulton KB, et al. Digoxin toxicity: an evaluation in current clinical practice. Arch Intern Med 1998; 158: 2444–9.

74. Gandhi AJ, Vlasses PH, Morton DJ, Bauman JL. Economic impact of digoxin toxicity. Pharmacoeconomics 1997; 12(2 Pt 1):175–81.

75. Antman EM, Wenger TL, Butler VP Jr, et al. Treatment of 150 cases of life-threatening digitalis intoxication with digoxin-specific Fab antibody fragments. Final report of a multicenter study. Circulation 1990; 81: 1744–52.

76. Gheorghiade M, Hall VB, Jacobsen G, et al. Effects of increasing maintenance dose of digoxin on left ventricular function and neurohormones in patients with chronic heart failure

treated with diuretics and angiotensin-converting enzyme inhibitors. Circulation 1995; 92:1801–7.

77. Yusuf S, Garg R, Held P, Gorlin R. Need for a large randomized trial to evaluate the effects of digitalis on morbidity and mortality in congestive heart failure. Am J Cardiol 1992; 69:64G–70G.

78. Adams KF Jr, Gheorghiade M, Uretsky BF, et al. Clinical benefits of low serum digoxin concentrations in heart failure. J Am Coll Cardiol 2002; 39:946–53.

79. Lindsay SJ, Kearney MT, Prescott RJ, et al. Digoxin and mortality in chronic heart failure. UK Heart Investigation. Lancet 1999; 354:1003.

80. Nolan J, Batin PD, Andrews R, et al. Prospective study of heart rate variability and mortality in chronic heart failure: results of the United Kingdom heart failure evaluation and assessment of risk trial (UK-heart). Circulation 1998; 98:1510–16.

81. Spargias KS, Hall AS, Ball SG. Safety concerns about digoxin after acute myocardial infarction. Lancet 1999; 354:391–2.

82. The Digitalis Investigation Group. The effect of digoxin on mortality and morbidity in patients with heart failure. N Engl J Med 1997; 336:525–33.

83. Vasan RS, Larson MG, Benjamin EJ, et al. Congestive heart failure in subjects with normal versus reduced left ventricular ejection fraction: prevalence and mortality in a population-based cohort. J Am Coll Cardiol 1999; 33:1948–55.

84. Soufer R, Wohlgelernter D, Vita NA, et al. Intact systolic left ventricular function in clinical conges-tive heart failure. Am J Cardiol 1985; 55: 1032–6.

85. Dougherty AH, Naccarelli GV, Gray EL, et al. Congestive heart failure with normal systolic function. Am J Cardiol 1984; 54:778–82.

86. Zile MR, Brutsaert DL. New concepts in diastolic dysfunction and diastolic heart failure. Part II: Causal mechanisms and treatment. Circulation 2002; 105:1503–8.

87. Setaro JF, Zaret BL, Schulman DS, et al. Usefulness of verapamil for congestive heart failure associated with abnormal left ventricular diastolic filling and normal left ventricular systolic performance. Am J Cardiol 1990; 66:981–6.

88. Hung MJ, Cherng WJ, Kuo LT, Wang CH. Effect of verapamil in elderly patients with left ventricular diastolic dysfunction as a cause of congestive heart failure. Int J Clin Pract 2002; 56:57–62.

89. Oren S, Grossman E, Frohlich ED. Reduction in left ventricular mass in patients with systemic hypertension treated with enalapril, lisinopril, or fosenopril. Am J Cardiol 1996; 77:93–6.

90. Hoffmann U, Globits S, Stefenelli T, et al. The effects of ACE inhibitor therapy on left ventricular myocardial mass and diastolic filling in previously untreated hypertensive patients: a cine MRI study. J Magn Reson Imaging 2001; 14: 16–22.

91. Warner JG Jr, Metzger DC, Kitzman DW, et al. Losartan improves exercise tolerance in patients with diastolic dysfunction and a hypertensive response to exercise. J Am Coll Cardiol 1999; 33:1567–72.

4

Heart failure in women

Wendy M Book, Brenda J Hott and Viola Vaccarino

Epidemiology of heart failure in women

Prevalence rates of heart failure overall are similar in women and in men across different study populations.[1–5] Women, however, have a lower prevalence of heart failure than men below the age of 70 or 75 years, and a higher prevalence at older ages. In absolute numbers, there are slightly more women than men with heart failure in the population.[1] Incidence rates of heart failure, however, are lower in women than in men in every age group.

Much of the information on the incidence of heart failure comes from the Framingham Study.[3,6] This study is based on a follow-up of a cohort assembled in 1948; therefore even latest updates of the Framingham data (up to 40 years of follow-up) may not be entirely contemporary. In this study, the average incidence of heart failure per 1000 population per annum among individuals ≥45 years was 4.7 in women and 7.2 in men. Incidence rates increased with age in both men and women, approximately doubling with each decade of age, and women lagged slightly behind men in incidence at all ages. Other community samples in the United States[2,7] and in Europe[8] also have found lower incidence rates in women.

The male predominance in incidence of heart failure appears to be due to the higher rate of coronary heart disease in men.[6]

However, once coronary heart disease has become manifest with a myocardial infarction, the risk of developing heart failure is higher in women than in men.[9–12] The reasons for the higher susceptibility of women towards heart failure after myocardial infarction are unclear.

It should be noted that the available incidence and prevalence data for heart failure are based on cases identified mostly on clinical criteria, occasionally with the aid of a chest radiograph or an echocardiogram. These data do not distinguish between different types of heart failure, e.g. systolic or diastolic dysfunction, or valvular heart disease. To date, information on the epidemiology of these subtypes of heart failure, overall and by gender, is largely unavailable.

Pathophysiology of heart failure in women

Risk factors and etiology

Our current understanding of risk factors for heart failure specific to women is limited and largely derived from the Framingham Study.[3,6,13,14] Major conditions predisposing to heart failure include coronary heart disease, hypertension, valvular heart disease, diabetes mellitus, and left ventricular hypertrophy.[3,7,14] Pulse pressure is also a strong risk factor for heart failure among the elderly.[15–17] These factors overall predict heart failure equally in men and in women; however, diabetes[14] and hypertension[18] are stronger risk factors for heart failure in women than in men. The risk of heart failure associated with diabetes is more than threefold higher in women than in men,[14] and the risk associated with hypertension also appears higher in women, about 50% higher[18] than in men, although this has not been an entirely consistent finding.[14]

Coronary heart disease and hypertension are the most common predisposing conditions both in men and women with heart failure, given the high prevalence of these risk factors.[3] In the Framingham Study, hypertension and coronary heart disease, alone or in combination, were present in 89% of men and 85% of women with heart failure.[3] The presence of these two factors combined represents the most common underlying cause of heart failure in both men and women. When present alone, however, coronary heart disease is a more common etiology of heart failure in men, whereas hypertension is a more common etiology in women.[3] Studies based on patient series,[19,20] as well as clinical trials of heart failure treatments,[21] have shown similar findings. Similarly, among hypertensive patients with heart failure, women are more likely than men to have hypertension as their primary underlying etiology of heart failure.[16] These disparities in etiology by gender may reflect, on the one hand, the lower prevalence of coronary heart disease and the higher prevalence of hypertension in women compared with men, and on the other hand, the greater impact of hypertension as a risk factor of heart failure in women, as described above.

Although ischemic heart disease is less common as a contributing factor to heart failure in women than in men, women who sustain a myocardial infarction are more likely to develop heart failure as a postinfarction complication,[9,11,12,22] an observation that is independent of their older age.[9] The reasons for these gender differences in susceptibility to heart failure after myocardial infarction have not been elucidated.

Systolic versus diastolic ventricular dysfunction

Although data are limited, women are thought to be more likely than men to have diastolic dysfunction as the underlying pathophysiological abnormality of heart failure.[16] This notion is mostly suggested by the finding – in those few studies of heart failure that were not restricted to patients with impaired left ventricular systolic function – that women have higher left ventricular ejection fraction and lower prevalence of left ventricular systolic dysfunction compared with men.[19,23,24] The lower prevalence of left ventricular systolic dysfunction in women with heart failure compared with men may be mostly (but not entirely) due to gender differences in the etiology of heart failure, with hypertension and diabetes being more common antecedents of heart failure in women and ischemic heart disease more common in men. In a sample of 557 symptomatic heart failure patients, Adams et al.[19] demonstrated that although women as a group had higher left ventricular ejection fraction than men, left ventricular ejection fraction did not differ between men and women when ischemic heart disease was the primary etiology of heart failure. However, in the nonischemic group, the finding of a higher left ventricular ejection fraction in women persisted,[19] and even among hypertensive patients with evidence of left ventricular hypertrophy, women were shown to have higher left ventricular systolic function than men.[25] These data suggest that gender differences in the etiology of heart failure should not explain entirely the gender differences in systolic function.

Pathology studies have indicated that during aging, there is a better preservation of myocardial structure in the female heart than in the male heart, including less extensive decrease in number, average cell diameter, and volume of myocytes in the left and right ventricles.[26] This reported less extensive loss of myocardial mass with aging in women than in men may in part depend on the cumulative protective effects of estrogen during women's lifetime (as discussed below), and may ultimately result in better preservation of systolic function in this subgroup.

Cardiovascular effects of estrogen

Estrogen exerts its many effects on different tissues via the estrogen alpha- and beta-receptors. Both vascular smooth muscle cells and the endothelium bind estrogen with high affinity at the estrogen alpha-receptor.[27] The beta-receptors are found in other tissues such as the prostate, uterus, bladder, lung, brain, ovary, and testis.

Effects on neurohormonal systems
Estrogen has numerous effects on the cardiovascular system that may have potential clinical implications for treatment of atherosclerosis, hypertension, and heart failure. For instance, estrogen regulates expression of nitric oxide synthase in the myocardium and the renin–angiotensin system. Oral conjugated estrogens are associated with an increase in angiotensinogen and a decrease in angiotensin-converting enzyme (ACE) activity.[28] As a result of the suppressive effect of estrogen on the renin–angiotensin system, in postmenopausal women taking estrogen therapy plasma renin levels are lower than those in men or postmenopausal women not on estrogen.[28] Similar suppression of renin levels is seen with estrogen alone versus an estrogen/progestin combination.[28] This decrease in renin levels may be related to estrogen-mediated suppression of beta-adrenergic activity, although lower circulating androgens in women might also play a role. Aldosterone levels do not appear to be significantly altered by estrogen therapy. Women have greater beta$_2$-receptor sensitivity than men, probably due to gender-related differences in post-receptor adenylate cyclase activity.[29]

Despite these effects of estrogen on the renin–angiotensin system, it is not known whether the clinical efficacy of ACE inhibitors is affected by estrogen status. However, these observations suggest that there may be gender-related differences in response to ACE inhibition and beta-blocker therapy.

Estrogen also decreases plasma endothelin-1 concentrations,[30] an effect that could be beneficial in women with heart failure. Endothelin-1 is a potent vasoconstrictor that is elevated in the plasma of patients with heart failure.

Effects on lipids
In addition, estrogen has effects on lipid profiles, coagulation and fibrinolytic systems, nitric oxide, and prostaglandins, all of which are important in the development of atherosclerosis and coronary syndromes. For example, when administered to postmenopausal women, estrogen decreases total cholesterol, low-density lipoprotein (LDL) cholesterol, increases high-density lipoprotein cholesterol, and decreases Lp(a).[31] However, estrogen replacement therapy also increases plasma triglyceride levels in some women, which may decrease LDL particle size.[32] Small LDL particles are associated with an increased risk of coronary atherosclerotic heart disease,

presumably due to increased susceptibility to oxidation. Therefore, the beneficial effects of estrogen may be offset by estrogen's adverse effect on triglyceride levels.

Clinical cardiovascular effects

Despite the wealth of data suggesting potentially beneficial effects of estrogen for the cardiovascular system, conflicting information has emerged regarding the benefits of estrogen on clinical cardiovascular events. An 18-year follow-up of women in the Nurses Health Study demonstrated a 53% risk reduction in coronary heart disease mortality among current hormone users,[33] a finding consistent with earlier observational studies.[34,35] However, a secondary prevention study of postmenopausal women with established coronary atherosclerotic heart disease demonstrated no advantage of an estrogen/progestin combination over placebo in reducing further cardiac events or stroke over a 4-year follow-up period.[36] In addition, there was a trend toward an increase in myocardial infarction after initiation of the estrogen/progestin combination.

Additional clinical trials are evaluating the cardiovascular effects of estrogens. The Raloxifene Use for The Heart (RUTH) trial is evaluating a selective estrogen agonist/antagonist (raloxifene) for primary prevention of cardiac events in women at risk. Another selective estrogen receptor modulator, tamoxifen, has been shown to improve endothelial function in men with atherosclerotic coronary artery disease.[37] Selective estrogen receptor modulators may have potential cardiovascular benefits without the need for concomitant progestin therapy.

Advances in the treatment of coronary disease and myocardial infarction have improved survival, but more survivors eventually develop heart failure. Therefore, therapies that prevent myocardial infarction should be most effective in reducing the future risk of heart failure related to atherosclerotic heart disease. Clinical trials are under way to define the role of estrogen for primary prevention of cardiovascular events. In addition, the specific effects of hormone replacement therapy on the development and progression of heart failure are yet to be determined.

Presentation of heart failure in women

Despite their lower prevalence of left ventricular systolic function, women with heart failure present with more symptoms and signs of decompensation than men, such as elevated respiratory rate, rales, and pulmonary edema, and higher New York Heart Association (NYHA) functional class.[20,24] Even in studies that included only patients with left ventricular dysfunction, such as the Studies of Left Ventricular Dysfunction (SOLVD),[38] and the Cardiac Insufficiency Bisoprolol Study (CIBIS II),[21] women had symptoms and signs indicating a more advanced disease stage than men. These included more often dyspnea at rest, fatigue, peripheral edema, third heart sound and elevated jugular pressure, and higher NYHA functional class. This tendency towards more symptoms and greater functional limitations among women was seen both in the treatment and in the prevention SOLVD studies. Similarly, among patients with idiopathic dilated cardiomyopathy, women were shown to report more symptoms, shorter exercise duration, and presented more frequently with signs of heart failure.[39] Although some of these differences in presentation might be due to the older age of the women, these findings overall indicate that women with heart failure suffer more limitations and lower quality of life compared with men.

Prognosis after heart failure in women

Studies based on community samples or patient registries

Despite general consensus on the poor prognosis of heart failure, there is considerable variability on mortality estimates across studies, and data on gender differences in mortality are conflicting. The Framingham Study has indicated that the prognosis of heart failure in women is significantly better than men; the median survival after diagnosis of heart failure is 1.7 years in men and 3.2 years in women, and the 1-year mortality rate is 43% in men and 36% in women.[40] Three other studies based on patient series also have reported lower mortality in women.[19,24,41] In one of these studies, of a large patient population in Connecticut,[24] the lower mortality rate in women at 6 months after hospital discharge was mostly accounted for by women's more favorable indicators of left ventricular function (higher left ventricular ejection fraction and systolic blood pressure). In two other patient registries, however, no gender differences in mortality were found at 1 year. These studies included a consecutive series of 435 heart failure patients hospitalized at the Brigham and Women's Hospital in Boston,[23] and the Italian Network Congestive Heart Failure Registry (IN-CHF).[20] In the IN-CHF, data

were collected on 6428 patients with heart failure who were seen by a cardiologist. Despite a similar incidence of heart failure in men and women, the registry included only 26% women, reflecting fewer cardiology referrals for women. The 1-year mortality was similar in women and men (15.9% vs 16.4%), regardless of etiology.

Studies based on clinical trials samples

A number of reports based on secondary analyses of randomized trials of heart failure treatment have also shown inconsistent results regarding gender differences in mortality. An analysis of the Flolan International Randomized Survival Trial (FIRST), which enrolled predominantly NYHA Class IV patients with severe cardiac dysfunction (left ventricular ejection fraction below 25%), demonstrated a trend towards improved survival in women,[42] as shown in Figure 4.1. This survival advantage persisted after adjustment for dobutamine use at randomization, mean pulmonary artery pressure, 6-minute walk distance, and treatment assignment.

The Cardiac Insufficiency Bisoprolol Study (CIBIS II), a study of the selective beta-blocker bisoprolol in NYHA class III–IV heart failure, also demonstrated a survival advantage for women compared with men.[21] The lower death rate in women was mostly due to a lower rate of cardiovascular mortality, in particular deaths due to pump failure (Figure 4.2). Rates of sudden death and fatal myocardial infarction were similar for men and women. The survival advantage of women over men was most pronounced in the group receiving beta-blockers, where women showed 50% lower mortality compared with men (6%

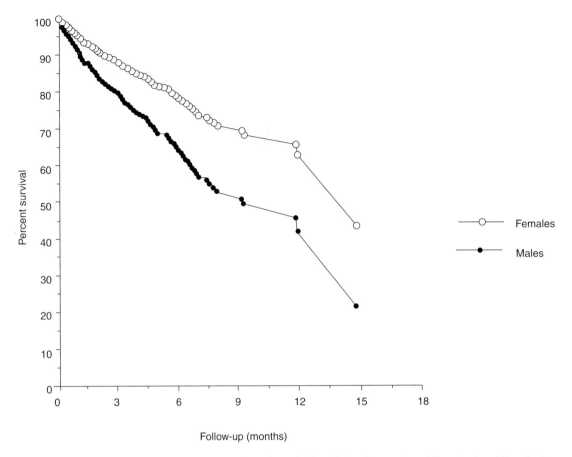

Figure 4.1   Survival curves for male vs female patients in the Flolan International Randomized Survival Trial (FIRST). Females had a statistically significant survival advantage over males in the study. (Reproduced with permission from Adams et al.[42])

vs 12%). There was a trend toward a lower mortality for women also in the placebo group (about 28% lower), but this difference was not statistically significant (Figure 4.3).

Conflicting results have been found in other large clinical heart failure trials. No gender-related mortality differences were seen in the US carvedilol studies,[43] the Italian Multicenter Cardiomyopathy Study (SPIC),[39] or the Metoprolol CR/XL Randomized Intervention Trial in Congestive Heart Failure (MERIT-

HF).[44] A higher 1-year mortality in women (22%) than in men (17%) was noted in the SOLVD trial.[45,46]

The common observation in all of these trials, which might play a role in the different results, is the low percentage of women who were included (22–30%), as well as differences in entry criteria and treatment modalities. In addition, there are fundamental differences in study sample between population-based studies, such as the Framingham Study, and

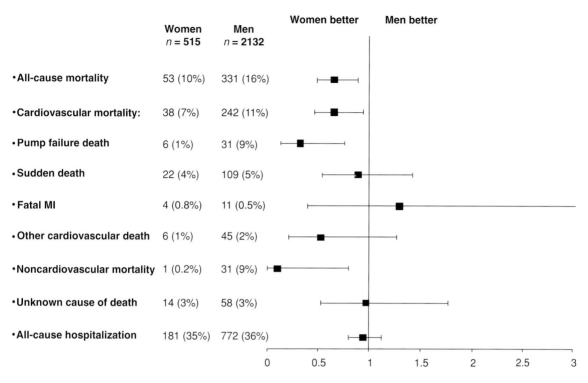

Figure 4.2 Comparison of cause of death and hospitalizations between males and females enrolled in the Cardiac Insufficiency Bisoprolol Study (CIBIS II). Women had lower all-cause mortality, heart failure death, noncardiovascular death, and hospitalization rates, but not fatal myocardial infarction (MI) and sudden death. (Reproduced with permission from Simon et al.[21])

clinical trial populations in which patients had to meet specific eligibility criteria and had to agree to participate in an intervention study. In this respect, community-based or registry-based studies provide more insight into the etiology and prognosis of women and men with heart failure followed by community cardiologists or practitioners. Another major difference with clinical trial samples is that, while clinical trials almost invariably included only patients with systolic dysfunction, as usually determined by reduced left ventricular ejection fraction, community-based studies or studies based on patient registries typically did not.

Role of heart failure etiology

Conflicting results have also been presented on whether the underlying etiology of heart failure (ischemic versus nonischemic) plays a role on the gender differences in outcome. Some studies have indicated that women survive longer than men when heart failure is due to nonischemic causes, but that survival is similar in men and women if heart failure is due to ischemic heart disease.[19,42] Other authors, however, have reported opposite findings, i.e. similar mortality in men and women with nonischemic heart failure, but

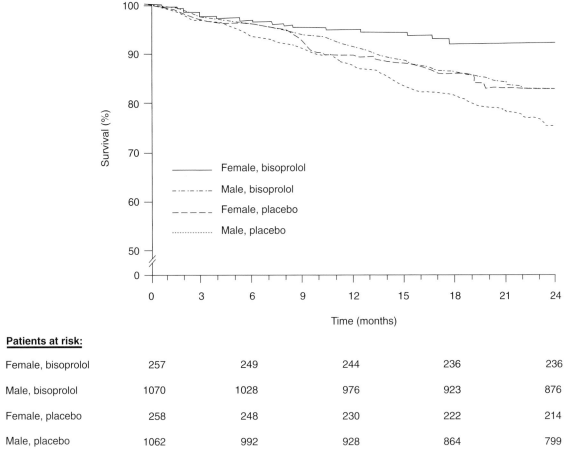

Patients at risk:

Female, bisoprolol	257	249	244	236	236
Male, bisoprolol	1070	1028	976	923	876
Female, placebo	258	248	230	222	214
Male, placebo	1062	992	928	864	799

Figure 4.3 Survival curves for male vs female patients based on treatment assignment in the Cardiac Insufficiency Bisoprolol Study (CIBIS II). Females treated with bisoprolol had a significant survival advantage over males in both treatment assignments and over women treated with placebo. (Reproduced with permission from Simon et al.[21])

lower mortality in women with ischemic heart failure.[21] Finally, other researchers have observed similar mortality in women and men regardless of the etiology of heart failure.[20] Therefore, the impact of the underlying cause of heart failure on gender differences in outcome remains unclear. There are also no data on whether differences in mortality according to gender depend on type of heart failure, i.e. heart failure due to systolic vs diastolic left ventricular dysfunction.

Functional status and quality of life in women with heart failure

Whereas most studies of heart failure have focused on survival, outcomes other than mortality are increasingly recognized as important.[47–49] Although data are sparse, it appears that heart failure has a major impact on functional status and quality of life.[23,41,50]

In the year after hospital discharge for heart failure, patients have been found to suffer on average complete dependence on one activity of daily living, and 35% are short of breath while walking less than one block.[41] Heart failure patients may suffer limitations to the point that they may prioritize enhancement in quality of life over surviving.[51] In the study by Burns et al.,[41] female and male heart failure patients surviving at 1 year had similar and substantial impairments in functional outcomes. However, in another patient series,[23] women had lower quality of life scores at 1 year after hospital discharge and less improvement in physical function relative to baseline compared with men.

Pharmacologic treatment of heart failure in women

Few studies have specifically examined the treatment of heart failure in women. Despite a similar prevalence of heart failure between men and women, most clinical trials have enrolled only 20–30% women (Table 4.1). The large-scale heart failure trials have included only patients with reduced left ventricular ejection fraction, typically 35% or less,[43,44,52–56] which may account for the lower enrollment of women who are more likely than men to have preserved systolic function, as described above. In addition, women with heart failure are less likely to be referred to a hospital and more likely to be treated by general practitioners than men.[57] Furthermore, once admitted to the hospital, women are less likely to be managed by a cardiologist than men.[58] Women are also less likely than men to undergo cardiac catheterization and other diagnostic tests after heart failure.[21,58] These gender differences referral and in evaluation may also contribute to the lower enrollment rates of women in heart failure trials.

Angiotensin-converting enzyme inhibitors

The ACE inhibitor trials all demonstrated a mortality reduction in women, but to a somewhat lesser degree than in men.[52–55] Despite this reduced benefit of ACE inhibitor therapy in women compared with men, ACE inhibitor therapy is associated with a clear mortality benefit in women, and therefore should be used for the treatment of heart failure due to left ventricular systolic dysfunction in women. Studies have shown that women are less likely than men to be treated with ACE inhibitors, although this difference might reflect the lower prevalence of left ventricular systolic dysfunction in women. For example, in the IN-CHF registry, which included patients with evidence of heart failure irrespective of left ventricular ejection fraction values,[21] women were 12% less likely than men to be treated with ACE inhibitors (74% vs 84%). However, in the CIBIS II trial, which included patients with left ventricular ejection fraction of 35% or less, women were only 2% less likely to be receiving ACE inhibitors (95% vs 97%).

Beta-blockers

The CIBIS II trial demonstrated improved survival associated with beta-blocker treatment in women, and this survival benefit was larger in women than in men.[21] The same benefit, however, was not observed with carvedilol or metoprolol.[43,44] Given the relatively small numbers of women in these trials, it is difficult to draw any definite conclusions about differential treatment effects in women between selective and nonselective beta-blockers. What we can conclude at this point is that women with mild to moderate heart failure have at least the same benefits from beta-blockade as men and should be treated with beta-blockers as part of standard heart failure therapy.

Spironolactone

Treatment of patients with recent or current Class IV congestive heart failure with an aldosterone antagonist (spironolactone) reduced all-cause mortality in the Randomized Aldactone Evaluation Study (RALES).[59] The RALES trial enrolled patients with both ischemic and non-ischemic etiologies for their heart failure. The patients were randomized to placebo or spironolactone 25 mg once daily in addition to standard therapy including ACE inhibitors in 95% and beta-blockers in 10%. Approximately 27% of participants in the trial were female. The 31% reduction in the risk of cardiac deaths was seen in both male and female participants. Therefore, spironolactone should be considered for all women with Class IV or recent Class IV heart failure. Hyperkalemia is a potential complication of treatment with spironolactone; therefore, caution should be exercised when administering spironolactone to patients with a serum creatinine above 2.5 mg/dl or baseline elevation of their potassium level.

Warfarin

Thromboembolic events occur in patients with reduced left ventricular ejection fraction and normal sinus rhythm at an incidence of approximately 1–5% per year.[60] Whereas the indication for Coumadin (warfarin) therapy is clear in patients with heart failure and atrial fibrillation or flutter, the use of Coumadin in low left ventricular ejection fraction with sinus rhythm remains controversial. A retrospective analysis of the SOLVD treatment and prevention trials found the annual incidence of thromboembolic events in normal sinus rhythm to be higher in women than in men (2.4% vs 1.8%).[60] In addition, the risk of a thromboembolic event increased as the ejection fraction fell in women but not in men. Women with a left ventricular ejection fraction less than 20% had an annual thromboembolic event incidence of nearly 4% compared with 2% for men. The estrogen status of the women evaluated in this retrospective analysis was not available; thus, further investigation into this issue is needed. When advising patients on anticoagulation, the risk

Trial	Year	No. of patients	Women (%)	Mean age (years)
Captopril–Digoxin	1988	300	51	57
SOLVD (prevention)	1992	4,228	11.5	59
SOLVD (treatment)	1991	2,569	23	61
CONSENSUS-I	1987	253	30	70
MDC	1993	383	27	49
PROMISE	1991	1,088	22	64
Vesnarinone	1993	477	13	58
RADIANCE	1993	178	24	60
DIG	1997	6,800	24	64
Carvedilol	1996	1,094	23	48
Total		17,370	19.7%	62

CONSENSUS = Cooperative North Scandinavian Enalapril Survival Study; DIG = Digitalis Investigation Group; MDC = Metoprolol in Dilated Cardiomyopathy; RADIANCE = Randomized Assessment of Digoxin on Inhibitors of the Angiotensin-Converting Enzyme; SOLVD = Studies of Left Ventricular Dysfunction. (From Lindenfeld et al.[62])

Table 4.1 Age and gender distribution in heart failure trials

of hemorrhagic stroke and serious bleeding events must be taken into account. Although the benefits of anticoagulation in patients with low left ventricular ejection fraction and sinus rhythm are controversial, women with very low left ventricular ejection fractions may obtain more benefit than men.

Estrogen replacement therapy

There are no studies examining the role of estrogen replacement in women with heart failure. Although there may be theoretical benefits of estrogen replacement therapy, the only role of estrogen replacement currently is osteoporosis prevention.

Heart failure with preserved systolic function

None of the large-scale clinical trials to date have included patients with preserved left ventricular ejection fraction. However, several ongoing large-scale clinical heart failure trials examining the effects of ACE inhibitors and angiotensin receptor blockers have included a preserved left ventricular function arm. The treatment of diastolic dysfunction, therefore, remains empiric. Since women are more likely than men to have heart failure with preserved left ventricular ejection fraction, inclusion of this group of patients is paramount to determine the most effective therapies for heart failure in women. The treatment of 'diastolic heart failure' is discussed in detail in Chapter 7.

Conclusions

In conclusion, due to the small number of women included in heart failure trials, it is difficult to ascertain if women truly respond differently to heart failure therapies than their male counterparts. However, from the available data there is no evidence to suggest that women, at least those with systolic dysfunction, require different therapy than men.

Cardiac transplantation

Transplantation has now become an accepted treatment option for patients with end-stage congestive heart failure. This is primarily due to the use of improved immunosuppressants, which has led to an improvement in survival. Currently the expected 1-year survival for orthotopic heart transplant is approximately 85%. However, the number of women undergoing transplantation remains lower than men. Although women represent approximately 40% of cadaveric donors, only approximately 25% of heart transplant recipients are female.[61] The reason for this disparity has not been well studied. Of interest is that these numbers also parallel the number of women involved in clinical congestive heart failure trials (Table 4.1).[62]

One explanation for the lower use of cardiac transplantation in women with heart failure compared with men might be the older age of the women. Although women are more likely than men to develop congestive heart failure after a myocardial infarction, they are more likely than men to develop coronary disease later in life and often past the acceptable age for heart transplant consideration. Also, severe left ventricular dysfunction on a nonischemic basis is more common in men than women.[63] Both of these facts may contribute to the lower numbers of women undergoing transplantation than men. In addition, women with heart failure are more likely to have hypertension[6,18,58,64] and diabetes[6,18,64,65] as risk factors. If women have retinopathy, neuropathy, or nephropathy they may be excluded from consideration for transplantation.

Referral patterns and patient preferences might also contribute to the gender disparity in cardiac transplantation. Philbin and DiSalvo have shown that women with heart failure are less likely than men to be referred to a specialist (cardiologist).[58] Therefore it would be expected that these women would also be less likely to be referred for transplantation. Additionally, women are less likely than men to accept transplant when offered to them as a treatment option.[66]

Few studies have looked at the survival of women after transplant. Most of these studies noted no difference in survival between women and men. However, Weslerch et al. found a decreased survival in women up to 3 years after transplant.[67] More consistent are the data on rejection post-transplant in women. Female transplant recipients have more episodes of rejection and are less likely to be successfully weaned off steroids than their male counterparts. Donor gender, however, also appears to play a role; transplants from female donors are associated with higher rates of rejection both in male and female recipients, but particularly so in female recipients (Figure 4.4).[68] However, despite these gender differences in rejection, and the fact that before transplant women often report more symptoms than men,[69] after transplantation there is no gender difference in quality of life.[70]

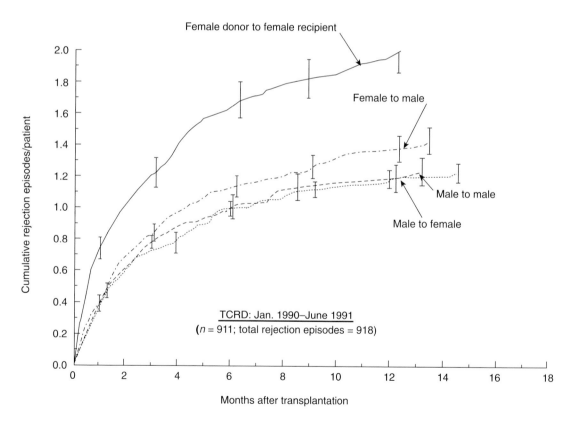

Figure 4.4 Cumulative rejection frequency over time, according to donor and recipient gender. (Reproduced with permission from Kobashigawa et al.[68])

Conclusion

Gender differences in the etiology, prognosis, and complications have been found between men and women with heart failure. While the pathophysiology behind these differences remains to be elucidated, these differences indicate the need to develop trials designed to study the efficacy of clinical therapies in women. Until these data become available, the existing evidence from large-scale clinical trials suggests that women benefit from the currently recommended therapies of heart failure and that these therapies, therefore, should be offered to women. Until more women are adequately represented in clinical trials, however, the most efficacious means of treating women with heart failure will remain unknown.

References

1. Schocken DD, Arrieta MI, Leaverton PE, Ross EA. Prevalence and mortality rate of congestive heart failure in the United States. J Am Coll Cardiol 1992; 20:301–6.
2. Rodeheffer RJ, Jacobsen SJ, Gersh BJ, et al. The incidence and prevalence of congestive heart failure in Rochester, Minnesota. Mayo Clin Proc 1993; 68:1143–50.
3. Ho KKL, Pinsky JL, Kannel WB, Levy DB. The epidemiology of heart failure: The Framingham Study. J Am Coll Cardiol 1993; 22(Suppl A):6A–13A.
4. Mittelmark MB, Psaty BM, Rautaharju PM, et al. Prevalence of cardiovascular diseases among older adults. The Cardiovascular Health Study. Am J Epidemiol 1993; 137:311–17.
5. McDonagh TA, Morrison CE, Lawrence A, et al. Symptomatic and asymptomatic left ventricular systolic dysfunction. Lancet 1997; 350:829–33.
6. Kannel WB, Belanger AJ. Epidemiology of heart failure. Am Heart J 1991; 121:951–7.
7. Gottdiener JS, Arnold AM, Aurigemma GP, et al. Predictors of congestive heart failure in the elderly: the Cardiovascular Health Study. J Am Coll Cardiol 2000; 35:1628–37.
8. Remes J, Reunanen A, Aromaa A, Pyorala K. Incidence of heart failure in eastern Finland: a population-based surveillance study. Eur Heart J 1992; 13:588–93.
9. Vaccarino V, Parsons L, Every NR, et al. Sex-based differences in early mortality after myocardial infarction. New Engl J Med 1999; 341:217–25.
10. Vaccarino V, Krumholz HM, Yarzebski J, et al. Sex differences in 2-year mortality after hospital discharge for myocardial infarction. Ann Int Med 2001; 134:173–81.
11. Marrugat J, Sala J, Masia R, et al. Mortality differences between men and women following first myocardial infarction. JAMA 1998; 280:1405–9.
12. Malacrida R, Genoni M, Maggioni AP, et al. A comparison of the early outcome of acute myocardial infarction in women and in men. New Engl J Med 1998; 338:8–14.
13. Kannel WB, Ho K, Thom T. Changing epidemiological features of cardiac failure. Br Heart J 1994; 72:S3–S9.
14. Kannel WB, D'Agostino RB, Silbershatz H, et al. Profile for estimating risk of heart failure. Arch Int Med 1999; 159:1197–204.
15. Chen Y, Vaccarino V, Williams CS, et al. Risk factors for heart failure in the elderly: a prospective community-based study. Am J Med 1999; 106:605–12.
16. Dunlap SH, Sueta CA, Tomasko L, Adams KF. Association of body mass, gender and race with heart failure primarily due to hypertension. J Am Coll Cardiol 1999; 34:1602–8.

17. Vaccarino V, Holford TR, Krumholz HM. Pulse pressure and risk of myocardial infarction and heart failure in the elderly. J Am Coll Cardiol 2000; 36:130–8.

18. Levy D, Larson MG, Vasan RS, et al. The progression from hypertension to congestive heart failure. JAMA 1996; 275:1604–6.

19. Adams KF, Dunlap SH, Sueta CA, et al. Relation between gender, etiology and survival in patients with symptomatic heart failure. J Am Coll Cardiol 1996; 28:1781–8.

20. Opasich C, Tavazzi L, Lucci D, et al. Comparison of one-year outcome in women versus men with chronic congestive heart failure. Am J Cardiol 2000; 86:353–7.

21. Simon T, Mary-Krause M, Funck-Brentano C, Jaillon P. Sex differences in the prognosis of congestive heart failure: results from the Cardiac Insufficiency Bisoprolol Study (CIBIS II). Circulation 2001; 103:375–80.

22. Gottlieb SS, Harpaz D, Avraham S, et al. Sex differences in management and outcome after acute myocardial infarction in the 1990s. A prospective observational community-based study. Circulation 2000; 102:2484–90.

23. Chin MH, Goldman L. Gender differences in 1-year survival and quality of life among patients admitted with congestive heart failure. Med Care 1998; 36:1033–46.

24. Vaccarino V, Chen Y, Wanf Y, et al. Sex differences in the clinical care and outcomes of congestive heart failure in the elderly. Am Heart J 1999; 138:835–42.

25. Gerdts E, Zabalgoitia M, Bjornstad H, et al. Gender differences in systolic left ventricular function in hypertensive patients with electrocardiographic left ventricular hypertrophy (the LIFE study). Am J Cardiol 2001; 87:980–3.

26. Olivetti G, Giordano G, Corradi D, et al. Gender differences and aging: effects on the human heart. J Am Coll Cardiol 1995; 26:1068–79.

27. Mendelsohn ME, Karas RH. The protective effect of estrogen on the cardiovascular system. New Engl J Med 1999; 340:1801–11.

28. Proudler AJ, Ahmed AI, Crook D, et al. Hormone replacement therapy and serum angiotensin-converting enzyme activity in postmenopausal women. Lancet 1995; 346:89–90.

29. Mills PJ, Ziegler MG, Nelesen RA, Kennedy BP. The effects of the menstrual cycle, race and gender on adrenergic receptors and agonists. Clin Pharmacol Ther 1996; 60:99–104.

30. Yikorkala O, Orphana A, Puolakka J, et al. Postmenopausal hormone replacement decreases plasma levels of endothelin-1. J Clin Endocrinol Metab 1995; 80:3384–7.

31. The Writing Group for the PEPI trial. Effects of estrogen/progestin regimens on heart disease risk factors in postmenopausal women. The Postmenopausal Estrogen/Progestin Interventions Trial. JAMA 1995; 273:199–208. (Erratum: JAMA 1995; 274:1676.)

32. Wakatsuki A, Ikenoue N, Okatani Y, Fukaya T. Estrogen-induced small low-density lipoprotein particles may be atherogenic in postmenopausal women. J Am Coll Cardiol 2001; 37:425–30.

33. Grodstein F, Stampfer MJ, Colditz GA, et al. Postmenopausal hormone therapy and mortality. New Engl J Med 1997; 336:1769–75.

34. Stampfer MJ, Colditz GA. Estrogen replacement therapy and coronary heart disease: a quantitative assessment of the epidemiologic evidence. Prev Med 1991; 20:47–63.

35. Grady D, Rubin SM, Petitti DB, et al. Hormone therapy to prevent disease and prolong life in postmenopausal women. Ann Int Med 1992; 117:1016–37.

36. Hulley S, Grady D, Bush T. Randomized trial of estrogen plus progestin for secondary prevention of coronary heart disease in postmenopausal women. JAMA 1998; 280:605–13.

37. Clarke SC, Schofield PM, Grace AA, et al. Tamoxifen effects on endothelial function and cardiovascular risk factors in men with advanced atherosclerosis. Circulation 2001; 103:1497–502.

38. Johnstone D, Limacher M, Rousseau M, et al. Clinical characteristics of patients in studies of left ventricular dysfunction (SOLVD). Am J Cardiol 1992; 70:894–900.

39. De Maria R, Gavazzi A, Recalcati F, et al. Comparison of the clinical findings in idiopathic dilated cardiomyopathy in women versus men. Am J Cardiol 1993; 72:580–5.

40. Ho KKL, Anderson KM, Kannel WB, et al. Survival after the onset of congestive heart failure in Framingham Heart Study subjects. Circulation 1993; 88:107–15.

41. Burns RB, McCarthy EP, Moskowitz MA, et al. Outcomes for older men and women with conges-

tive heart failure. J Am Geriatr Soc 1997; 45:276–80.

42. Adams KF, Sueta CA, Gheorghiade M, et al. Gender differences in survival in advanced heart failure. Insights from the FIRST study. Circulation 1999; 99:1816–21.

43. Packer M, Bristow MR, Cohn JN, et al. The effect of carvediolol on morbidity and mortality in patients with chronic heart failure. US Carvedilol Heart Failure Study Group. New Engl J Med 1996; 334:1349–55.

44. MERIT-HF Investigators. Effects of controlled-release on total mortality, hospitalizations, and well-being in patients with heart failure: Metoprolol CR/XL randomized intervention trial in congestive heart failure. JAMA 2000; 283: 1295–302.

45. Limacher MC, Yusuf S (for the SOLVD Investigators). Gender differences in presentation, morbidity and mortality in the Studies of Left Ventricular Dysfunction (SOLVD): a preliminary report. In: Wenger NK, Speroff L, Packard B, eds, Cardiovascular Health and Disease in Women. Greenwich, CT: Le Jacq Communications, 1993:345–8.

46. Bourassa MG, Gurne O, Bangdiwala SI, et al. Natural history and patterns of current practice in heart failure. The Studies of Left Ventricular Dysfunction (SOLVD) investigators. J Am Coll Cardiol 1993; 22:14A–19A.

47. Fergus I, Demopoulos LA, LeJemtel TH. Quality of life in older patients with congestive heart failure. Effects of ACE inhibitors. Drugs and Aging 1996; 8:23–8.

48. Konstam V, Salem D, Pouleur H, et al. Baseline quality of life as predictor of mortality and hospitalization in 5,025 patients with congestive heart failure. SOLVD Investigators. Am J Cardiol 1996; 78:890–5.

49. Taylor SH. Congestive heart failure. Towards a comprehensive treatment. Eur Heart J 1996; 17:43–56.

50. Dracup K, Walden JA, Stevenson LW, Brecht M. Quality of life in patients with advanced heart failure. J Heart Lung Transplant 1992; 11:273–9.

51. Rector TS, Tschumperlin LK, Kubo SH, et al. Use of living with heart failure questionnaire to ascertain patients' perspectives on improvement in quality of life versus risk of drug-induced death. J Card Fail 1995; 1:201–6.

52. Pfeffer MA, Braunwald E, Moye LA, et al. Effect of captopril on mortality and morbidity in patients with left ventricular dysfunction after myocardial infarction: results of the Survival and Ventricular Enlargement Trial. New Engl J Med 1992; 327:669–77.

53. The SOLVD Investigators. Effect of enalapril on survival in patients with reduced left ventricular ejection fraction and congestive heart failure. New Engl J Med 1991; 325:293–302.

54. The CONSENSUS trial study group. Effects of enalapril on mortality in severe congestive heart failure: results of the Cooperative North Scandinavian Enalapril Survival Study (CONSENSUS). New Engl J Med 1987; 316: 1429–35.

55. The SOLVD Investigators. Effect of enalapril on mortality and the development of heart failure in asymptomatic patients with reduced left ventricular ejection fraction. New Engl J Med 1992; 327:685–91.

56. CIBIS II Investigators and Committees. The Cardiac Insufficiency Bisoprolol Study II (CIBIS II): a randomized trial. Lancet 1999; 353:9–13.

57. Clarke KW, Gray D, Hampton JR. Evidence of inadequate investigation and treatment of patients with heart failure. Br Heart J 1994; 71:584–7.

58. Philbin EF, DiSalvo TG. Influence of race and gender on care process, resource use, and hospital-based outcomes in congestive heart failure. Am J Cardiol 1998; 82:76–81.

59. Pitt B, Zannad F, Remme WJ, et al. The effect of spironolactone on morbidity and mortality in patients with severe heart failure. Randomized Aldactone Evaluation Study Investigators. New Engl J Med 1999; 341:709–17.

60. Dries DL, Rosenberg YD, Waclawiw MA, Domanski MJ. Ejection fraction and risk of thromboembolic events in patients with systolic dysfunction and sinus rhythm: evidence for gender differences in the studies of left ventricular dysfunction trials. J Am Coll Cardiol 1997; 29:1074–80.

61. Transplant Patient DataSource 2001 Sept. 6. Richmond, VA: United Network for Organ Sharing. Retrieved September 6th from the world wide web: http://www.patients.unos.org/data. htm.

62. Lindenfeld J, Krause-Steinrauf H, Salerno J. Where are all the women with heart failure? J Am Coll Cardiol 1997; 30:1417–19.

63. Smith AS, Bronzena S. Cardiac transplantation in women. In: Julian DG, Wenger NK, eds, Women and Heart Disease. London: Martin Dunitz, 1997:392–404.

64. Petrie MC, Dawson NF, Murdoch DR, et al. Failure of women's hearts. Circulation 1990; 99:2334–41.

65. Shindler DM, Kostis JB, Yusuf S, et al. Diabetes mellitus, a predictor of morbidity and mortality in the Studies of Left Ventricular Dysfunction (SOLVD) Trials and Registry. Am J Cardiol 1996; 77:1017–20.

66. Aaronson KD, Schwartz JS, Goin JE, Mancini DM. Sex differences in patient acceptance of cardiac transplant candidacy. Circulation 1995; 91:2753–61.

67. Wechsler ME, Giardina EV, Sciacca RR, et al. Increased early mortality in women undergoing cardiac transplantation. Circulation 1995; 91:1029–35.

68. Kobashigawa JA, Kirklin JK, Naftel DC, et al. Pretransplantation risk factors for acute rejection after heart transplantation: a multiinstitutional study. The Transplant Cardiologists Research Database Group. J Heart Lung Transplant 1993; 12:355–66.

69. Mendes LA, Davidoff R, Cupples LA, et al. Congestive heart failure in patients with coronary artery disease: the gender paradox. Am Heart J 1997; 134:207–12.

70. Bunzel B, Grundbock A, Laczkovics A, et al. Quality of life after orthotopic heart transplantation. J Heart Lung Transplant 1991; 10:455–9.

5

Heart failure in pregnancy
Patrizia Presbitero and Tullia Todros

Introduction

Heart disease is present in 0.5% of all pregnant women and accounts for about 10% of all maternal mortality.[1] Rheumatic heart disease, although declining, remains the most prevalent. In the last decade congenital heart disease, which is usually corrected surgically, i.e. prior to pregnancy, is emerging as the leading cause of heart failure in pregnancy.

Cardiac failure can sometimes occur during pregnancy, even if the underlying cardiac disease is moderate, because of the significant hemodynamic changes that are present during gestation.

Hemodynamic changes during pregnancy

The most important change is the increase in blood volume, which almost doubles by the end of the pregnancy.[2] It starts to increase from 6 weeks, increases rapidly in the second trimester, and slows in the third trimester, becoming stable in the last 8 weeks. The red cell mass increases but less in comparison to the plasmatic volume, so that there is a fall in the hemoglobin concentration, with hematocrit levels about 33–34%, and hemoglobin around 11–12 g/dl.[3] Serum aldosterone increases in the last trimester, causing sodium and water retention. This hemodynamic change, which was conceived to protect the mother from blood loss at delivery, is one of the most important causes of heart failure; it can complicate pregnancy in many patients who were well compensated before.

The increase in cardiac output is another important hemodynamic change. This is partly due to the increase in blood volume and partly to the increase in heart rate. Heart rate starts to increase in the first weeks of pregnancy by 10–12 beats/min until the first half of the third trimester. Finally, there is a fall in peripheral vascular resistance due to the low resistance of the utero–placental circulation and to the increased level of circulating prostaglandin.[4] Because of these changes, even in a physiological pregnancy, dyspnea, palpitation, peripheral edema, and systolic heart murmur can occur, mimicking heart failure.

Therefore it can be difficult to make the differential diagnosis between physiological and pathological changes occurring in patients with previous heart disease. Pain and anxiety cause an increase in sympathetic tone, which is responsible for increased cardiac output and increased blood pressure. One of the main objectives during labor and delivery in patients with heart disease is to control pain with the use of analgesics. During uterine contractions, blood volume is increased due to the diversion of blood from the uterus to the systemic circulation. The increase in blood volume during the second stage of labor is due to increased venous return caused by compression of the vena cava. The amount of blood loss during delivery is about 500–700 ml. Because of the hemodynamic changes, the periods of greatest concern for the occurrence of heart failure are between 28 and 34 weeks' gestation, during labour and immediately postpartum, when physiological load on the heart is maximized.[5]

Conditions that cause heart failure during pregnancy

All the cardiac conditions in which valvular regurgitation or left to right shunts is present benefit from the decrease in arterial resistance during pregnancy and rarely lead to heart failure. Only when ventricular function is severely impaired can heart failure occur.

When valvular stenosis (mitral valve as well as aortic stenosis) is present, the increased cardiac output cannot be accommodated because of the decreased orifice, and heart failure can occur.

Mitral stenosis

Mitral stenosis is the most common (90%) of valvular heart diseases that can give problems during pregnancy. In mitral stenosis, pulmonary wedge pressure increases constantly during pregnancy, delivery (particularly during uterine contractions), and up to 15 min after delivery. Even moderate mitral stenosis can give rise to severe heart failure during pregnancy, requiring medical treatment or surgery.[6] When the stenosis is severe (valvular area less than 1 cm), tachycardia, with a decrease in the diastolic filling time, and the increase in blood volume cause a significant rise in pulmonary wedge pressure with resulting pulmonary edema.

Aortic stenosis

Aortic stenosis, although much more rare, is even more dangerous because heart failure can occur suddenly. In the presence of fixed cardiac output the patient is unable to face a sudden increase in volume without increasing left ventricular pressure and, consequently, pulmonary capillary pressure.

Death has been reported in patients with severe aortic stenosis.[7] A patient with moderate aortic stenosis (gradient of 50–70 mmHg) should be followed carefully. Most important is the appearance of electrocardiogram (ECG) changes of left ventricular overload not present before pregnancy, which often require aggressive treatment.

The gradient cannot be a guide to treatment, because during pregnancy it increases significantly due to the increase in cardiac output.

Left ventricular systolic dysfunction

All cardiac diseases with decreased left ventricular function are at risk of cardiac failure during pregnancy. The risk increases not only with the decrease of the ejection fraction but also with the occurrence of symptoms. With a left ventricular ejection fraction less than 40%, heart failure can be expected during the second to third trimester. The increased blood volume and stroke volume may be tolerated if the left ventricle dilates to accommodate it. This may vary within the different diseases and cannot be predicted.

Congenital heart disease

Among congenital heart diseases, the cyanotic heart diseases can manifest heart failure during pregnancy in up to 60% of cases. Even if cyanosis decreases, because of hemodilution that occurs during pregnancy, dyspnea, peripheral edema, and a decrease in oxygen saturation occur frequently, needing treatment and premature delivery.[8]

In taking care of pregnant women who have had surgery for congenital heart disease, there are two conditions that must be followed carefully because they are likely to cause heart failure. These conditions are now considered.

Transposition of the great arteries after Mustard or Senning intra-atrial repair

In this condition the right ventricle supports the systemic circulation. Up to 20% of these patients reaching adulthood have a decrease in right ventricular function that can worsen during pregnancy because of the overloaded right ventricle (two cases of heart failure in pregnancy in such patients have been reported in the literature).

After Fontan procedure

After the *Fontan procedure* all the systemic venous return is directed to the pulmonary artery directly or through the right atrium. In this case, the high output during pregnancy cannot be accommodated and right heart failure can occur. Even after surgical repair, there is a high number of spontaneous abortions (40%).

Prosthetic valve

Heart failure in patients with a prosthetic valve can be due to a malfunction of the valve or to left ventricular dysfunction. A biological valve can experience an accelerated degeneration during pregnancy, becoming stenotic or insufficient; this occurs in 10–50% of the cases often very rapidly, requiring valve replacement. In a mechanical valve, thrombosis can occur, even with anticoagulant treatment, requiring thrombolysis or surgery.[9]

Peripartum cardiomyopathy

Peripartum cardiomyopathy describes unexplained heart failure that occurs within 1 month before and up to 6 months after delivery in women who did not have a previous history of heart disease.[10] Peripartum cardiomyopathy presents with all degrees of severity, from mild left ventricular dysfunction to fulminating edema. Congestive heart failure can develop in the first days after delivery with severe dyspnea, orthopnea, tachycardia, hypotension, fluid overload, and sometimes mitral regurgitation. Ventricular tachycardia may precede the onset of clinical heart failure. Mortality, when heart failure is present, is very high.

Peripartum cardiomyopathy is common in women with multiple pregnancies and this may be caused by greater hemodynamic burden – higher stroke volume and stroke output – than in single pregnancies.

Differential diagnosis includes pre-existing dilated cardiomyopathy, peripartum myocardial infarction, which is rare, and pulmonary embolism.

Diagnosis of heart failure during pregnancy

Most cases of heart disease are diagnosed before pregnancy and very few become apparent for the first time during gestation. The symptoms of patients at risk of cardiac failure because of their cardiac disease should be watched carefully. If heart failure is suspected, a chest X-ray should be performed, regardless of the stage of gestation. The radiation dose of a chest X-ray is 0.07–0.15 rad, which is well below the dangerous level for the fetus.[11] This method is still the most reliable used to evaluate and follow pulmonary congestion. The echocardiogram is very important to confirm the diagnosis, to assess the severity of valvular disease, and to check ventricular function. When cardiac failure is present, there is a risk of hypoxia for the fetus; therefore, intensive fetal monitoring by means of two-dimensional and Doppler ultrasound and cardiotocography should be performed.

The management of heart failure in pregnancy

In assessing a pregnant woman with cardiac disease and heart failure, it is important to:
- carefully evaluate the underlying cardiac disease.
- recognize and treat factors that can trigger heart failure. Infections, particularly pulmonary infections in patients with high pulmonary pressure, can result in heart failure. Diuretics should be prescribed in these cases in order to prevent the occurrence of pulmonary edema. Arrhythmia, more often atrial fibrillation with high ventricular rate response, can cause heart failure, particularly in patients with mitral stenosis. In these patients, the shortened diastolic filling time may suddenly increase pulmonary wedge pressure, causing pulmonary edema. It is vital to treat the atrial fibrillation either by controlling the heart rate with beta-blocking agents, calcium antagonists, digoxin, or conversion to sinus rhythm with DC shock.
- consider the stage of pregnancy, because the fetal survival has to be taken into account. In fact, during heart failure, the utero–placental circulation is mostly impaired and the risk of death of the fetus is very high. Bed rest is essential in order to minimize oxygen consumption. It is also important to restrict water and salt intake.

Medications

Most of the drugs used to treat heart failure can be prescribed safely during pregnancy.

Diuretics are the first drugs to be employed in order to reduce hypervolemia.

Furosemide
Furosemide is the drug of choice because it does not have any contraindications during pregnancy. Collateral effects to be controlled are hypovolemia and hypokalemia. Particular caution should be taken in cyanotic patients.

Spironolactone
Spironolactone can be used for heart failure in pregnancy, especially in cases of hypokalemia. No adverse events have been reported on patients treated with spironolactone during pregnancy.

Digoxin
As there are no reports of teratogenicity associated with the use of digoxin, considering its long use and availability, one would consider it a drug of choice in treating congestive heart disease in pregnancy, especially when supraventricular arrhythmias and systolic dysfunction are present. Digoxin levels may be lower during pregnancy because of the increased renal clearance, so the dose should be increased. In the presence of decreased renal function or concomitant administration of amiodarone, the maintenance may require reduction. In the third trimester, serum digoxin levels may appear falsely elevated because of the presence of digoxin-like substances interfering with radioimmunoassays. Hence, the monitoring of digoxin levels would not be helpful in guiding treatment.

Angiotensin-converting enzyme inhibitors
Angiotensin-converting enzyme inhibitors should be withdrawn during pregnancy because of teratogenic effects.[12,13] In patients that need these drugs because of cardiomyopathy with systemic hypertension, hydrazaline,

perhaps in combination with a long-acting nitrate, should be substituted. Caution should be taken not to lower the blood pressure too much or too suddenly because this could impair the utero–placental blood flow and cause fetal hypoxia.

Angiotensin type 1 receptor blockers
There are no data available at this time about angiotensin type 1 receptor blockers in pregnancy.

Beta-blockers
No increased risk of fetal malformations has ever been reported with the use of beta-blockers during pregnancy. The prolonged administration of these drugs increases the risk of fetal growth restriction,[14] because they alter the utero–placental blood flow.[15,16] Theoretically, they could induce uterine contractions; however, an increase in preterm labors has not been demonstrated in patients treated with beta-blockers.

Antiarrhythmic agents
Ectopic beats are present in one-third of pregnant women. However, when arrhythmias occur during heart failure they can worsen the clinical status. Any antiarrhythmic drugs can be prescribed in pregnancy. Quinidine and verapamil have been used for long-term treatment of supraventricular and ventricular arrhythmias without any evidence of teratogenic effects.[17]

However, all these drugs have a depressive effect on myocardial contractility, so they should not be used in the presence of an impaired left ventricle. The only antiarrhythmic drug that should be used in this case is amiodarone;[18] in chronic administration, this drug can have side effects on the mother in 3–5% of cases, including thyroid malfunction, photosensitivity, and corneal deposition. In the fetus, long-term treatment with amiodarone can cause neonatal hypothyroidism; however, this is reversible.

Percutaneous and surgical treatment of heart failure in pregnancy
Heart surgery is considered in valvular disease when medical treatment fails to control heart failure, or in the presence of signs of persistent pulmonary hypertension.

Percutaneous valvotomy
Recently, balloon valvotomy procedures to widen the mitral valve have made nonsurgical treatment an option for treating mitral valve stenosis. The results of the percutaneous procedure are excellent if the valve is pliable, noncalcific, and the subvalvular apparatus is not too compromised.[18] The procedure, which is performed under X-ray guidance, should be performed in the second trimester, when embryogenesis is accomplished. This will avoid the negative effect on the fetal thyroid, which can be caused by ionic contrast agents late in gestation. There are no immediate detrimental effects of radiation on the fetus[19] because during percutaneous valvuloplasty, the radiation dose is between 0.05 and 0.2 rad, which is lower than the maximum acceptable dose of radiation for pregnant women (0.5–5 rad). Risk for the mother and particularly for the fetus is lower than previously reported when surgical commissurotomy was performed. Percutaneous aortic valvotomy has been reported in four cases in the literature with good results.[20] In these patients, a reduction of the gradient is the aim of the procedure in order to tide over the pregnancy until aortic valve replacement can be performed.

Open-heart surgery
Open-heart surgery is not an easy decision to take for a pregnant woman, as the risks to the

fetus are considerable, mainly due to hypotension and hypothermia during cardiopulmonary bypass. It should only be considered in serious cases that involve life-threatening pulmonary edema, which cannot be managed medically.

The second trimester of pregnancy is usually preferred for any heart operation. Maternal outcome has been good in several series, with a risk of death of 1%, which is similar to the risk of valve replacement in non-pregnant women. Fetal loss is about 20–30%.[21,22]

Timing of delivery

A major problem when heart failure develops is the timing of delivery. The risk for the mother of continuing the pregnancy must be balanced with the risk for the fetus of a preterm birth. Moreover, in patients needing surgery, continuing the pregnancy may be a risk for the fetus as well. A fetal death rate of 6% is reported for mitral commissurotomy (open or closed) and a 20% rate for mitral valve replacement.[23] The survival rate for preterm neonates is very high after 32 weeks (95%) and the risk of neurologic sequelae is low.[24] Therefore, if the pregnancy is ≥ 32 weeks, delivery should be expedited. Since the survival rate is low before 28 weeks ($<75\%$)[24] and the risk of brain damage in the surviving neonates is high (10–14%),[25,26] at this stage of pregnancy surgery should be undertaken without delivering the fetus.

The choice may be more difficult between 28 and 32 weeks, and decisions must be individualized. If the fetus is going to be delivered up to 34 weeks, lung maturation must be induced with betamethasone administration to the mother. The management of these patients requires a multidisciplinary approach in a tertiary care center. Cardiologists, obstetricians, midwives, anesthetists, and pediatricians must be involved.

As to the mode of delivery, we believe that cesarean section should be preferred. Although cardiac output is increased during general or epidural anesthesia, the increase is lower (30%) than during spontaneous delivery (50%).[27,28] Moreover, induction of labor at an early gestational age often fails, or may take a long time, making it more difficult to optimize the care of the mother and neonate. If heart surgery is chosen, the cesarean section can be performed at the same time.

Breast-feeding

Breast-feeding should be avoided in patients who have had heart failure during pregnancy in order to avoid the transmittal of the drug to the fetus via the breast milk and also to avoid any additional stress on the mother.

Cardioversion

Cardioversion can be performed safely at any time during pregnancy.

References

1. Presbitero P, Contrafatto I. Pregnancy and the heart cardiology. Clinical Medicine Series. London: McGraw-Hill, 1999.

2. Robson SC, Hunter S, Boys RJ, Dunlop W. Serial study of factors influencing changes in cardiac output during human pregnancy. Am J Physiol 1989; 256:H1060–5.

3. Letsky E. Haematological changes during pregnancy. In: Heart Disease in Pregnancy. London: BMJ Publishing Group, 1997.

4. Hunter S, Robson S. Adaptation of the cardiovascular system to pregnancy. In: Heart Disease in Pregnancy. London: BMJ Publishing Group, 1997.

5. Elkayam Gleicher. Cardiac problems in pregnancy. In: Diagnosis and Management of Maternal and Fetal Disease, 2nd edn. New York: Alan R Liss.

6. Avila WS, Grinberg M, D'Ecourt LV, et al. Clinical course of women with mitral valve stenosis during pregnancy and puerperium. Arq Bras Cardiol 1992; 58:359.

7. Lao TT, Sermer M, MaGee L, et al. Congenital aortic stenosis and pregnancy – a reappraisal. Am J Obstet Gynecol 1993; 169:540–5.

8. Presbitero P, Somerville J, Stone S, et al. Pregnancy in cyanotic congenital heart disease. Outcome of mother and fetus. Circulation 1994; 89:2673–6.

9. Sbarouni E, Oakley CM. Outcome of pregnancy in women with valve prostheses. Br Heart J 1994; 71:196–201.

10. Hibbard JU, Lindheimer M, Lang RM. A modified definition for peripartum cardiomyopathy and prognosis based on echocardiography. Obstet Gynecol 1999; 94:311–16.

11. Wakeford R. The risk of childhood cancer from intrauterine and preconceptional exposure to ionizing radiation. Environ Health Perspect 1995; 103:1018–23.

12. Rosa FW, Bosco LA, Graham CF, et al. Neonatal anuria with maternal angiotensin converting enzyme inhibition. Obstet Gynecol 1989; 74:371–4.

13. Buttar HS. An overview of the influence of ACE inhibitors on fetal–placental circulation and peri-natal development. Mol Cell Biochem 1997; 176:61–71.

14. Eliahou HE, Silverberg DS, Reisen E, et al. Propranolol for the treatment of hypertension in pregnancy. Am J Obstet Gynaecol. 1978; 85:431–436.

15. Pruyn SC, Phelan JP, Buchann GC. Long-term propranolol therapy in pregnancy: Maternal and fetal outcome. Am J Obstet Gynecol. 1979; 135:485–489.

16. Tcherdakoff PH, Colliard M, Berrard R, et al. Propranolol in hypertension during pregnancy. Br Med J, 1978; 2:670.

17. Tan HL, Lie KI. Treatment of tachyarrhythmias during pregnancy and lactation. Eur Heart J 2001; 22:458–64.

18. Penn IM, Barrett PA, Pannikote V, et al. Amiodarone in pregnancy. Am J Cardiol 1985; 56:196–197.

19. Abouzied AM, Al Abbady M, Al Gendy MF, et al. Percutaneous balloon mitral commissurotomy during pregnancy. Angiology 2001; 52:205–9.

20. Presbitero P, Prever SB, Brusca A. Interventional cardiology in pregnancy. Eur Heart J 1996 17: 182–8.

21. Pomini F, Mercogliano D, Cavalletti C, et al. Cardiopulmonary bypass in pregnancy. Ann Thorac Surg 2000; 61:259–68.

22. Mahli A, Izdes S, Coskun D. Cardiac operations during pregnancy: review of factors influencing fetal outcome. Ann Thorac Surg 2000; 69:1622–6.

23. Parry AJ, Westaby S. Cardiopulmonary bypass during pregnancy. Perf Rev 1994; 3:8–13.

24. Draper ES, Manktelow B, Field DJ, James D. Prediction of survival for preterm births by weight and gestational age: retrospective population based study. Br Med J 1999; 319: 1093–7.

25. Veen S, Ens-Dokkum MH, Schreuder AM, et al. Impairments, disabilities, and handicaps of very preterm and low-birth weight infants at five years of age. The collaborative Project of Preterm and Small for Gestational Age Infants (POPS) in the Netherlands. Lancet 1991; 338:511–12.

26. Kok JH, den Ouden AL, Verloove-Vanhorick SP, Brand R. Outcome of very preterm small for gestational age infants: the first nine years of life. Br J Obstet Gynaecol 1998; 105:162–8.

27. Robson S, Dunlop W, Boys R, Hunter S. Cardiac output during labour. Br Med J 1987; 295: 1169–73.

28. James C, Banner T, Caton D. Cardiac output in women undergoing cesarean section with epidural or general anesthesia. Am J Obstet Gynecol 1989; 160:1178–82.

6

Heart failure therapy in blacks: same or different illness?

Clyde W Yancy

Introduction

Heart failure is rapidly becoming a disease of epidemic proportions, with over 5 million Americans affected and many more patients affected worldwide.[1] The burgeoning choices of effective medical therapy for heart failure have been gratifying to both patients and physicians, but important questions are being raised as to whether or not the disease is expressed in the same manner in all patients and whether or not all of the available medical therapies are effective in all patients. The most poignant questions have been raised about the natural history and response to medical therapy in black patients with heart failure.

The emphasis for this discussion is on African-Americans, i.e. blacks living in the United States. It is possible that the amalgamation of persons of African descent with a European lineage within a Western society yielded a peculiar environment for the development of heart disease, thus creating a unique milieu for the African-American. Any discussion on race and disease must not only reflect potential physiological differences but also certain sociopolitical influences that almost assuredly impact on health. These anthropological issues are intriguing, but are beyond the scope of this discussion and have

been reviewed elsewhere.[2] It is not clear if all patients of African descent are similar in disease expression and in their response to medical therapy. In particular, the bulk of available data in heart failure, especially regarding therapy, has come from clinical trials with larger contingents of African-Americans. Thus, the majority of information is pertinent to the African American group and may not be applicable to others of African descent. This important potential difference will need to be explored in future trials. For simplicity, the term 'black' will be utilized for the remainder of this chapter.

The natural history of hypertension in blacks has been characterized by a striking incidence of end-organ pathology and purported (but not definitively proven) differences in the response to standard medical therapy.[3] As the experience in the contemporary management of heart failure becomes a more robust and mature database, concern has been expressed regarding the natural history of heart failure in major subsets of patients, especially those who are self-characterized as black. Blacks represent a significant cohort of the patients affected by heart failure and important questions have been raised regarding whether or not heart failure is a different illness in blacks (as suspected in hypertension) or the same illness.[4]

Natural history of heart failure in blacks

Mortality

In the United States, heart failure affects 3% of the black population.[5] When blacks are affected with heart failure, the disease appears to occur at an earlier age, is more likely to be associated with worse left ventricular (LV) function, is manifest as a more severe functional limitation, is associated with higher rates of hospitalization and, most worrisome of all, a higher risk of death.[6-8] Blacks are also at higher risk for heart failure, perhaps developing this disease twice as often as whites. Older databases have suggested that the population-based mortality rate for heart failure is 1.8 times higher for black men and 2.4 times higher for black women.[9] That would represent an increase of at least 80% and as much as 140% over the norm. More recent data extracted from clinical trials would suggest a less striking difference in mortality, approximately a 43% increase, but this still remains a dramatic disparity in the natural history of this disease (Figure 6.1).[6]

Socioeconomic status

Data from an older survey done at Cook County Hospital in Chicago established many of the features currently ascribed to heart failure in blacks. In that survey of 301 black patients with heart failure, the average age was 56 ± 13. In the United States, the average age for patients with heart failure is above 70 years. Eighty-seven percent were unemployed with over one-half of the unemployment not due to medical illnesses. Forty-nine percent had an educational level less than 9th grade.[8] In a more recent evaluation of educational status done within the SOLVD

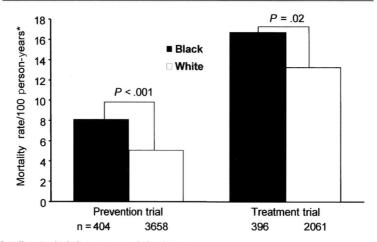

SOLVD studies: racial differences in mortality rates

Mortality rates include treatment and placebo arms.
Adapted from Dries DL etal. *N Engl J Med.* 1999;340:609-616

Figure 6.1

(Studies of Left Ventricular Dysfunction) trials, 34.5% of black patients had an educational level of 8 or fewer years compared with 21.9% in white patients within the SOLVD prevention trial and 42.4% and 25.2% respectively, in the treatment trial. Economic misfortune was also evaluated in SOLVD, with 35.6% of black patients reporting major financial stress vs 22.8% of white patients in the prevention trial and 38.4% vs 23.1% respectively, in the treatment trial. In univariate analysis, a lower educational level was associated with an increased risk of death (relative risk=1.59). However, financial distress was not associated with an increased risk of death. In a multivariate analysis that included clinical factors such as LV function assessment and functional class as determined by New York Heart Association criteria, black patients remained at increased risk of death even after adjusting for socioeconomic factors.[6]

Thus, despite the striking socioeconomic differences between black and white patients in the SOLVD trial, the explanation for the excess mortality seen in black patients appears to involve factors other than the easily presumed adverse socioeconomic environment.

Etiology of heart failure in blacks

Clear differences between black and white patients begin to emerge when the typical etiologies of heart failure are reviewed. A consistent finding in virtually all databases is the presence of hypertension as a potential sole putative cause of left ventricular dysfunction leading to heart failure.

Hypertension has long been associated with heart failure and is a major risk factor for the development of heart failure, as noted in the Framingham database. In 72,422 person-years

of follow-up, 392 cases of heart failure were identified in the original cohort of 5143 subjects. In 91% of all cases of heart failure, hypertension predated the onset of clinical heart failure. After adjusting for myocardial infarction, diabetes, LV hypertrophy, and valvular heart disease, hypertension was still responsible for a twofold increased risk of developing heart failure in men and a threefold increased risk in women.[10–12] However, the Framingham database does not identify subjects with hypertension alone as a cause of heart failure and the demographics and socioeconomics of that New England community are vastly different from the black community.

In the Cook County database, hypertension was identified as the cause of heart failure if there was no evidence of concomitant ischemic heart disease. If multiple etiological factors were present, coronary artery disease took precedence over hypertension and hypertension over alcohol-related LV dysfunction. Using these strategies, there was a 61% incidence of hypertension as the sole cause of heart failure among blacks.[8] In the SOLVD registry report, only 4% of white patients were felt to have hypertension as the sole etiology of heart failure, whereas 32% of black patients were felt to have LV dysfunction on the basis of hypertension alone (Figure 6.2).[13,14]

More contemporary reports of disease etiology are available from recent major clinical trials in heart failure. As noted in Table 6.1, a consistent observation is readily made. In all of the major heart failure trials that reported data according to race, black patients were much more likely to have hypertension as the potential sole etiology of LV dysfunction leading to heart failure. Figure 6.3 demonstrates the incidence of coronary artery disease as a cause of heart failure in blacks vs whites in the major clinical trials and Figure 6.4

Etiology of heart failure

	Framingham*	SOLVD†	
		Black	White
Hypertension	77%	32%	4%
CAD	39–50%	36%	73%
Rheumatic/Valvular	2–20%	11%	10%
Idiopathic	5–15%	13%	12%

*Kannel and Belanger[14]
† Bourassa et al.[13]

Figure 6.2

Study	Total number of patients	Number of black patients	Percentage of black patients	Coronary artery disease (percentage black/non-black)	Hypertension (percentage black/non-black)
V-HeFT I	630	180	28.5	21/53	47/37
V-HeFT II	789	215	27	28/62	65/41
SOLVD	5719	800	14	53/83	62/35
US HF	1094	217	20	32/52	66/48
BEST	2708	627	23	43/63	57/37
MERIT-HF	3991	207	5	27/65	82/35

V-HeFT = Veterans Administration Vasodilator Heart Failure Trials
SOLVD = Studies of Left Ventricular Dysfunction
US HF = United States Carvedilol Heart Failure Trials program
BEST = Beta-blocker Evaluation of Survival Trial
MERIT-HF = Metoprolol CR/XL Randomized Intervention Trial in Heart Failure

Table 6.1 Disease etiology of heart failure in black patients studied in major heart failure trials

demonstrates the same relationship for hypertension. Taken together, the aggregate data from these major trials demonstrate that hypertension is the likely cause of heart failure in about 60% of black patients with ischemic heart disease accounting for most of the remaining 40%. Other conditions such as idiopathic dilated cardiomyopathy and alcohol-induced LV dysfunction are important causes of LV dysfunction but the exact percentage incidence of these causes is difficult to determine from published data. The inescapable conclusion is that heart failure in blacks differs most significantly from that seen in non-blacks based on a stronger association of hypertension with LV dysfunction.

An important observation must be acknowledged. Despite the strong association of hyper-

Heart failure in African Americans: incidence of coronary artery disease

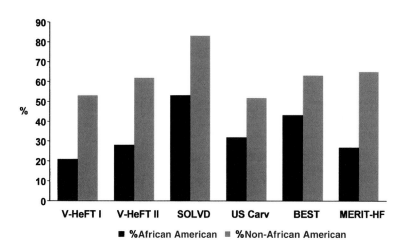

Figure 6.3

Heart failure in African Americans: incidence of hypertension

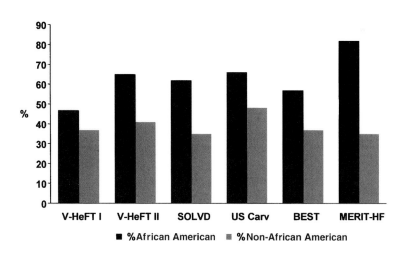

Figure 6.4

tension with LV dysfunction and subsequent heart failure in black patients, 30–40% of black patients with heart failure have coronary artery disease as the most likely etiology.[13] One should not avoid the search for ischemic heart disease with the potential for intervention in lieu of a presumption that hypertension is the sole cause of heart failure in black patients.

Such an approach is not supported by the literature and would be deemed inappropriate.

Review of clinical trials

Prior to reviewing any of the major clinical trials with regard to outcomes of black patients, it must be noted that no trial yet completed has prospectively evaluated black patients with the statistical power to demonstrate either a survival advantage or a survival decrement due to a given medical regimen. As such, all available data represent post hoc retrospective analyses of subgroups in major clinical trials, and thus the data are qualified as being suggestive or 'hypothesis generating' but not definitive. Nevertheless, the insight gained from these trials has been invaluable and perhaps even informative with regard to best approaches in the management of heart failure in black patients.

The V-HeFT trials

The first trials to raise the question of differential outcomes between blacks and whites with heart failure were the V-HeFT trials I and II (Vasodilator Heart Failure Trials). V-HeFT I was a landmark trial that established the clinical utility of vasodilator therapy for heart failure.[15,16] An evaluation of the black patients in the trial corroborates earlier statements that blacks with heart failure have a higher incidence of hypertension as a disease etiology and that they are more likely to have more advanced LV dysfunction based on larger cardiothoracic ratios on chest radiograph. Of note, plasma norepinephrine levels in the V-HeFT trials were similar for both blacks and non-blacks despite the presence of more severe LV dysfunction in blacks.[17] On retrospective review, an important finding was observed. The benefit of vasodilator therapy appeared to

have been present only in the black patients within the trial and not in the white patients. The annual mortality rate in the placebo group of black patients was 17.3%, which was reduced to 9.7% ($P = 0.04$). For the non-black group, the placebo mortality rate was 18.8% vs 16.9% for the active vasodilator arm of isosorbide dinitrate and hydralazine ($P = $ NS).[17] V-HeFT II evaluated the benefit of direct vasodilator therapy vs. angiotensin-converting enzyme (ACE) inhibitor therapy for chronic heart failure. Based on retrospective review, the advantage of ACE inhibitor therapy was seen only in the non-black group. The annual mortality rate in the non-black patients on vasodilator therapy was 14.9% which was reduced to 11.0% with ACE inhibitor therapy ($P = 0.02$). In the black patients, the corresponding values were 12.9% vs 12.8% (Figure 6.5).[17] The intriguing conclusion based on these analyses was that direct vasodilator therapy is preferred in blacks and ACE inhibitor therapy in non-blacks.

Such a conclusion is thought provoking but not of sufficient statistical merit to change the current treatment paradigms for heart failure. Even though the univariate statistics in both retrospective analyses achieved significance, the between-group differences, i.e. black vs white, did not reach statistical significance, perhaps because of sample size, meaning that despite the suggestive analyses, a more rigorous test of between-group differences (measured as an interactive P value) did not show sufficient difference in outcomes between the two groups in either trial to be significant.

The SOLVD trial

The SOLVD database has since been re-analysed to determine the outcomes in the treatment of heart failure with ACE inhibitor therapy as a function of race. Preliminary

V-HeFT I & II results: annual mortality rate analysed by race (Carson et al.[17])

	n	Annual mortality rate		*P*
		Placebo	**Active**	
V-HeFT I				
AA	180	17.3%	9.7%	0.04
Non-AA	450	18.8%	16.9%	NS
V-HeFT II				
AA	215	12.9%	12.8%	NS
Non-AA	574	14.9%	11.0%	0.02

These findings will be further evaluated in the pending A-HeFT trial.
AA, African American
Non-AA, non-African American.

Figure 6.5

analyses of the SOLVD database suggested that black patients were 28% more likely to die from any cause and 37% more likely to die from any cause or be hospitalized for heart failure.[6] Not only was this a retrospective review but also the patient populations differed considerably at baseline, especially with regard to measures of LV function. Matched cohorts of black and white patients were extracted from the SOLVD database with the matching based on the trial in which they participated (i.e. treatment or prevention), LV function assessment, randomization to ACE inhibitor or placebo, gender, and age. After matching the populations, black patients still had a higher rate of death from any cause, 12.2 vs 9.7 per 100 person-years, and a higher rate of hospitalization for heart failure, 13.2 vs 7.7 per 100 person-years. Enalapril therapy was associated with a 44% decrease in the risk of hospitalization for heart failure in white patients but with no significant reduction in hospitalization for black patients (Figure 6.6).[18] There was no change in blood pressure response on enalapril in the black patients vs a 5.0 mmHg decrease in systolic blood pressure and a 3.6 mmHg decrease in diastolic blood pressure in white patients on enalapril.[18] There was no change in the risk of death in response to enalapril therapy in either group.[18] The data were interpreted as representing a lesser response to ACE inhibitor therapy in black patients with LV dysfunction.

Once again, the findings are thought provoking, but are limited by two observations. Even though the groups were matched according to the listed variables, there were still differences between the two groups of patients, especially with regard to disease etiology: black patients in this cohort once again had a higher incidence of hypertension and a lower incidence of ischemia. An additional observa-

Lesser response to ACE inhibitor in black compared with white patients with LV dysfunction (Exner et al.[18])

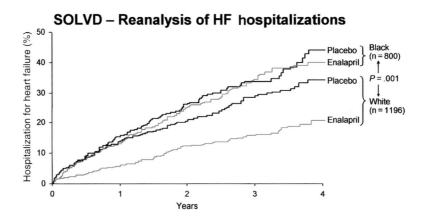

Figure 6.6

tion is that there was no change in blood pressure in the black cohort compared with the white cohort. In addition to suggesting a lesser response to ACE inhibitor therapy, this observation is also evidence that higher doses of ACE inhibitor therapy may be required in black patients to effect the same outcome. This has been suggested in the treatment of hypertension and may be relevant in the treatment of heart failure as well.

The BEST trial

The concerns regarding differential outcomes in heart failure management as a function of race were punctuated by the release of data from the BEST trial (Beta-Blocker Evaluation of Survival Trial).[19] In this trial, bucindolol, a nonselective beta-blocker, was evaluated in a group of patients with advanced heart failure. Among this group of 2708 patients, 627 were black, representing the largest cohort of black patients yet studied in a clinical trial. Survival

benefit was demonstrated only in the non-black patients, with a trend toward a 17% increased mortality rate in black patients.[19] It is noted that the survival advantage seen in the non-black patients was an 18% improvement, which is markedly lower than that seen for any other positive beta-blocker trial (Figure 6.7). This finding would suggest that perhaps some of the observations in the BEST database are drug-specific and may not reflect the response to all beta-blockers used for heart failure. Data are also available from the BEST database showing that there was a striking reduction (19%) in plasma norepinephrine levels in all patients at 3 months after therapy was initiated:[19] this finding would suggest a significant sympatholytic effect of the drug in addition to its beta-blocking properties. A reduction in plasma norepinephrine of this magnitude is similar to that seen in the MOXCON trial (unpublished data), which was halted prematurely due to a 50% increase

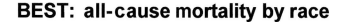

BEST: all-cause mortality by race

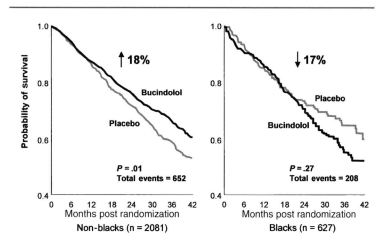

The Beta-blocker Evaluation of Survival Trial Investigators[19].

Figure 6.7

in sudden death episodes. It is suggested that bucindolol exerts too much withdrawal of adrenergic support and thus is not ideal in the treatment of heart failure. Further investigation will be required to see if this is equally applicable to both black and non-black patients.

The US Carvedilol trials program

Data from the US Carvedilol Trials program vary from the BEST database and suggest a favorable outcome using beta-blocker therapy, i.e. carvedilol, to treat heart failure in black patients with responses that are similar in magnitude to those seen in non-black patients.

In the US Carvedilol Heart Failure Trials program, 1094 patients were enrolled in four concurrent trials testing the efficacy of carvedilol, a nonselective, vasodilating beta-blocker, in the management of chronic heart failure of mild to moderate severity. The results have been previously reported.[20] Two-hundred and seventeen black patients were included. The black patients were more likely to have hypertension and less likely to have ischemic heart disease. The addition of carvedilol to a regimen that included an ACE inhibitor yielded a similar increase in measures of LV function, similar but minimal reductions in blood pressure, and a greater decrease in heart rate in the black patients vs. the non-black patients. Carvedilol was associated with a 48% reduction in the combined endpoint of death from any cause or hospitalization for any reason and a 51% reduction in the progression of heart failure. Progression of heart failure was defined as death due to heart failure, hospitalization for heart failure, and a sustained increase in medical therapy for heart failure.[21] These findings were of a similar magnitude to that seen in non-black patients and suggest that the regimen of ACE inhibitor therapy plus

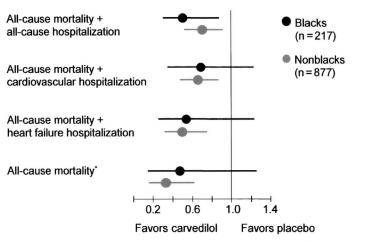

US Carvedilol program: effect of race on outcomes (Yancy et al.[21])

*Not a primary endpoint.   Mean duration 6.5 months.

Figure 6.8

carvedilol was beneficial in both groups of patients (Figures 6.8 and 6.9).

The COPERNICUS trial

The COPERNICUS (Carvedilol Prospective Randomized Cumulative Survival Study Group) trial evaluated the effect of carvedilol on survival in severe chronic heart failure. The major finding was that of a 35% decrease in the risk of death in patients treated with carvedilol.[22] A preliminary analysis of the black subgroup (121 patients of 2289 studied) appears to corroborate the US Carvedilol Heart Failure Trials program data with a similar effect on the combined endpoint of death from any cause or hospitalization for any reason.[23] Although these are once again retrospective reviews, the consistency of the data in both trials suggests that this regimen appears to have efficacy in the management of heart failure in black patients (Figure 6.10).

The MERIT-HF trial

Corroborating data are likewise available from the MERIT-HF (Metoprolol CR/XL Randomized Intervention Trial in Heart Failure) trial.[24] Of the nearly 4000 patients with chronic heart failure studied, 5% were black. Once again, the black population was primarily African-American, even though 75% of all patients studied were European. The relatively small number of black patients studied precludes sufficient events to reach statistical significance. Yet, an analysis of the data by race demonstrates encouraging trends. In 207 black patients, total mortality or hospitalization for any cause had an identical point estimate as the non-black patients ($n = 3784$), but the confidence intervals overlapped the line of neutrality. The data were less impressive for total mortality or hospitalization for heart failure, with the point estimate approximating the line of neutrality.[25] Certainly these

US Carvedilol trials: effect of race on death or hospitalization for any cause[21]

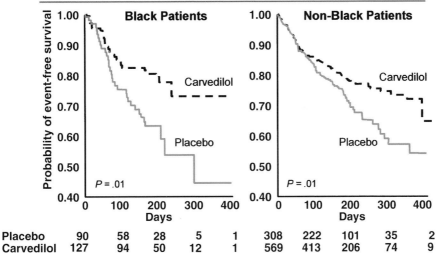

Placebo	90	58	28	5	1	308	222	101	35	2
Carvedilol	127	94	50	12	1	569	413	206	74	9

Figure 6.9

Effect of Carvedilol in Black patients with heart failure

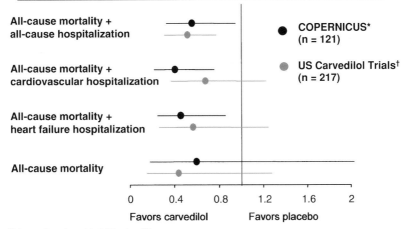

*Mean duration 10.5 (Packer[23])
†Mean duration 6.5 (Yancy et al.[21])

Figure 6.10

data do not send a message to avoid beta-blocker therapy in black patients with heart failure; rather, the findings are consistent with a treatment strategy in black patients with heart failure not dissimilar from that for all patients with heart failure.

Current recommendations and future trials

The foregoing review of the clinical trials demonstrates the difficulty of retrospective subgroup analyses of large multicenter investigations to answer questions for which they were not originally powered to determine. Until definitive data can be determined from well-designed prospective trials, the foregoing data will have to guide therapy. A US-based trial, A-HeFT (African American Heart Failure trial), is being commenced; this trial will evaluate the specific efficacy of a novel nitric oxide donor given to black patients as adjunctive therapy upon a background medical regimen that will include ACE inhibitor and beta-blocker therapy (pers comm).

Currently, it would seem that sufficient data are not available to warrant withholding ACE inhibitor therapy or beta-blocker therapy from black patients. The combination of ACE inhibitor therapy and beta-blocker therapy has yielded the best clinical results yet seen in the treatment of heart failure in black patients. The findings using beta-blockers appear to be drug-specific, as not all agents appear to work similarly, and thus treatment decisions will need to be guided by the results of clinical trials.

Any observations according to race and the response to medical therapy need to be cautiously interpreted. There is considerable heterogeneity in the black population and no finding can be considered to be universally applicable. In addition, there are likely to still be certain nonphysiological variables that will influence health outcomes in people who are arbitrarily identified with a certain race. The racial designation of 'black' merely provides a convenient grouping which allows for the observation of a certain phenotype of heart failure that may be a different illness. Ultimately, the identification of more precise genetic profiles of disease states will supersede the crude designations of race to stratify people with clinical illnesses, and decisions regarding therapy will be made on a genetic/physiological basis.

Plausible physiologic mechanisms of heart failure in blacks

The foregoing discussion demonstrates that heart failure in blacks is an enigmatic disease characterized by a unique natural history, worrisome prognosis, and variable responsiveness to neurohormonal antagonism. If these observations are cogent, a physiological basis must be present to explain these differing manifestations of heart failure. Several candidate biological systems appear to be different in blacks and may in fact contribute to a unique milieu in the black patient with heart failure.

The vasodilatory response

One of the prevailing hypotheses accounting for hypertension in blacks is an altered vasodilatory response. Data supporting this hypothesis demonstrate that in response to the arterial infusion of either nitroprusside or methacholine, the resultant increase in forearm blood flow is reduced in blacks with hypertension compared with whites (Figure 6.11).[26] It is important to note that nitroprusside is a direct nitric oxide donor, which results in an increase in nitric oxide via an endothelium-independent manner. Methacholine results in an increase in nitric oxide via an endothelium-dependent pathway. This would suggest that the response to nitric oxide is blunted in blacks. It is intriguing to rec-

Vasodilator reserve in hypertension (Stein et al.[26])

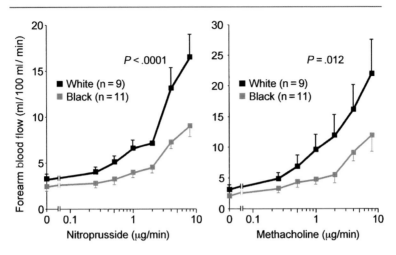

Figure 6.11

ognize that the benefit of nitrate therapy for heart failure in blacks (e.g. direct vasodilator therapy used in the V-HeFT trials) may have been due in part to the use of high-dose nitric oxide donors. ACE inhibitors work in part by raising bradykinin levels through inhibition of kininases. The increased level of bradykinin in turn stimulates inducible nitric oxide synthase resulting in increased nitric oxide production. If there is a blunted response to nitric oxide in blacks, this would negate one of the important properties of ACE inhibitor therapy and perhaps result in the described lesser response to ACE inhibitors.

The renin–angiotensin aldosterone system

The renin–angiotensin–aldosterone system appears to contribute to an altered neurohormonal milieu in black patients. Circulating levels of renin are lower in blacks, and angiotensin levels may be similarly lower.[15–17]

Natriuretic peptide levels have been described to be higher in low-renin essential hypertension.[27,28] Much promise was held for variations in the ACE genotype as an explanation for subsensitive responses in the renin–angiotensin–aldosterone system. The DD genotype has been associated with LV hypertrophy, myocardial infarction, and heart failure.[29] However, there has not been a consistent description of the overexpression of this genotype in blacks, and other mechanisms appear responsible for the attenuated response of the renin–angiotensin–aldosterone system. Recently, a genetic polymorphism of the angiotensinogen promoter has been described in blacks but its relationship to clinical disease is not yet clear.[30]

The sympathetic nervous system

Two observations suggest that the response of the sympathetic nervous system to LV dysfunction is attenuated in blacks. The findings of similar norepinephrine levels despite more severe LV dysfunction in the black population in the V-HeFT trials suggest that the responsiveness of the sympathetic nervous system is attenuated in blacks.[15-17] Moreover, the failure of black patients to respond to the beta-blocker bucindolol also suggests that the sympathetic nervous system may be different in blacks.[19] An emerging database is beginning to document the presence of genetic polymorphisms in the beta-adrenergic receptors. A genetic polymorphism at position 164 of the β_2-receptor (Ile-164) has been associated with less favorable outcomes in heart failure due to a more aggressive natural history and worse LV dysfunction.[31] Whether this polymorphism is overexpressed in blacks is not known. A genetic polymorphism at position 389 in the β_1-receptor (wild type: Arg389 vs. Gly389) has been described.[32] It is associated with a significant decrease in coupling to the stimulatory G proteins and, when exposed to an isoproterenol bath, the resultant activity of adenyl cyclase is sharply reduced compared with the wild type (Figure 6.12).[32] This genetic polymorphism has been described as being over-

expressed in blacks and could represent the basis for either a subsensitive adrenergic response to LV dysfunction or impaired responsiveness to beta-blockers.

Within the cytochrome P450 system, CYP2D6 is an enzyme responsible for the metabolism of beta-blockers. It is absent in only 1% of Asians and 8% of whites but is absent and/or less active in a much larger population of blacks.[33] This, too, might be operative in the response of black patients to beta-blockers.

Transforming growth factor beta-1 and endothelin

Angiotensin II is known to stimulate the production of transforming growth factor beta-1 (TGF-β_1), which is associated with an increase in collagen synthesis and has been linked to the development of end-stage renal disease.[34] It is also known to be associated with LV hypertrophy and thus represents a plausible mechanism that might be operative in hypertension with end-organ dysfunc-

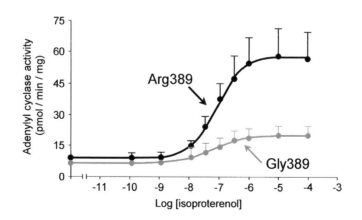

Figure 6.12

tion.[35] Additionally, TGF-β_1 stimulates mRNA for endothelin-1 which, among its many properties, causes an increase in blood pressure due to its significant vasoconstrictor function. Levels of TGF-β_1 have been measured in the setting of hypertension. The highest levels are noted to be present in black hypertensives (Figure 6.13).[36] Of note, a genetic polymorphism (proline allele at codon 10 in the TGF-β_1 gene resulting in 40% higher TGF-β_1 mRNA levels) has been described in blacks that leads to the overexpression of TGF-β_1.[36]

Endothelin is stimulated by TGF-β_1, angiotensin II, ischemia, hypoxia, and hypertension (especially, salt-sensitive hypertension).[37] Endothelin acts via an interface with either endothelin-A (ET-A) or endothelin-B (ET-B) receptors. ET-A mediates vasoconstriction and is a growth promoter, especially of smooth muscle cells. ET-B mediates vasodilation and is growth inhibitory.[37] The use of ET-A receptor antagonists in salt-sensitive hypertension results in significant

reduction of blood pressure.[37] The levels of pre-proendothelin-1 mRNA have been measured in animals that are spontaneously hypertensive and are either salt resistant or salt sensitive. Both models develop LV hypertrophy with indistinguishable pre-proendothelin-1 mRNA. However, when heart failure ensues, levels of the progenitor of endothelin-1 are dramatically elevated in the salt-sensitive animals and remain normal in the salt-resistant animals.[38] The suggestion is that endothelin-1 is operative in the conversion from LV hypertrophy to LV failure in salt-sensitive hypertension. It is intriguing to postulate that an elaborate biological mechanism may be operative in blacks with salt-sensitive hypertension who develop hypertensive heart disease. Angiotensin II may stimulate the production of TGF-β_1, which is overexpressed in blacks. This, in turn, leads to end-stage renal disease and LV hypertrophy while stimulating the production of endothelin-1, which exacerbates hypertension and, in the setting of salt-sensitive

TGF-β_1 levels in hypertension (Suthanthiran et al.[36])

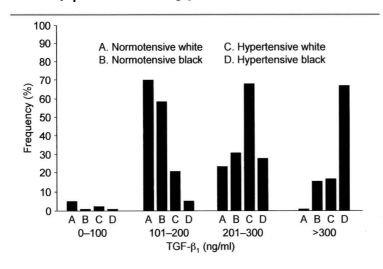

Figure 6.13

hypertension, results in the conversion from ventricular hypertrophy to ventricular failure. This is only a postulated mechanism and needs to be further investigated.

Summary

Heart failure in blacks appears to be a different cardiac malady from heart failure in non-blacks. The natural history is characterized by the earlier onset of disease, with more advanced LV dysfunction at the time of diagnosis. Hypertension is associated with LV dysfunction in black patients in the majority of cases of heart failure studied in recent clinical trials. However, ischemic heart disease as an etiology of LV dysfunction should not be overlooked. The prognosis is worrisome, given higher mortality and hospitalization rates.

A review of major clinical trials reveals an inconsistent response to medical therapy, especially neurohormonal antagonists. These data must be interpreted cautiously because, to date, a prospective trial of heart failure management in blacks has not been done and blacks have been underrepresented in the majority of clinical heart failure trials.

Encouraging data do suggest that ACE inhibitor therapy plus beta-blockers, especially carvedilol, work in black patients. Thus, current treatment algorithms for heart failure should not be altered based on the race of the patient.

Given that blacks represent an extremely heterogeneous population, it is difficult to identify consistent perturbations in biological systems that may contribute to hypertensive heart disease. However, novel biological mechanisms have been described that may be operative in the pathogenesis of hypertensive heart disease and thus may present new and unique treatment targets in the future. Much work remains to be done.

References

1. National Heart, Lung and Blood Institute. Morbidity and Mortality: 1996 Chartbook on Cardiovascular, Lung, and Blood Diseases. Bethesda, MD: National Institutes of Health, May 1996.
2. Schwartz RS. Racial profiling in medical research. New Engl J Med 2001; 344:1392–3.
3. Saunders E. Hypertension in minorities: blacks. Am J Hypertens 1995; 8(12 pt 2):115S–119S.
4. Yancy CW. Heart failure in African Americans: a cardiovascular enigma. J Card Fail 2000; 6: 183–6.
5. American Heart Association: Biostatistical Fact Sheet. African Americans and Cardiovascular Diseases. Dallas, TX: American Heart Association, 1999.
6. Dries DL, Exner DV, Gersh BJ, et al. Racial differences in the outcome of left ventricular dysfunction. New Engl J Med 1999; 340:609–16.
7. Afzal A, Ananthasubramaniam K, Sharma N, et al. Racial differences in patients with heart failure. Clin Cardiol 1999; 22:791–4.
8. Mathew J, Davidson S, Narra L, et al. Etiology and characteristics of congestive heart failure in blacks. Am J Cardiol 1996; 78:1447–50.
9. Gillum RF. The epidemiology of cardiovascular disease in black Americans. New Engl J Med 1996; 335:1597–9.

10. Kannel WB. The natural history of congestive heart failure; the Framingham Study. New Engl J Med 1971; 285:1441–6.

11. Kannel WB, Castelli WP, McNamara PM, et al. Role of blood pressure in the development of congestive heart failure: the Framingham Study. New Engl J Med 1972; 287:781–7.

12. Levy D, Larson MG, Ramachandran SV, et al. The progression from hypertension to congestive heart failure. JAMA 1996; 275:1557–63.

13. Bourassa MG, Gurne O, Bangdiwala SI, et al. Natural history and patterns of current practice in heart failure. J Am Coll Cardiol 1993; 22(Suppl A):14A–19A.

14. Kannel WB, Belanger AJ. Epidemiology of heart failure. Am Heart J 1991; 121(3 pt 1):951–7.

15. Cohn JN, Archibald DG, Ziesche S, et al. Effect of vasodilator therapy on mortality in chronic congestive heart failure; results of a Veterans Administration Cooperative Study. New Engl J Med 1986; 314:1547–52.

16. Cohn JN, Johnson G, Ziesche S, et al. A comparison of enalapril with hydralazine-isosorbide dinitrate in the treatment of chronic congestive heart failure. New Engl J Med 1991; 325:303–10.

17. Carson P, Ziesche S, Johnson G, Cohn JN. Racial differences in response to therapy for heart failure; an analysis of the Vasodilator–Heart Failure Trials. J Card Fail 1999; 5: 178–87.

18. Exner DV, Dries DL, Domanski MJ, Cohn JN. Lesser response to angiotensin-converting-enzyme inhibitor therapy in black as compared with white patients with left ventricular dysfunction. New Engl J Med 2001; 344:1351–7.

19. The Beta-Blocker Evaluation of Survival Trial Investigators. A trial of the beta-blocker bucindolol in patients with advanced chronic heart failure. New Engl J Med 2001; 344:1659–67.

20. Packer M, Bristow MR, Cohn JN, et al. The effect of carvedilol on morbidity and mortality in patients with chronic heart failure. New Engl J Med 1996; 334:1349–55.

21. Yancy CW, Fowler MB, Colucci WS, et al. Race and the response to adrenergic blockade with carvedilol in patients with chronic heart failure. New Engl J Med 2001; 344:1358–65.

22. Packer M, Coats AJ, Fowler MB, et al. Effect of carvedilol on survival in severe chronic heart failure. New Engl J Med 2001; 344:1651–8.

23. Packer M. Data presented at the American Heart Association Annual Scientific Sessions, 2000.

24. MERIT-HF Study Group. Effect of Metoprolol CR/XL in chronic heart failure: Metoprolol CR/XL randomised intervention trial in congestive heart failure (MERIT-HF). Lancet 1999; 353:2001–7.

25. Goldstein S. Data presented at the American Heart Association Annual Scientific Sessions, 2000.

26. Stein CM, Lang CC, Nelson R, et al. Vasodilation in black Americans: attenuated nitric oxide mediated responses. Clin Pharmacol Therap 1997; 62: 436–43.

27. Norton GR, Woodiwiss AJ, Hartford C, et al. Sustained antihypertensive actions of a dual angiotensin-converting enzyme neutral endopeptidase inhibitor, sampatrilat, in black hypertensive subjects. Am J Hypertens 1999; 12: 563–71.

28. MacGregor GA, Sagnella GA, Markandu ND, et al. Raised plasma levels of atrial natrituretic peptide in subjects with untreated essential hypertension. J Hypertens 1986; 4(Suppl 6):S567–9.

29. Schunkert H, Hense HW, Holmer SR, et al. Association between a deletion polymorphism of the angiotensin-converting-enzyme gene and left ventricular hypertrophy. New Engl J Med 1994; 330:1634–8.

30. Semin Nephrol 1996; 3:83–93.

31. Liggett SB, Wagoner LE, Craft LL, et al. The Ile 164 beta2-adrenergic receptor polymorphism adversely affects the outcome of congestive heart failure. J Clin Invest 1998; 102:1534–9.

32. Mason DA, Moore JD, Green SA, Liggett SB. A gain of function polymorphism in a G-protein coupling domain of the human beta-1 adrenergic receptor. J Biol Chem 1999; 274:12670–4.

33. Xie HG, Kim RB, Wood AJ, Stein CM. Molecular basis of ethnic differences in drug disposition and response. Ann Rev Pharmacol Toxicol 2001; 41:815–50.

34. Ketteler M, Noble NA, Border WA. Increased expression of transforming growth factor-beta in renal disease. Curr Opin Nephrol Hypertens 1994; 3:446–52.

35. Villareal FJ, Dillmann WH. Am J Physiol 1992; 262:H1861–6.

36. Suthanthriran M, Baogui L, Song JO, et al. Transforming growth factor-beta-1 hyperexpression in African-American hypertensives: a novel

mediator of hypertension and/or target organ damage. Proc Nat Acad Sci 1999; 97:3479–84.

37. Kirchengast M, Munter K. Endothelin-1 and endothelin receptor antagonists in cardiovascular remodeling. A minireview. Proc Soc Exp Biol Med 1999; 221:312–25.

38. Iwanaga Y, Kihara Y, Hasegawa K, et al. Cardiac endothelin-1 plays a critical role in the functional deterioration of left ventricles during the transition from compensatory hypertrophy to congestive heart failure in salt-sensitive hypertensive rats. Circulation 1998; 98:2065–73.

7

The treatment of diastolic heart failure

Karen Hogg and John McMurray

What are we trying to treat in the patient with diastolic heart failure

Although there are many reports of different agents improving indices of diastolic function, the significance of such observations is doubtful. First, it is very difficult to know what exactly many noninvasive indices actually measure.[1–4] Second, the relationship between these and symptoms, functional capacity, or clinical outcome is unclear.[1–4] Third, drugs such as phosphodiesterase inhibitors, which increase mortality, can be shown to improve noninvasive measures of diastolic function.[5,6]

Consequently, as with heart failure associated with systolic dysfunction, it is improvement in patient well-being and outcome, rather than in ejection fraction, that is important. In other words, we are looking for treatments that improve symptoms, increase functional capacity, reduce the need for hospital admission, and lower mortality. Symptom and morbidity reduction may be particularly important in patients with diastolic heart failure as some (but not all) studies show a better survival than in patients with poor systolic function.[7–9]

Evidence-based treatment of diastolic heart failure

In striking contrast to heart failure associated with left ventricular systolic dysfunction, there is a paucity of evidence on which treatments should be used in patients with heart failure and preserved left ventricular (LV) systolic function. Although there are many overviews of the theoretical benefits or hazards of particular treatments,[10–14] a thorough review of the literature reveals only five completed randomized controlled trials.[15–20] These are worth reviewing in detail.

Heart rate limiting calcium channel blockers

Conceptually, a drug that slows heart rate and reduces myocardial contractility is therapeutically attractive in patients with diastolic dysfunction.[21] Setaro et al.[15] carried out a small, prospective, randomized crossover comparison of verapamil and placebo in well-characterized patients with diastolic heart failure.

Twenty-two patients were studied. Patients with symptomatic or occult myocardial ischemia and asymmetrical LV septal hypertrophy were not enrolled. We are not told if atrial fibrillation was an exclusion criterion.

Diuretic dose was kept constant but digoxin was withdrawn 7 days before randomized treatment was started. Digoxin withdrawal may be associated with clinical deterioration and we are not told what proportion of patients were receiving digoxin at baseline (and how many of these were randomized to placebo and verapamil in the initial treatment period).

A baseline exercise treadmill exercise test (modified Naughton protocol), congestive heart failure (CHF) score, and cardiac radionuclide study were obtained. The radionuclide study included measurement of left ventricular ejection fraction (LVEF) and peak filling rate.

Patients were then randomized to placebo or verapamil. The initial dose of verapamil was 80 mg three times daily for 1 week and, if tolerated, this was increased to 120 mg three times daily (if the initial dose was not tolerated it could be decreased to 80 mg twice daily). The mean daily dose of verapamil taken was 256 mg (range 160–360 mg).

After 2 weeks of treatment, patients were re-evaluated by a blinded investigator, with repeat clinical examination, CHF scoring, exercise testing, and radionuclide scanning.

There was then a 4-day 'wash-out' period, followed by crossover to the second treatment period with similar re-evaluation.

Twenty of the 22 patients completed the study (one did not comply and a second developed a supraventricular tachycardia during the placebo phase, requiring open-label verapamil treatment).

Effect of verapamil on measures of systolic and diastolic function

LVEF did not change (baseline $60 \pm 9\%$, placebo $60 \pm 10\%$, verapamil $62 \pm 8\%$, respectively). Peak filling rate increased from baseline (1.85 ± 0.45 edv/s) with verapamil (2.29 ± 0.54 edv/s, $P < 0.05$), but did not change during placebo treatment (2.16 ± 0.48 edv/s), although the between-treatment group comparison was not statistically significant. There was also a suggestion of a 'carry-over' effect of verapamil on peak filling rate in patients receiving this treatment before placebo.

Effect of verapamil on blood pressure and heart rate

Average systolic blood pressure did not differ significantly between groups. Diastolic blood pressure at baseline was 84 ± 6 mmHg, 79 ± 6 mmHg during treatment with verapamil ($P < 0.05$), and 82 ± 8 mmHg at the end of the placebo period. The corresponding mean heart rates were baseline 79 ± 11, verapamil 71 ± 11 ($P < 0.05$), and placebo 78 ± 9 beats/min. Verapamil did not reduce peak heart rate or systolic blood pressure during exercise.

Effect of verapamil on congestive heart failure score and functional capacity (Figure 7.1)

The mean baseline CHF score was 6.7 ± 1.7. After treatment with verapamil this decreased, significantly, to 3.8 ± 1.6, whereas, following placebo treatment, the score increased to 6.1 ± 1.9 ($P < 0.01$).

In the 12 patients capable of exercise, the mean treadmill time (min) was 10.7 ± 3.4 at baseline, 13.9 ± 4.3 after verapamil ($P < 0.05$), and 12.3 ± 4 after placebo. The between-treatment group comparison was also significant ($P < 0.01$).

Recently, Hung et al. have reported a very similar study comparing verapamil to placebo in a cross-over design.[20] 15 patients were studied and each treatment period lasted 3 months. Verapamil increased exercise time compared to placebo and improved the CHF score. Verapamil also improved Doppler indices of diastolic function.[20]

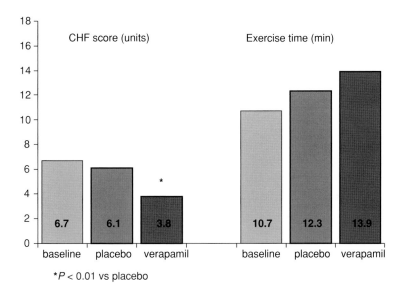

Figure 7.1 Effects of verapamil in diastolic heart failure. CHF = congestive heart failure: a lower CHF score means better symptom status.

Beta-blockers

As with verapamil, beta-blockers – drugs with heart rate slowing and negatively inotropic actions – might be expected to improve diastolic function. Aronow et al.[19] examined the effect of propanolol on outcome in 158 elderly ($\geq$62 years) patients with heart failure and an LVEF $\geq$0.40. In contrast to the study of Setaro et al.[15] with verapamil, patients with coronary heart disease were not excluded and, in fact, all patients had a prior Q-wave infarction. Another important difference in enrolment criteria was that all patients were receiving baseline diuretic and beta-blocker therapy. One-third of patients were in atrial fibrillation; 79 patients were randomized to receive propranolol and 79 patients did not receive propranolol. This open design is clearly a crucial issue. Follow-up was for 32 months.

The initial dose of propranolol was 10-mg/day. The dose was increased by 10-mg

increments at 10-day intervals until the target dose of 30 mg three times daily was reached.

Two-dimensional echocardiography was carried out at baseline, before randomization, and after 1 year of treatment. LVEF and LV mass were measured by a blinded echocardiographer.

Mortality and the composite endpoint of death or nonfatal myocardial infarction (MI) were also assessed by intention to treat.

Propranolol was discontinued by 11 of 79 patients (14%) because of adverse effects (worsening CHF in seven and hypotension in four).

Figure 7.2 shows the effect of 1 year's treatment with and without propranolol on LVEF and LV mass (66 patients in the former and 65 patients in the latter group). There was a significantly greater increase in LVEF and greater reduction in LV mass with propranolol.

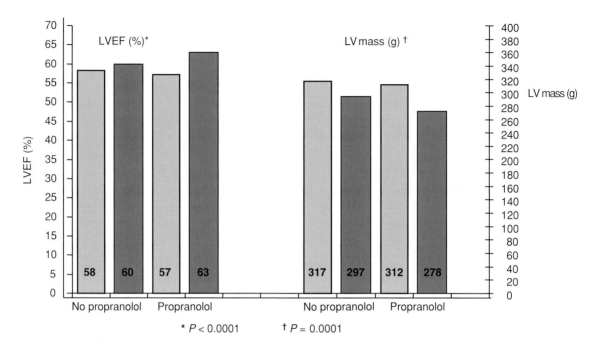

Figure 7.2 Effects of propranolol in diastolic heart failure: left ventricular ejection fraction (LVEF) and left ventricular (LV) mass. Left bars refer to baseline and right bars to 1-year data in each panel for each intervention.

Figure 7.3 shows the effects of propranolol, compared with no propranolol, on death and death or nonfatal MI after 2.7 years: 44 out of 79 (56%) propranolol-treated patients died, compared with 60 out of 79 randomized to no propranolol (76%, $P = 0.007$). The respective figures, rates for death or nonfatal MI, were 47 (59%) and 65 (82%), with $P = 0.002$.

These are clearly favorable results, although the lack of placebo control and highly selected patient group must be noted. The beneficial action of beta-blockers in post-MI patients is well recognized and the findings of this study might have been anticipated. Similarly, the composite death or MI endpoint, while important, is perhaps not the most relevant one in the more general population of patients with normal LVEF heart failure. The place of beta-blockers in the treatment of diastolic heart failure will be clarified. A large prospective,

randomized controlled morbidity/mortality trial, comparing placebo to nebivolol, is presently enrolling patients with CHF, a large proportion of whom are expected to have a 'preserved' LVEF (see below).

Angiotensin-converting enzyme inhibitors

One small trial has compared treatment with enalapril to no treatment with enalapril in 21 elderly patients (mean age 80 years) with New York Heart Association (NYHA) class III CHF associated with prior Q-wave MI but a 'preserved' LVEF (>0.50).[16] All patients were in sinus rhythm and treated with furosemide but no other cardiac drug. The target dose of enalapril was 10 mg twice daily (by week 5 of titration). A chest X-ray, echocardiogram, and

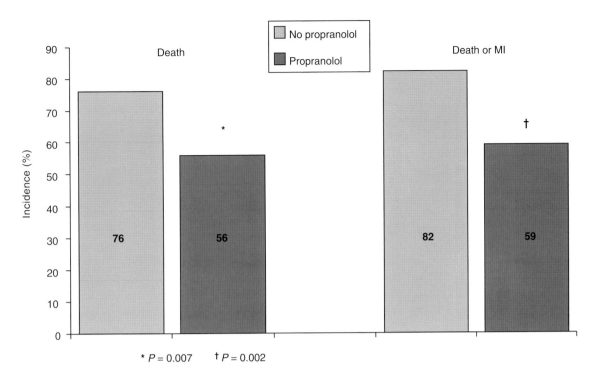

Figure 7.3 Effects of propranolol in diastolic heart failure: incidence of death and death or nonfatal myocardial infarction (MI).

modified Bruce protocol treadmill exercise test were performed at baseline and after 3 months of treatment.

Figures 7.4 and 7.5 show the effects of enalapril on NYHA class, exercise time, radiographic cardiothoracic ratio, and echocardiographic LVEF.

All of these measures improved, significantly, in the enalapril group but not the control (no enalapril) group. Similarly, LV mass fell after enalapril treatment (from 313 ± 43 g to 280 ± 46 g, $P < 0.001$) but not in the control group (306 ± 51 to 309 ± 55 g). Peak mitral Doppler E/A ratio increased with enalapril (from 0.6 ± 0.1 to 0.7 ± 0.1, $P < 0.001$) but not in the control group (0.6 ± 0.2 to 0.6 ± 0.2). Resting systolic and diastolic blood pressure fell during enalapril treatment (but not in the control group).

Again, while encouraging, these findings must be treated with caution: first, *within*-group rather than *between*-group differences are described; second, only 21 patients were studied; and third, the study had an open design although the chest X-ray and echocardiographic measures were made by a blinded observer.

Of course, there is reason to believe that, in patients with prior MI, an angiotensin-converting enzyme ACE inhibitor is of benefit in reducing the risk of future vascular events. However, a more recent comparison of outcome in patients with diastolic heart failure receiving and not receiving ACE inhibitors suggests these treatments may reduce heart failure re-hospitalization.[21] Clearly, the nonrandomized nature of this comparison means that firm conclusions cannot be

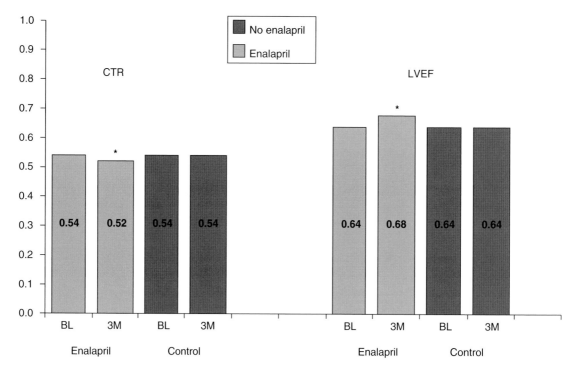

Figure 7.4   Effects of enalapril in diastolic heart failure: cardiothoracic ratio (CTR) and echocardiographic left ventricular ejection fraction (LVEF). BL = baseline; 3M = 3 months

drawn. Whether ACE inhibitors (or angiotensin receptor blockers) reduce morbidity/mortality in patients with diastolic heart failure is a question currently addressed in two large ongoing and one planned randomized controlled trials (see below).

Digoxin

Surprisingly, the largest trial experience with any antifailure therapy in patients with diastolic heart failure is with digoxin.[17,18] At first sight, digoxin would seem an unsuitable treatment for this form of heart failure. Classically, digitalis glycosides are thought of as agents which increase cytosolic calcium concentrations, which, if not rapidly reversed, should, if anything, impair myocardial relaxation. It is possible, however, that the sympathetico-

inhibitory, pro-parasympathetic and renin–angiotensin–aldosterone suppressing actions of digoxin are beneficial in CHF.[23]

The Digitalis Investigation Group (DIG) ancillary trial in patients with CHF and a preserved LVEF represents the largest randomized controlled trial in diastolic heart failure to date. As part of the overall DIG program, 988 patients with a clinical diagnosis of CHF and an LVEF >0.45 were randomized to receive placebo ($n = 496$) or digoxin ($n = 492$). By comparison, 3403 patients with CHF and an LVEF of ≤0.45 were randomized to placebo and 3397 to digoxin in the main trial. There were 116 deaths (23.4%) in the placebo group and 115 deaths (23.4%) in the digoxin group in the ancillary trial. For the combined endpoint of death or CHF hospitalization, the results in the ancillary trial (risk ratio with digoxin 0.82,

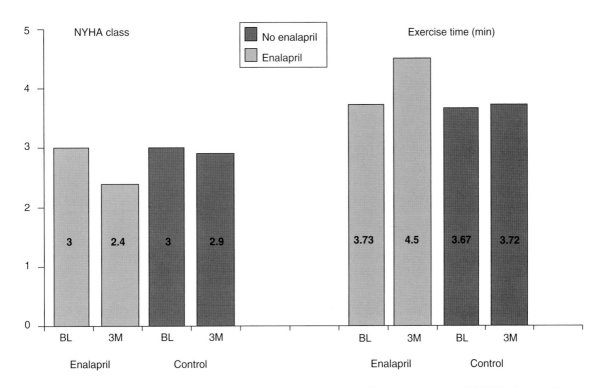

Figure 7.5 Effects of enalapril in diastolic heart failure: New York Heart Association (NYHA) class and exercise time. BL = baseline; 3M = 3 months

95% CI 0.63–1.07) were consistent with the findings in the main trial (risk ratio 0.85, 95% CI 0.79–0.91; $P<0.001$). Unfortunately, no further information on outcome in the preserved LVEF ancillary trial is available. The findings of the DIG trial are supported, to some extent, by those of the rather curious German and Austrian Xamoterol Study Group trial.[23] This study compared the effects of placebo, xamoterol, and digoxin on symptoms, signs, and exercise capacity in patients with a spectrum of CHF. LVEF was not reported, but 80–90% of patients were in NYHA class I or II CHF, about one-half had angina pectoris, only one-quarter were taking diuretics, and just over one-third had radiological cardiomegaly (a cardiothoracic ratio ≥0.52). In other words, it is highly likely that many of these patients had diastolic heart failure. Digoxin significantly im-

proved breathlessness, tiredness, chest pain, edema, and lung crackles.[24] Digoxin also reduced weight and cardiothoracic ratio more than placebo.

New studies in diastolic heart failure

Recently, the unsatisfactory state of affairs regarding adequate clinical trials in patients with diastolic heart failure has begun to improve. Three trials or trial programs including such patients are underway and a fourth is planned. The Candesartan in Heart Failure: Assessment of Reduction in Mortality and Morbidity (CHARM) program has three component trials, one of which has enrolled 3024 patients with an LVEF >0.40 (study 0007 or 'CHARM Preserved').[22] In all three trials candesartan is compared to placebo and the primary end-point of each individual trial is cardiovascular death or CHF hospitalization.

The Perindopril for Elderly People with Chronic Heart Failure (PEP–CHF) study is recruiting 1000 patients >70 years with CHF and no major LV systolic dysfunction (LVEF <0.40 or wall motion index <1.4). Patients must also have echocardiographic evidence of left atrial enlargement, LV hypertrophy, or diastolic dysfunction (Doppler criteria).[26] The primary endpoint is death or CHF hospitalization.

The third ongoing trial is the Study of Effects of Nebivolol Intervention on Outcomes and Rehospitalisation in Seniors with heart failure (SENIORS).[27] SENIORS is randomizing 2000 patients ≥70 years with CHF and either a documented LVEF ≤0.35 *or* a hospital admission for CHF within 12 months. It is expected that about one-half of

patients have CHF and a 'preserved' LVEF. The treatment comparison is the beta-blocker nebivolol versus placebo. The primary endpoint is death or cardiovascular hospitalization.

Lastly, another major morbidity/mortality trial comparing placebo to irbesartan is underway in patients with CHF and preserved LV systolic function. This study, know as I-PRESERVE, is enrolling patients ≥60 years with typical signs and symptoms, a LVEF ≥0.45 and either a CHF hospitalization within the preceding 6 months plus a current NYHA class II-IV symptoms or current NYHA class III-IV symptoms and 'corroborative evidence' (echocardiographic, ECG or radiological abnormalities). It is hoped to enroll 3600 patients and the primary end point is the composite of death or cardiovascular hospitalization. The active therapy compared to placebo is irbesartan.

References

1. Brutsaert DL. Diagnosing primary diastolic heart failure. Eur Heart J 2000; 21:94–6.
2. Caruana L, Petrie MC, Davie AP, McMurray JJ. Do patients with suspected heart failure and preserved left ventricular systolic function suffer from 'diastolic heart failure' or from misdiagnosis? A prospective descriptive study. BMJ 2000; 321: 215–18.
3. Vasan RS, Levy D. Defining diastolic heart failure: a call for standardized diagnostic criteria. Circulation 2000; 101:2118–21.
4. Caruana L, Davie AP, Petrie M, McMurray J. Diagnosing heart failure. Eur Heart J 1999; 5:393.
5. Binkley PF, Shaffer PB, Ryan JM, Leier CV. Augmentation of diastolic function with phos-

phodiesterase inhibition in congestive heart failure. J Lab Clin Med 1989; 3:266–71.
6. Monrad ES, McKay RG, Baim DS, et al. Improvement in indexes of diastolic performance in patients with congestive heart failure treated with milrinone. Circulation 1984; 6:1030–7.
7. Vasan RS, Benjamin EJ, Levy D. Prevalence, clinical features and prognosis of diastolic heart failure: an epidemiologic perspective. J Am Coll Cardiol 1995; 7:1565–74.
8. Senni M, Tribouilloy CM, Rodeheffer RJ, et al. Congestive heart failure in the community: a study of all incident cases in Olmsted County, Minnesota, in 1991. Circulation 1998; 21:2282–9.
9. Vasan RS, Larson MG, Benjamin EJ, et al. Congestive heart failure in subjects with normal

versus reduced left ventricular ejection fraction: prevalence and mortality in a population-based cohort. J Am Coll Cardiol 1999; 7:1948–55.

10. Weinberger HD. Diagnosis and treatment of diastolic heart failure. Hosp Pract 1999; 3:115–18,121–2,125–6.

11. Cody RJ. The treatment of diastolic heart failure. Cardiol Clin 2000; 3:589–96.

12. Remme WJ. How to treat diastolic heart failure: a personal point of view. Rev Port Cardiol 1999; 5:V117–23.

13. Garcia MJ. Diastolic dysfunction and heart failure: causes and treatment options. Cleve Clin J Med 2000; 10:727–9,733–8.

14. Vasan RS, Benjamin EJ. Diastolic heart failure – no time to relax. N Engl J Med 2001; 1:56–9.

15. Setaro JF, Zaret BL Schulman DS, et al. Usefulness of verapamil for congestive heart failure associated with abnormal left ventricular diastolic filling and normal left ventricular systolic performance. Am J Cardiol 1990; 12:981–6.

16. Aronow WS, Kronzon I. Effect of enalapril on congestive heart failure treated with diuretics in elderly patients with prior myocardial infarction and normal left ventricular ejection fraction. Am J Cardiol 1993; 7:602–4.

17. No authors listed. Rationale, design, implementation, and baseline characteristics of patients in the DIG trial: a large, simple, long-term trial to evaluate the effect of digitalis on mortality in heart failure. Control Clin Trials 1996; 1:77–97.

18. No authors listed. The effect of digoxin on mortality and morbidity in patients with heart failure. The Digitalis Investigation Group. N Engl J Med 1997; 8:525–33.

19. Aronow WS, Ahn C, Kronzon I. Effect of propranolol versus no propranolol on total mortality plus nonfatal myocardial infarction in older patients with prior myocardial infarction, congestive heart failure, and left ventricular ejection fraction

> or = 40% treated with diuretics plus angiotensin-converting enzyme inhibitors. Am J Cardiol 1997; 80:207–9.

20. Hung MJ, Cherng WJ, Kuo LT, Wang CH. Effect of verapamil in elderly patients with left ventricular diastolic dysfunction as a cause of congestive heart failure. Int J Clin Pract 2002; 56: 57–62.

21. Vasan RS, Benjamin EJ, Levy D. Congestive heart failure with normal left ventricular systolic function. Clinical approaches to the diagnosis and treatment of diastolic heart failure. Arch Intern Med 1996; 2:146–57.

22. Philbin EF, Rocco TA Jr. Use of angiotensin-converting enzyme inhibitors in heart failure with preserved left ventricular systolic function. Am Heart J 1997;(2 Pt 1):188–95.

23. Massie BM, Abdalla I. Heart failure in patients with preserved left ventricular systolic function: do digitalis glycosides have a role? Prog Cardiovasc Dis 1998; 4:357–69.

24. No authors listed. Double-blind placebo-controlled comparison of digoxin and xamoterol in chronic heart failure. The German and Austrian Xamoterol Study Group. Lancet 1988; i:489–93.

25. Swedberg K, Pfeffer M, Granger C, et al. Candesartan in heart failure – assessment of reduction in mortality and morbidity (CHARM): rationale and design. Charm-Programme Investigators. J Card Fail 1999; 3:276–82.

26. Cleland JG, Tendera M, Adamus J, et al. Perindopril for elderly people with chronic heart failure: the PEP–CHF study. The PEP investigators. Eur J Heart Fail 1999; 3:211–17.

27. Shibata MC, Flather MD, Bohm M, et al. Study of the Effects of Nebivolol Intervention on Outcomes and Rehospitalisation in Seniors with Heart Failure (SENIORS). Rationale and design. Int J Cardiol 2002; 86: 77–85.

8

Heart failure due to cardiomyopathy (nonischemic primary cardiomyopathy)

Anjan Gupta and Jeffrey D Hosenpud

Introduction

In the late 19th century, Krehl first suggested the concept of primary myocardial disease when he described several cases of 'chronic myocarditis' in which myocardial degeneration, hypertrophy, and inflammation were found in autopsied hearts.[1] But it was not until 1957 that Brigden introduced the term 'cardiomyopathy' to describe myocardial disease of unknown etiology in the absence of coronary disease.[2] In 1968, the World Health Organization specifically defined 'myocardial disease' as pathology of the heart that excluded vascular, hypertensive, or valvular diseases and stated that the pathology should be categorized as 'primary' when the etiology was unknown and 'secondary' when it was known.[3] Despite these more precise definitions, the term 'cardiomyopathy' is generally used to mean primary myocardial disease of either a specific or unknown etiology. Unfortunately, it is also widely used as a synonym for ventricular dysfunction of any cause (e.g. ischemic cardiomyopathy, valvular cardiomyopathy).

Traditionally, classification systems for the cardiomyopathies have been based on anatomic and physiologic characteristics (i.e. dilated, hypertrophic, and restrictive) rather than on etiologic ones (Figure 8.1). Although this classification disregards underlying etiologies, more often than not, specific etiologies do tend to fall into anatomic categories. Furthermore, as will be described later, this anatomic classification is helpful in the medical management of patients who have cardiomyopathy. Prognosis, also, is generally more closely linked to anatomic and physiologic characteristics than to specific etiology.

Dilated cardiomyopathy

Pathophysiology and mechanisms of disease

In patients who have dilated cardiomyopathy, the primary myocardial defect is abnormal contraction. Responding to reduced myocardial contractility, the heart dilates out of proportion to the degree of hypertrophy, resulting in enlargement in all four chambers, which develop relatively thin cardiac walls.[4]

Despite 20 years of research, the relationship in humans between inflammation and cardiomyopathy is still elusive. Some forms of dilated cardiomyopathy have been suggested to be secondary to small vessel disease, specifically to microvascular spasm.[5] Direct myocardial toxicity is the suggested cause for alcohol-induced cardiomyopathy[6] and is clearly present in anthracycline-induced dilated cardiomyopathy.[7,8]

The genetic etiology of dilated cardiomyopathy has been investigated. In a recent

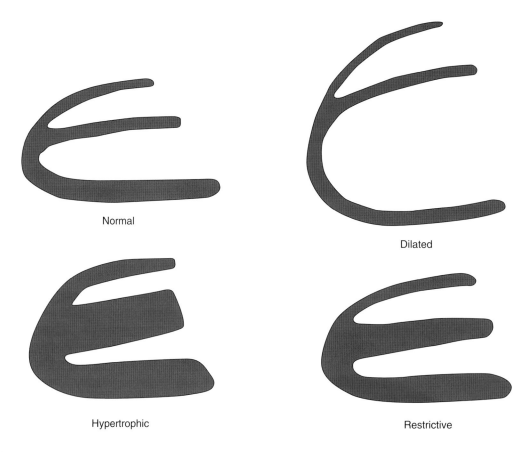

Normal

Dilated

Hypertrophic

Restrictive

Figure 8.1 Anatomic classification of cardiomyopathy. In dilated cardiomyopathy (upper right) both ventricular chambers increase beyond normal dimensions (upper left) and chamber walls become relatively thin (i.e. the ratio of radius to wall thickness increases). In hypertrophic cardiomyopathy (lower left), walls thicken but usually the septal wall is thickest. In restrictive cardiomyopathy (lower right), ventricular cavities are relatively smaller and walls are relatively thick, but to a lesser extent than in hypertrophic cardiomyopathy.

study, 445 consecutive patients with a left ventricular ejection fraction below 50% and no coronary artery disease were documented in Germany.[9] Familial dilated cardiomyopathy was confirmed in 10.8% of the original patients and suspected in an additional 24.2%.

Clinical features of dilated cardiomyopathy

Irrespective of underlying etiology, most patients present in similar fashion, albeit in a continuum of heart failure. Especially in the acute setting, physical findings typically include traditional findings of heart failure.

The vast majority of patients have no obvious associated cause for their disease (Table 8.1). Approximately 10–15% can be expected to present with a clinical dilated cardiomyopathy and evidence of a chronic myocarditis on endomyocardial biopsy.[10]

Alcohol-induced cardiomyopathy

Alcohol abuse is a common condition, but cardiomyopathy is uncommon with abuse.

Idiopathic	Granulomatous disease	Neuromuscular disease
Infectious	Idiopathic	Duchenne's
Viral disease	Sarcoidosis	Friedreich's ataxia
Coxsackievirus	Giant cell	Limb girdle
Echovirus	Wegner's	Neurofibromatosis
Adenovirus	Metabolic/endocrine	Myasthenia gravis
Arbovirus	Acromegaly	Toxins
Bacterial	Hypothyroidism	Alcohol
Diphtheria	Pheochromocytoma	Arsenic
Tuberculosis	Diabetes	Cobalt
Leptospirosis	Beriberi	Lead
Rickettsia	Selenium deficiency	Carbon tetrachloride
Typhus	Kwashiorkor	Carbon monoxide
Q fever	Collagen vascular disease	Catecholamines
Protozoal	Lupus erythematosus	Amphetamines
Chagastic	Dermatomyositis	Cocaine
Malarial	Polyarteritis nodosa	Anthracyclines
Leishmaniasis	Scleroderma	Cyclophosphamide

Table 8.1 Reported causes and associations with dilated cardiomyopathy

The reported incidence of alcohol as a significant risk factor is 20–30%.[11,12] When seen, in a clinical sense both in its histology and its overt response to general medical therapy, this event is not significantly different from that in patients who have idiopathic cardiomyopathy.[11,12]

Excessive alcohol consumption is likely to precede the onset of heart failure by a minimum of 10 years.[13,14] Males are more susceptible than females,[15] and concurrent smoking, hypertension, and malnutrition may be contributing factors. Furthermore, because individuals who develop cardiomyopathy are unlikely to develop chronic cirrhosis, there appears to be a differential organ susceptibility to alcohol.[16]

Abstaining from alcohol may improve the prognosis. In one study of 64 patients, in the roughly one-third who abstained the mortality rate was 9% over the next 4 years, contrasted with 57% in those who continued drinking.[6] A second study of 31 patients supported these findings.[17]

Diabetic cardiomyopathy

Diabetic cardiomyopathy as a unique entity was first recognized by Rubler et al. in 1972.[18] These findings were supported in a retrospective analysis from the Framingham Study, which showed that patients who had diabetes mellitus had a 2.4-fold higher incidence of developing heart failure on insulin.[19]

Potential pathogenetic mechanisms are increased vascular permeability resulting in increased glycosylation of collagen,[20] alterations in intracellular Ca^{2+} kinetics,[21] and microvascular damage[22] akin to diabetic retinopathy and nephropathy.

Peripartum cardiomyopathy

The syndrome of unexplained heart failure in women postpartum was detailed in the mid-1930s by a number of investigators[23,24] but had been suggested even earlier. It is clear now that onset ranges from the middle of the third trimester through several months following delivery. Most commonly, however, signs and symptoms of heart failure appear postpartum.[25]

Recently published clinical and research recommendations based on a workshop and review conducted jointly by the National Heart, Lung, and Blood Institute and by the Office of Rare Diseases of the National Institutes of Health are as follows:

- Diagnosis of peripartum cardiomyopathy should follow the criteria in Table 8.2,[26] especially for the timing and demonstration of ventricular systolic dysfunction by echocardiography.
- Once the diagnosis is made, it is essential for specialists in obstetrics, perinatology, and cardiology to collaborate. Any diagnosis made before birth should include specialists in anesthesiology and neonatalogy, and consideration of transfer to a high-risk perinatal center should be considered.
- Family history should be obtained for these patients.
- Standard heart failure protocols should be initiated, but use of angiotensin-converting

enzyme inhibitors should be avoided before birth; otherwise, these drugs are a mainstay of therapy.

- If endomyocardial biopsy indicates myocarditis and there is no improvement after 2 weeks of standard heart failure therapy, immunosuppressive therapy can be considered.
- Subsequent pregnancies should be managed in a high-risk perinatal center if not avoided, as this is a controversial issue.

Anthracycline-induced cardiomyopathy

Depending on a variety of risk factors and total dose, this form of toxin-induced cardiomyopathy may affect 5–20% of patients.[27–31] Clinical presentation resembles that of dilated cardiomyopathy of other etiologies. It may manifest between 1 week and years after chemotherapy.[27] It has been suggested that the shorter the latency period, the worse the severity and ultimate prognosis.[27]

The most sensitive study to detect cardiac toxicity appears to be endomyocardial biopsy.[32] Despite significant histologic evidence of toxicity, most studies (e.g. echocardiography, radionuclide angiography, and systolic time intervals) can fail to detect toxicity because they rely on systolic cardiac function, which may not fall.[33] Conceivably, diastolic function might provide more sensitive data in following these patients.

Therapy for dilated cardiomyopathy

Therapy for dilated cardiomyopathy focuses on treatment of congestive heart failure, including general information about the disease, self-monitoring, therapeutic strategies, risk

---

Classic
Development of cardiac failure in the last month of pregnancy or within 5 months of delivery
    Absence of an identifiable cause for the cardiac failure
    Absence of recognizable heart disease prior to the last month of pregnancy

Additional
Left ventricular systolic dysfunction demonstrated by classic echocardiographic criteria, e.g. depressed shortening fraction or ejection fraction

Source: reprinted with permission from Pearson et al.[26]

Table 8.2   Definition of peripartum cardiomyopathy

factor modification, infection prophylaxis, and nonpharmacologic therapy. In addition to general management of heart failure, different types of dilated cardiomyopathy require specific treatment strategies.

Viral and other inflammatory myocarditis

Although early clinical studies were optimistic about results of immunosuppressive therapy in viral myocarditis,[34–37] two prospective randomized trials involving prednisone failed to demonstrate similar results.[38,39] Nonetheless, immunosuppressive therapy has been successful in a subset of patients who have peripartum myocarditis, resulting in histological evidence of improvement in 90% of patients.[40] Similarly, biopsy evidence of inflammation associated with sarcoidosis is a marker for significant improvement in response to corticosteroids.[41–43] In cases of documented viral persistence, antiviral therapy or immunoaugmentation with interferon has been beneficial,[44] a novel approach under study in large-scale clinical trials.

In the Myocarditis Treatment Trial, patients who had active myocarditis by 'Dallas criterion' were randomly assigned to receive prednisone and azathioprine, prednisone and ciclosporin, or no immunosuppression for 6 months.[45] There was no difference in cumulative mortality among the treatment groups. A similar rise in 10% in both groups suggested a high likelihood of spontaneous improvement. Despite the trial's several shortcomings it undoubtedly showed that immunosuppressive therapy is not useful in all patients with myocarditis and that not every patient who has new onset heart failure needs endomyocardial biopsy.

Tachycardia-induced cardiomyopathy

Gossage and Braxton Hicks were the first to suggest that atrial fibrillation might be responsible for left ventricular dilatation and hypertrophy.[46] It is now understood that chronic tachycardia, one of the most easily reversible causes of ventricular dysfunction, induces a major form of cardiomyopathy.

Controlling the heart rate is vital in ameliorating heart failure states associated with tachycardias. Attempts should be made to restore normal sinus rhythm by either pharmacologic means or by electrical cardioversion. If this is not possible, the next option is to attempt control of ventricular rates by either pharmacologic means or by atrioventricular junction nodal ablation with permanent pacemaker implantation. Other supraventricular arrhythmias may respond to electrophysiologic ablation techniques. The last option to control dysrhythmia and ameliorate heart failure might be a Maze operation or other surgical ablation technique.

Diabetic cardiomyopathy

In patients who have diabetes, tight control of glucose may serve a purpose beyond standard treatment of heart failure; it may be beneficial for cardiac functioning. In a study of diabetic rats, chronic addition of propionyl-L-carnitine to the diet overcame the induced myocardial dysfunction,[47] an approach that might be explored as a treatment in humans.

Cardiomyopathy due to nutritional deficiency

In Northeast China, selenium deficiency has been reported as sometimes leading to a particular form of dilated cardiomyopathy. Selenium deficiency leads to decreased activity of glutathione peroxidase, which results in increased free-radical formation, which can cause direct myocyte injury. Similar cases have also been reported in HIV-positive patients on parenteral nutrition. Selenium replacement can reverse the ventricular dysfunction.

Patients who contract beriberi, a thiamine (vitamin B_1) deficiency, present with high-output cardiac failure and dilated cardiomyopathy with symptoms of edema, polyneuritis, and cardiac pathology. Thiamine is necessary for carbohydrate metabolism and thiamine replacement can rapidly restore cardiac function to normal, although long-term deficiency may make the condition irreversible.

Carnitine deficiency, which may be familial, may lead to dilated cardiomyopathy and cardiac lesions associated with endocardial fibroelastosis. In carnitine deficiency, impaired oxidation and mitochondrial transport of fatty acids lead to lipid accumulation in the cytoplasm.[48] Oral therapy with L-carnitine can be quite effective.[49]

Peripartum cardiomyopathy

Treatment of peripartum cardiomyopathy differs substantially from that for dilated cardiomyopathy because of risk to the fetus during pregnancy and to nursing mothers and an increased incidence of thromboembolism during pregnancy. Anticoagulation should be seriously considered. Hydralazine may be safely used for afterload reduction. Digoxin, diuretics, Food and Drug Administration Class C drugs, should be seriously considered. Simple sodium restriction may be enough to prevent fluid accumulation. Angiotensin-converting enzyme inhibitors are relatively contraindicated, and warfarin should never be used prenatally because of its severe teratogenic effects.

If symptoms and ventricular function do not improve, cardiac transplantation should be contemplated. Moreover, if left ventricular function is not fully recovered after delivery, the mother should be warned to avoid future pregnancies, as the rate of maternal mortality and morbidity is unacceptably high. Those who have completely recovered and are con-templating another pregnancy should be advised that recurrence is certainly possible, and warned that it is usually more severe the second time.[50]

Prognosis of dilated cardiomyopathy

In general, irrespective of underlying etiology, the prognosis of patients who have dilated cardiomyopathy depends on cardiac function. Exceptions are patients with peripartum cardiomyopathy (where prognosis is more favorable), anthracycline-induced cardiomyopathy with rapid onset (where prognosis is poor), and alcoholic cardiomyopathy with continued alcohol consumption (where prognosis is generally poor). As Figure 8.2 shows, the difference in actuarial survival in the two adult series was probably related to differing severity of illness.[50–52] Even in the group that had better outcome, the rate of survival at 1 year was 83% and only 72% at 2 years. Children who present after the age of 2 years appear to have a dismal prognosis, although this series is quite small.

As seen in Table 8.3, a variety of factors may influence prognosis. Most consistently powerful determinants are ejection fraction[10,53] and functional class.[54] Other factors are filling pressures,[10,53,54] cardiac output,[53] age at both extremes,[44,52] ventricular arrhythmias,[51] atrial fibrillation,[53] ventricular conduction delay,[53] interstitial fibrosis,[53] and ventricular hypertrophy.[10,53]

Restrictive cardiomyopathy

Pathophysiology

The primary myocardial defect in the restrictive form of cardiomyopathy is abnormal dias-

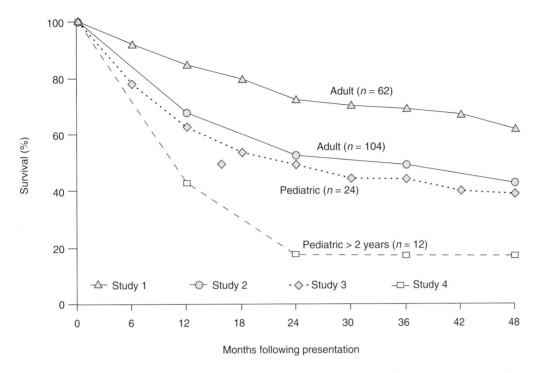

Figure 8.2 Rates of actuarial survival in patients with dilated cardiomyopathy in four separate series. Depending on the series and underlying patient characteristics, 1-year survival ranges from just below 90% to as low as 45%. Overall, pediatric patients appear to have the worst overall prognosis.

Ejection fraction
Functional class
Alcohol
Ventricular arrhythmias
Elevated filling pressures
Reduced cardiac output
Degree of ventricular hypertrophy
Degree of interstitial fibrosis
Intraventricular conduction abnormalities
Maximum oxygen consumption
Pediatric age group

Table 8.3 Predictors of outcome in dilated cardiomyopathy

tolic relaxation that restricts ventricular filling, creates high filling pressures and, despite normal or near-normal systolic function, reduces stroke volume secondary to reduction in total ventricular volume.[55] Consequently, regardless of diastolic volume, diastolic pressure increases abnormally. In addition to the left-sided shift in the pressure–volume ratio, restrictive cardiomyopathy accelerates the rate of rise in pressure for any given change in volume.[56]

Depending on the specific disease process, the mechanisms responsible for reducing ventricular compliance vary: an intrinsically abnormal myocardium, infiltration of the myocardium by such nonmyocardial materials as collagen or abnormal protein, endomyocardial disease, and space-occupying lesions (thrombus or tumor) that reduce the total ventricular volumes.

From the comprehensive list (Table 8.4) of reported causes of restrictive cardiomyopathy,

Primary (idiopathic)	Tumor infiltration
Amyloidosis	Storage diseases
Endocardial fibrosis	Anthracyclines
Eosinophilic heart disease	Radiation
Hemochromatosis	Cardiac transplant
Sarcoidosis	

Source: reprinted with permission from Hosenpud JD.

Table 8.4 Reported causes of restrictive cardiomyopathy

Age 39 years (mean) 1–77 years (range)	
Sex 19 (56%) male; 15 (44%) female	
Symptomatology:	
Chest pain	56%
Fatigue	50%
Dyspnea	61%
Clinical findings:	
Jugular venous distension	62%
Rale	19%
S3	48%
S4	32%
Ascites	25%
Edema	32%
Hemodynamics:[b]	
Right atrial pressure (mmHg)	12±6
Pulmonary wedge pressure (mmHg)	21±7
Cardiac index (L/min/m^2)	2.9±1.0
LVEDVI (ml/m^2)[c]	67±18
LV ejection fraction	68%±10%

[a] Data from seven studies.[117,121,122,124–127]
[b] Results expressed as mean ± 1 SD.
[c] LVEDVI = left ventricular end-diastolic volume index.

Table 8.5 Clinical and hemodynamic characteristics of 34 patients with primary restrictive cardiomyopathy[a]

idiopathic restrictive cardiomyopathy, amyloidosis, and endocardial fibrosis will be expanded upon; other etiologies will be mentioned briefly.

Idiopathic restrictive cardiomyopathy

Some patients have no specific etiology.[54,57] In such cases of primary or 'idiopathic' restrictive cardiomyopathy, histopathologic findings are nonspecific and generally include myocardial cell hypertrophy and an increase in interstitial fibrosis. Presumably, there may be a primary defect in myocardial cell relaxation.

Clinical and hemodynamic findings of patients who have idiopathic restrictive cardiomyopathy (Table 8.5) show a very large age range at presentation and an almost equal distribution between males and females.[54,57–60]

In spite of frequent complaints of dyspnea, only a few patients will have any objective evidence of pulmonary interstitial edema or alveolar edema. Chest pain is the second most frequent complaint, followed by fatigue. Filling pressures are elevated, but resting cardiac output tends to be normal. Ejection fractions are normal, ventricular volumes tend to be small, ventricular wall thickness is normal or mildly in-

creased, and atria are moderate to severely enlarged (Figure 8.3). Histopathologically, a salient finding is prominent interstitial fibrosis (Figure 8.4).[55,61]

In contrast with the extremely high 1- and 2-year mortality rates seen in patients who have dilated cardiomyopathy, patients with primary restrictive cardiomyopathy appear to have a better early prognosis: approximately 10% mortality at 1 year. Ultimately, however, the prognosis is poor: only 10% of patients survive at 10 years.

Amyloidosis

The second most frequently reported cause of restrictive cardiomyopathy is associated with amyloid protein deposition into the myocar-

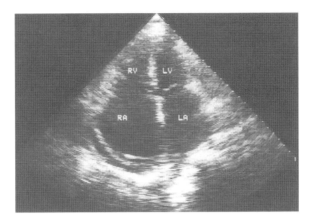

Figure 8.3 Echocardiogram (apical four-chamber view) from a patient with restrictive cardiomyopathy shows small left ventricular (LV) and right ventricular (RV) chamber sizes and relatively normal wall thicknesses. The left atrium (LA) and right atrium (RA) are both markedly enlarged. (Reprinted with permission from Hosenpud JD)

dial interstitium. 'Amyloid' is a generic term for deposition of a variety of fibrous proteins that are arranged spatially in a beta-pleated sheet configuration, a configuration that gives amyloid its characteristic staining properties in tissue.

Gross anatomic findings in amyloid heart disease are similar to those in primary restrictive cardiomyopathy with notable differences. On echocardiography, both left and right ventricular wall thicknesses tend to be symmetrically increased, and the intraventricular septum is hypokinetic. The atrioventricular valves can appear thickened and there is a par-

ticular granular and speckled pattern in the myocardium.[62–64]

The prognosis is poor for patients who have restrictive cardiomyopathy secondary to amyloidosis. Many do not survive beyond 2 years of symptom onset. In a large study of patients who had amyloid heart disease and congestive heart failure the median time of survival was 6 months.[65]

Endomyocardial fibrosis

In 1930, Loeffler described endomyocardial fibrosis with or without eosinophilia.[66] Since

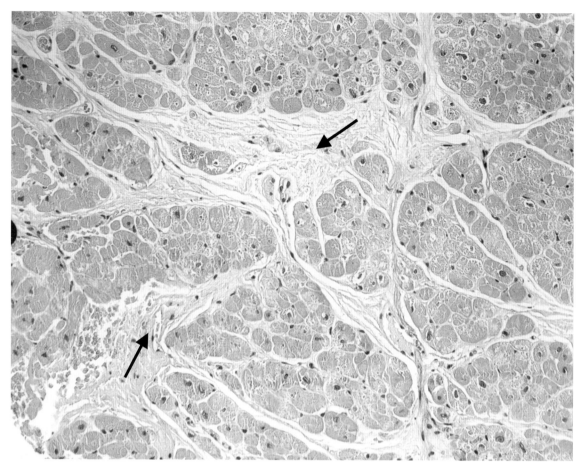

Figure 8.4 Endomyocardial biopsy (hematoxylin–eosin × 255) from a patient with primary restrictive cardiomyopathy shows extensive interstitial fibrosis (arrows) and relatively normal myocytes. (Reprinted with permission from Hosenpud JD)

Loeffler's original two patients, over 100 cases have been reported. The suggested primary etiology is eosinophilic damage to the endocardium and it is thought that patients who do not present with documented eosinophilia are at a later stage of the disease.[67] The mechanism of injury appears to be a direct toxic effect of eosinophilic secretory products (granule basic proteins) on the myocardium.[68]

Depending on the stage of the disease process, the hemodynamic findings of restriction may have different mechanisms. During the thrombotic stage, in addition to endomy-

ocardial damage, ventricular thrombi may be so large that the remaining ventricular chamber volume cannot sustain cardiac output. In the fibrotic stage, presumably the thick endocardial peel prevents normal diastolic relaxation.

The cardiovascular clinical findings are essentially similar to those found in other forms of restrictive cardiomyopathy and include symptoms and signs of biventricular congestive heart failure.[69–72] Again, the prognosis is variable, perhaps depending on the underlying disease process. Although a patient may have eosinophilia long before cardiac symptoms develop,[73] once symptoms develop, the prognosis is poor.[73–75] Studies have shown that the outcome can be modified when aggressive therapy is directed simultaneously to reducing the total eosinophil count, treating congestive heart failure, and in some cases, resorting to surgical endomyocardial stripping and valve replacement.[69,71]

Other causes

Other reported causes of restrictive cardiomyopathy include sarcoidosis and other granulomatous diseases of the myocardium,[67,76] hemochromatosis,[77] cardiac tumors,[78,79] radiation,[80] anthracycline toxicity,[81] collagen vascular diseases,[82] genetic connective tissue diseases,[83] and coronary arteritis.[84] It has been suggested recently that the cardiac allograft exhibits 'restrictive' physiology.[85,86] It remains to be determined whether this is an intrinsic myocardial abnormality or an artifact of a discrepancy between the size of a donor's heart and the size of the recipient's (i.e. problems with matching or with recipient volume regulation, or both).

Specific therapy for restrictive cardiomyopathy

Primary restrictive cardiomyopathy
In primary restrictive cardiomyopathy, obviously when there is no known specific etiology, there is no specific treatment.

Amyloid cardiomyopathy
Typically, it is difficult and not effective to attempt to manage amyloid cardiomyopathy. Low-dose diuretics and vasodilators are the most useful of the drug options but their many side effects require close supervision. Calcium channel blockers have been disappointing.

Nifedipine (and other calcium channel blockers), which is bound by amyloid fibrils may exacerbate symptoms of heart failure by a negative inotropic mechanism.[87–89] Digoxin may be selectively bound to the fibrils, resulting in increased sensitivity and toxicity, making it relatively contraindicated.[89–91] Pacemakers help treat underlying conduction abnormalities.

Modest evidence now suggests that the treatment of myeloma and plasma cell dyscrasias may alter the course of cardiac amyloidosis. In a study on 220 patients with primary amyloidosis,[92] melphalan plus prednisone was superior to colchicine alone, and adding colchicine did not enhance the benefits of melphalan plus prednisone. Of patients treated with melphalan plus prednisone, 28% had a favorable response (at least 50% reduction in serum and urine monoclonal protein) compared with 3% of those treated with colchicine alone. Those who had major cardiac involvement had the shortest times of survival (5 months) compared with those who had nephrotic syndrome (16 months) or neuropathy (34 months). Cardiac causes accounted for 51% of deaths.[92]

Skinner et al. reported that, in patients with cardiac amyloidosis and congestive heart failure, melphalan and prednisone significantly improved median survival compared with controls: 12 vs 5 months.[93]

Endomyocardial fibrosis
Patients who have endomyocardial fibrosis, characterized by thickening and scarring of the endocardium, can expect a poor overall prognosis. However, the damage of eosinophilic systemic disease may be ameliorated by use of aggressive therapy,[70] and cardiac performance improved by aggressive surgical therapy, including endocardiectomy and valvular replacement/repair.[71] In Loffler's endocardial fibrosis, corticosteroids and cyto-

toxic agents (hydroxyurea) can improve symptoms and survival.[94]

Hemochromatosis

In patients with hemochromatosis, cardiac function may improve by means of aggressive total body iron removal,[77] either repeated phlebotomy or chelation therapy.

Generic therapy for restrictive cardiomyopathy

Diuretics

Once cardiovascular compromise is severe, generic therapy for restrictive cardiomyopathy is extremely difficult. The diastolic ventricular pressure–volume relationship is quite steep, demanding that diuretics, a mainstay of therapy, be used cautiously, because small changes in volume can produce large changes in filling pressures. Further complicating treatment, a reduction in filling pressures to alleviate symptoms of congestion may produce dramatic falls in cardiac output, because any decrease in myocardial compliance requires higher filling pressures for adequate ventricular filling.

Inotropic agents

Patients who have restrictive cardiomyopathy usually have normal systolic function, in some patients even at the upper range of normal, limiting the use of inotropic agents. Therefore, digitalis may be the only drug that can be prescribed; it is needed for rhythm control in the many patients who have atrial arrhythmia along with restriction and atrial dilation.

Vasodilators

A mainstay for most forms of heart failure, vasodilator therapy may have a small role in treating restrictive cardiomyopathy. In these patients, stroke volume depends upon high filling pressures and is usually fixed at peak pressures. Because cardiac dilation is rare, this component of wall stress is insignificant. Thus, vasodilator therapy will reduce preload, as well as both filling pressures and stroke volume, profoundly reducing arterial pressure secondary to both arteriolar dilation and the fall in cardiac output.

Calcium channel blockers

Calcium channel blockers, effective in hypertrophic cardiomyopathy, have not proven to be so in restrictive cardiomyopathy.[95] In patients whose stroke volume is fixed and whose cardiac output depends on heart rate, use of calcium channel blocking agents could be more disastrous than beneficial.

For all practical purposes, therapy for restrictive cardiomyopathy is limited to diuretic therapy for patients who have mild-to-moderate symptoms and to cardiac transplantation for patients who have severe disease.

Hypertrophic cardiomyopathy

Pathophysiology and mechanisms of disease

Initially described by Teare in 1958,[96] hypertrophic cardiomyopathy has always been surrounded by controversy and is still poorly understood. Most clinicians who study primary myocardial disease feel that although there may be outflow tract obstruction, the principal abnormality is impaired ventricular compliance, which is probably due to the inappropriate myocardial hypertrophy. Hence, the most accurate and most commonly used term for this form of the disease is 'hypertrophic cardiomyopathy'.

Clearly, most patients with this disease have a distinctive pattern of hypertrophy that affects the ventricular septum much more than it does the other ventricular walls, a pattern termed 'asymmetric septal hypertrophy'. Microscopy reveals disorganized myocardial fibers with no evidence of any remaining normal orientation parallel to lines of stress, i.e. 'myofibril disarray.'

Most patients have 'systolic anterior motion' or SAM: a pressure gradient across the aortic outflow tract caused primarily by the mitral valve moving anteriorly during systole and abutting the septum (Fig. 8.5).[97]

In 50–75% of patients, the disease appears to be inherited as an autosomal dominant trait and in the remaining patients the cause seems to be sporadic.[98,99] As with other autosomal dominant diseases, even within a given family, penetrance and phenotype are quite variable.

Clinical features of hypertrophic cardiomyopathy

Symptoms

The principal symptoms are dyspnea, chest pain, and syncope.[100–103] Exertional dyspnea is the most common symptom (in upwards of 90% of patients). The etiology of dyspnea is probably high filling pressures combined with reduced myocardial compliance, especially with exercise.[104–109] This symptom, along with chest pain and syncope, correlates with neither the presence nor the amount of the outflow tract gradient.[110,111]

Up to 50% of patients report syncope or near syncope.[101–103] No relationship is apparent between syncopal symptoms and the severity of outflow tract gradients.[101–103,111,112] Holter monitor and treadmill exercise studies indicate that, in most cases, the etiology of the syncope is arrhythmic, as these studies reveal frequent ventricular and atrial arrhythmias and overt ventricular tachycardia in up to 40% of patients.[113–116]

Finally, usually late in the disease, systolic ventricular function deteriorates in a few patients, and more characteristic symptoms of heart failure supervene. If patients lose both sinus rhythm and atrioventricular synchrony, signs and symptoms of both left and right ventricular dysfunction can quickly follow.[101,110]

Clinical findings

With or without measurement of resting or exercise outflow tract gradients clinical findings can either be entirely normal or confined to signs of elevated left ventricular filling pressures (fourth heart sound). In more advanced stages, signs of both systemic and pulmonary venous congestion appear. When a resting or provoked outflow tract gradient is measured, clinical examination can be diagnostic.

Medical management

Beta-blockers

As early as 1964, Harrison et al. reported that beta-blocking agents improved the hemodynamics of patients who have hypertrophic cardiomyopathy.[117] Several studies have since confirmed the efficacy of these agents in reducing symptoms and improving hemodynamics. Most hemodynamic studies found that beta-blockade reduced the gradient of the outflow tract and suggested that this reduction improved symptoms.[118,119]

Initial studies suggesting that beta-blockade might improve diastolic function[120,121] have not been supported by careful studies of diastolic indices.[122,123] Finally, beta-blockers may affect generation of ventricular arrhythmias, especially during exercise and stress when catecholamine levels are elevated. Although many patients have a good initial response to beta-blockers, the long-term response (especially with high doses) by many patients is one of complaints of fatigue and depression.

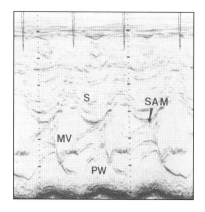

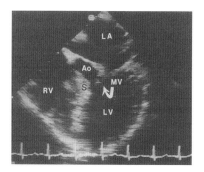

Figure 8.5 The typical M-mode (top) and transesophageal (bottom) echocardiograms in patients with hypertrophic cardiomyopathy. With the onset of systole, the mitral valve (MV) exhibits systolic anterior motion (SAM) and abuts the ventricular septum (S), causing an outflow tract gradient. Ao = aorta, LA = left atrium, LV = left ventricle, PW = posterior wall, RV = right ventricle.

Calcium channel blockers

Substantial data show that patients experience high efficacy and sustained response to treatment with calcium channel blockers.[124–127] Although many calcium channel blockers have proven efficacious, the one most studied has been verapamil. In 19 patients who had hypertrophic cardiomyopathy, verapamil improved exercise performance by an average of 45%,[128] but there was no correlation between this improvement and change in outflow tract gradient, which was reduced by an average of 35 mmHg.

Amiodarone

Although recent studies have demonstrated that the antiarrhythmic agent amiodarone has hemodynamic benefits,[129] the mechanisms responsible for this are unclear. Possible mechanisms are the drug's negative inotropic effects, vascular dilation, and suppression of ventricular arrhythmias. Amiodarone improves symptoms in patients who are refractory to both beta-blockers and calcium channel blockers.[130]

Disopyrimide

Disopyrimide also effectively reduces gradients and improves symptoms,[131–133] probably through negative inotropic action, but the hemodynamic and clinical benefits decrease with time.[134]

Diuretics

Diuretics need to be used carefully in patients who have elevated filling pressures. As with restrictive cardiomyopathy, one must balance the reduction of resting filling pressures enough to eliminate symptoms of congestion but not enough to reduce ventricular filling. This is particularly difficult in patients who have chronic atrial fibrillation, as the atrial contraction can be responsible for as much as 50% of ventricular filling.

Arrhythmia management

Arrhythmia management is a major concern in treating patients who have hypertrophic cardiomyopathy, because loss of atrioventricular synchrony can quickly make symptoms worse. In the event that synchrony is lost, it is reasonable to attempt to convert atrial arrhythmias, either electrically or pharmacologically, and to maintain sinus rhythm. In patients who have hypertrophic cardiomyopathy, amiodarone effectively controls both atrial and ventricular arrhythmias.

Treatment of comorbid conditions

Finally, comorbid conditions must be addressed. Systemic anticoagulation is indicated in patients whose atrial fibrillation is either intermittent or persistent, and endocarditis prophylaxis is indicated in patients who have a systolic murmur consistent with SAM.

Pacing

In 1992, Jeanrenaud et al. reported that dual-chamber A–V sequential pacing improved symptoms in drug refractory patients.[135] The proposed mechanism for this improvement was that changing the contraction sequence in the ventricles ultimately decreased the outflow tract gradient. Subsequently, Fananapazir et al. suggested that long-term pacing resulted in ventricular remodeling, in reduced left ventricular hypertrophy, and in improved exercise capacity and hemodynamics.[136] However, in a recent randomized and prospective crossover study, there were no demonstrable results from dual-chamber pacing.[137]

Alcohol septal ablation

Transcoronary septal reduction is a new approach to gradient reduction in hypertrophic cardiomyopathy that uses injection of alcohol into the first septal perforator branch of the left anterior descending artery.[138–140] Worldwide, preliminary data from several series show significant gradient reduction and improvement of symptoms.

Surgical management

In 1961, Morrow and Brockenbrough presented the first report of surgical therapy for hypertrophic cardiomyopathy in which they performed subaortic ventriculomyotomy on two patients, which resulted in reduced outflow tract gradient and clinical improvement.[141] The procedure has been since modified, and used to treat many patients who are refractory to medical management.[142] Depending on the series with additional late mortality, overall operative mortality ranges from 0% to 26%.[143] In Maron et al.'s report of 124 patients who underwent septal myotomy– myectomy at the National Institutes of Health, operative mortality was 8%. In the first 6 months postoperation, 88% of these patients had clinical improvement and this improvement persisted in 70% of the initial group.[144]

Septal myotomy–myectomy is currently recommended only for patients who are refractory to medical management and who have an outflow tract gradient of at least 50 mmHg. Symptom reduction is the sole justification for the procedure, as there is no evidence that surgical therapy prolongs survival or alters arrhythmias.

Prognosis of hypertrophic cardiomyopathy

In three studies of four patient groups, including both adults and children,[144–146] the overall 10-year rate of actuarial survival in a large cohort in the United Kingdom was up to 80% in 184 adults and up to 60% in 27 children.[131] In a large surgical series from the National Institutes of Health, survival was slightly worse.[144]

In their meta-analysis of both surgical and medical approaches to this disease, Canedo and Frank could demonstrate no differences in outcome between groups when they compared 255 surgically treated and 184 medically treated patients who had hypertrophic cardiomyopathy.[143] In a selected series of 33 patients who had experienced cardiac arrest and were successfully resuscitated, outcome was substantially poorer than the general adult experience: 10-year actuarial survival was up to 65%.[146]

The difficulty of determining the natural history of a disease when using data from recognized referral centers for that disease was pointed out by Spirito et al. in their interesting study of 25 outpatients who had hypertrophic cardiomyopathy. When these patients were followed for a mean period of 4.4 years, there were no deaths or any documented evidence of clinical deterioration.[147] Therefore, the prognosis appears particularly good in such relatively asymptomatic patients.

Aside from considering mortality, significant concerns in patients who have hypertrophic cardiomyopathy are that approximately 5% develop endocarditis, 5–10% develop systemic emboli, approximately 10–15% eventually develop atrial fibrillation, and 5–10% experience myocardial decompensation and symptoms of heart failure. It is hoped that in recognizing these comorbid events and, when available, directing preventive therapy (e.g. antibiotic prophylaxis, anticoagulation), we will be able to reduce these complications in this population.

Conclusions

Cardiomyopathies are a heterogeneous group of diseases that have multiple associations but largely unknown disease mechanisms. Although anatomic classification of cardiomyopathies is rudimentary, it is affording insight into such issues as etiology and associations and, especially, into medical management and prognosis. Although there is currently no available direct therapy for almost all of these diseases, and generic heart failure management is certainly limited, the use of beta-blockade therapy is much more encouraging. Where prognosis is poor, strong consideration should be given to cardiac replacement therapy.

References

1. Krehl L. Beitrag zur Kentniss der idiopathischen Herzmuskelerkrankungen. Dtsch Arch F Klin Med 1891; 48:414–31.
2. Brigden W. Uncommon myocardial diseases: the noncoronary cardiomyopathies. Lancet 1957; 2:1243–9.
3. Fejfar Z. Accounts of international meetings: idiopathic cardiomegaly. Bull WHO 1968; 28:979–92.
4. Douglas PS, Morrow R, Ioli A, Reichek N. Left ventricular shape, afterload and survival in idiopathic dilated cardiomyopathy. J Am Coll Cardiol 1989; 13:311–15.
5. Factor SM, Minase T, Cho S, et al. Microvascular spasm in the cardiomyopathic Syrian hamster: a preventable cause of focal myocardial necrosis. Circulation 1982; 66:342–54.
6. Demakis JG, Proskey A, Rahimtoola SH, et al. The natural course of alcoholic cardiomyopathy. Ann Intern Med 1974; 80:293–7.
7. Kantrowitz NE, Bristow MR. Cardiotoxicity of antitumor agents. Prog Cardiovasc Dis 1984; 27:195–200.
8. Bristow MR, Mason JW, Billingham ME, Daniels JR. Dose–effect and structure–function relationships in doxorubicin cardiomyopathy. Am Heart J 1981; 102:709–18.
9. Gruenig E, Tasman JA, Kuecherer H, et al. Frequency and phenotypes of familial dilated cardiomyopathy. J Am Coll Cardiol 1998; 31:186–94.
10. Schwarz F, Mall G, Zebe H, et al. Determinants of survival in patients with congestive cardiomyopathy: quantitative morphologic findings and left ventricular hemodynamics. Circulation 1984; 70:923–8.
11. Regan TJ, Levinson GE, Oldewurtel HA, et al. Ventricular function in noncardiacs with alcoholic fatty liver: role of ethanol in the production of cardiomyopathy. J Clin Invest 1969; 48:397–407.
12. Lang RM, Borow KM, Neumann A, Feldman T. Adverse cardiac effects of acute alcohol ingestion in young adults. Ann Intern Med 1985; 102:742–7.
13. Burch GE, Giles, TD. Alcoholic cardiomyopathy: concept of the disease and its treatment. Am J Med 1971; 50:141–5.
14. McDonald CD, Burch GE, Walsh JJ. Alcoholic cardiomyopathy managed with prolonged bed rest. Ann Intern Med 1971; 74:681–91.
15. Wu CF, Sudhakar M, Jaferi G, et al. Preclinical cardiomyopathy in chronic alcoholics: a sex difference. Am Heart J 1976; 91:281–6.
16. Lefkowitch JH, Fenoglio JJ Jr. Liver disease in alcoholic cardiomyopathy: evidence against cirrhosis. Hum Pathol 1983; 14:457–63.
17. Shugoll GI, Bowen PJ, Moore JP, Lenkin ML. Follow-up observations and prognosis in primary myocardial disease. Arch Intern Med 1972; 129:67–72.
18. Rubler S, Dglugash J, Yuceoglu YZ, et al. New type of cardiomyopathy associated with diabetic glomerulosclerosis. Am J Cardiol 1972; 30:595–602.
19. Kannel WB, Hjortland M, Castelli WP. Role of diabetes in congestive heart failure: the Framingham study. Am J Cardiol 1974; 34:29–34.

20. Brownlee M, Cerami A, Viassara H. Advanced glycosylation end products in tissue and the biochemical basis of diabetic complications. N Engl J Med 1988; 318:1315–21.

21. Ganguly PK, Pierce GN, Dhalla KS, Dhalla NS. Defective cardiac sarcoplasmic reticular calcium transport in diabetic cardiomyopathy. Am J Physiol 1983; 244:E528–35.

22. Factor SM, Minase T, Cho S, et al. Coronary microvascular abnormalities in the hypertensive-diabetic rat, a primary cause of cardiomyopathy? Am J Pathol 1984; 116:9–20.

23. Hull E, Hafkesbring E. Toxic post-partal failure. New Orleans Med Surg J 1937; 89:556–7.

24. Gouley BA, McMillan TM, Bellet S. Idiopathic myocardial degeneration associated with pregnancy and especially the puerperium. Am J Med Sci 1937; 194:185–99.

25. Homans DC. Peripartum cardiomyopathy. N Engl J Med 1985; 312:1432–7.

26. Pearson GD, Veille J-C, Rahmitoola S, et al. Peripartum cardiomyopathy: National Heart, Lung, and Blood Institute and Office of Rare Diseases (National Institutes of Health) Workshop Recommendations and Review. JAMA 2000; 283:1183–8.

27. Saltiel E, McGuire W. Doxorubicin (Adriamycin) cardiomyopathy. West J Med 1983; 139:332–41.

28. Minow RA, Benjamin RS, Lee ET, Gottlieb JA. Adriamycin cardiomyopathy – risk factors. Cancer 1977; 39:1397–402.

29. Billingham ME, Bristow MR, Glatstein E, et al. Adriamycin cardiotoxicity: endomyocardial biopsy evidence of enhancement by irradiation. Am J Surg Path 1977; 1:17–23.

30. Billingham ME. Endomyocardial changes in anthracycline-treated patients with and without irradiation. Front Radiat Ther Onc 1979; 13:67–81.

31. Torti FM, Bristow MR, Howes AE, et al. Reduced cardiotoxicity of doxorubicin delivered on a weekly schedule. Ann Int Med 1983; 99:745–56.

32. Mason JW, Bristow MR, Billingham ME, Daniels JR. Invasive and noninvasive methods of assessing Adriamycin cardiotoxic effects in man: superiority of histopathologic assessment using endomyocardial biopsy. Cancer Treat Rep 1978; 62:857–64.

33. Bristow MR, Lopez MB, Mason JW, et al. Efficacy and cost of cardiac monitoring in patients receiving doxorubicin. Cancer 1982; 50:32–41.

34. Ainger LE. Acute aseptic myocarditis: corticosteroid therapy. J Pediatr 1964; 64:716–23.

35. Stogman VW. Die Grippenmyokarditis beim sangling und kleinkind. Wien Klin Wochenschr 1971; 84:502–4.

36. Wimmer M, Proll E, Salzer-Muhar U, et al. Immunosuppressive behandlung der chronischen myocarditis. Wien Med Wochenschr 1988; 19:658–63.

37. Kishimoto C, Thorp KA, Abelmann WH. Immunosuppression with high doses of cyclophosphamide reduces the severity of myocarditis but increases the mortality in murine Coxsackievirus B3 myocarditis. Circulation 1990; 82:982–9.

38. Latham RD, Mulrow JP, Virmani R, et al. Recently diagnosed idiopathic dilated cardiomyopathy; incidence of myocarditis and efficacy of prednisone therapy. Am Heart J 1989; 117:876–958.

39. Parrillo JE, Cunnion RE, Epstein S, et al. A prospective, randomized, controlled trial of prednisone for dilated cardiomyopathy. N Engl J Med 1989; 321:1061–80.

40. Midei MG, DeMent SH, Feldman AM, et al. Peripartum myocarditis and cardiomyopathy. Circulation 1990; 81:922–8.

41. Lorell B, Alderman EL, Mason JW. Cardiac sarcoidosis: diagnosis with endomyocardial biopsy and treatment with corticosteroids. Am J Cardiol 1978; 42:143–6.

42. Valentine HA, Tazelaar HD, Macoviak J, et al. Cardiac sarcoidosis: response to steroids and transplantation. J Heart Transplant 1987; 6:244–50.

43. Lemery R, McGoon MD, Edwards WD. Cardiac sarcoidosis: a potentially treatable form of myocarditis. Mayo Clin Proc 1985; 60:549–54.

44. Miric M, Vasiljevic J, Bojic M, et al. Long-term follow-up of patients with dilated heart muscle disease treated with human leucocytic interferon alpha or thymic hormones: initial results. Heart 1996; 75:596–601.

45. Hahn EA, Hartz VL, Moon TE. The myocarditis treatment trial: design methods and patient enrollment. Eur Heart J 1995; 16:162–7.

46. Gossage AM, Braxton Hicks JA. On auricular fibrillation. Q J Med 1913; 6:435–40.

47. Pasini E, Comini L, Ferrari R, et al. Effect of propionyl-L-carnitine on experimental induced cardiomyopathy in rats. Am J Cardiovasc Pathol 1992; 4:216–22.

48. Waber LJ, Valle D, Neill C. Carnitine deficiency presenting as familial cardiomyopathy: a treatable defect in carnitine transport. J Pediatr 1982; 101:700–5.

49. Tripp ME, Katcher ML, Peters HA. Systemic carnitine deficiency presenting as familial endocardial fibroelastosis: a treatable cardiomyopathy. N Engl J Med 1984; 310:142–8.

50. Elkayam U, Ostrzega EL, Shotan A. Peripartum cardiomyopathy. In: Gliecher N, ed., Principles and Practice of Medical Therapy in Pregnancy, 2nd edn. Norwalk: Appleton and Lange, 1992.

51. Figulla HR, Rahlf G, Nieger M, et al. Spontaneous hemodynamic improvement or stabilization and associated biopsy findings in patients with congestive cardiomyopathy. Circulation 1985; 71:1095–104.

52. Taliercio CP, Seward JB, Driscoll DJ, et al. Idiopathic dilated cardiomyopathy in the young: clinical profile and natural history. J Am Coll Cardiol 1985; 6:1126–31.

53. Griffin ML, Hernandez A, Martin TC, et al. Dilated cardiomyopathy in infants and children. J Am Coll Cardiol 1988; 11:139–44.

54. Unverferth DV, Magorien RD, Moeschberger ML, et al. Factors influencing the one-year mortality of dilated cardiomyopathy. Am J Cardiol 1984; 54: 147–52.

55. Wilson JR, Schwartz JS, St John Sutton M, et al. Prognosis in severe heart failure: relation to hemodynamic measurements and ventricular ectopic activity. J Am Coll Cardiol 1983; 2:403–10.

56. Chew CYC, Ziady GM, Raphael MJ, et al. Primary restrictive cardiomyopathy non-tropical endomyocardial fibrosis and hypereosinophilic heart disease. Br Heart J 1977; 39:399–413.

57. Benotti JR, Grossman W. Restrictive cardiomyopathy. Ann Rev Med 1984; 35:113–25.

58. Siegel RJ, Shah PK, Fishbein MC. Idiopathic restrictive cardiomyopathy. Circulation 1984; 70:165–9.

59. Mehta AV, Ferrer PL, Pickoff AS, et al. M-mode echocardiographic findings in children with id-

iopathic restrictive cardiomyopathy. Pediatr Cardiol 1984; 5:273–80.

60. Sapire DW, Casta A, Swischuk LE, Casta D. Massive dilatation of the stria and coronary sinus in a child with restrictive cardiomyopathy and persistence of the left superior vena cava. Cathet Cardiovasc Diagn 1983; 9:47–53.

61. Erath HG, Graham TP Jr, Smith CW, Boucek RJ Jr. Restrictive cardiomyopathy in an infant with massive biatrial enlargement and normal ventricular size and pump function. Cathet Cardiovasc Diagn 1978; 4:289–96.

62. Arbustini E, Buonanno C, Trevi G, et al. Cardiac ultrastructure in primary restrictive cardiomyopathy. Chest 1983; 84:236–8.

63. Child JS, Krivokapich J, Abbasi AS. Increased right ventricular wall thickness on echocardiography in amyloid infiltrative cardiomyopathy. Am J Cardiol 1979; 44:1391–5.

64. Child JS, Levisman JA, Abbasi AS, MacAlpin RN. Echocardiographic manifestations of infiltrative cardiomyopathy. Chest 1976; 70:726–31.

65. Pierard L, Verheugt FWA, Meltzer RS, Roelandt J. Echocardiographic aspects of cardiac amyloidosis. Acta Cardiol 1981; 36:455–61.

66. Kyle RA, Greipp PR. Amyloidosis (AL): clinical and laboratory feature in 229 cases. Mayo Clin Proc 1983; 58:665–83.

67. Loeffler W. Endocarditis parietalis fibroplastica mit bluteosinophiline. Schweiz Med Wchnscr 1930; 66:817–20.

68. Roberts WC, Ferrans VJ. Pathologic anatomy of the cardiomyopathies. Idiopathic dilated and hypertrophic types, infiltrative types, and endomyocardial disease with and without eosinophilia. Hum Pathol 1975; 6:287–342.

69. Spry CJF, Tai P-C, Davies J. The cardiotoxicity of eosinophils. Postgrad Med J 1983; 59:147–51.

70. Cherian G, Vijayaraghavan G, Krishnaswami S, et al. Endomyocardial fibrosis: report on the hemodynamic data in 29 patients and review of the results of surgery. Am Heart J 1983; 105:659–66.

71. Olsen EGJ, Spry CJF. Relation between eosinophilia and endomyocardial disease. Prog Cardiovasc Dis 1985; 27:241–54.

72. Parrillo JE, Borer JS, Henry WL, et al. The cardiovascular manifestations of the hypere-

osinophilic syndrome. Am J Med 1979; 67:572–82.

73. Kudenchuk PJ, Hosenpud JD, Fletcher S. Eosinophilic endomyocardiopathy. Clin Cardiol 1986; 9:344–8.

74. Solley GO, Maldonado JE, Gleich GJ Jr, et al. Endomyocardiopathy with eosinophilia. Mayo Clin Proc 1976; 51:697–708.

75. Benvenisti DS, Ultmann JE. Eosinophilic leukemia? Report of 5 cases and review of the literature. Ann Intern Med 1969; 71:732–6.

76. Chusid MJ, Dale DC, West BC, Wolff SM. The hypereosinophilic syndrome: analysis of 14 cases and review of the literature. Medicine 1975; 54:1–27.

77. Ratner SJ, Fenoglio JJ Jr, Ursell PC. Utility of endomyocardial biopsy in the diagnosis of cardiac sarcoidosis. Chest 1986; 90:528–33.

78. Cutler DJ, Isner JM, Bracey AW, et al. Hemochromatosis heart disease: an unemphasized cause of potentially reversible restrictive cardiomyopathy. Am J Med 1980; 69:923–8.

79. Kaplan A, Cohen J. Restrictive cardiomyopathy as the presenting feature of reticulum cell sarcoma. Am Heart J 1969; 77:307–14.

80. Landau E, Reisin LH. LV myxoma resembling restrictive cardiomyopathy. Am Heart J 1986; 112:1356.

81. Westerhof PW, van der Putte SCJ. Radiation pericarditis and myocardial fibrosis. Eur J Cardiol 1976; 4/2:213–18.

82. Mortensen SA, Olsen HS, Baandrup U. Chronic anthracycline cardiotoxicity: haemodynamic and histopathological manifestations suggesting a restrictive endomyocardial disease. Br Heart J 1986; 55:274–82.

83. Doherty NE, Siegel RJ. Cardiovascular manifestations of systemic lupus erythematosus. Am Heart J 1985; 110:1257–65.

84. Navarro-Lopez F, Llorian A, Ferrer-Roca O, et al. Restrictive cardiomyopathy in pseudoxanthoma elasticum. Chest 1980; 78:113–15.

85. Papapietro SE, Rogers LW, Hudson NL, et al. Intramyocardial coronary arteritis and restrictive cardiomyopathy. Am Heart J 1987; 114:175–8.

86. Humen DP, McKenzie FN, Kostuk WJ. Restricted myocardial compliance one year following cardiac transplantation. J Heart Transplant 1984; 3:341–5.

87. Young JB, Leon CA, Short D III, et al. Evolution of hemodynamics after orthotopic heart and heart–lung transplantation: early restrictive patterns persisting in an occult fashion. J Heart Transplant 1987; 6:34–43.

88. Pollak A, Falk RH. Left ventricular systolic dysfunction precipitated by verapamil in cardiac amyloidosis. Chest 1993; 104:618–20.

89. Gertz MA, Falk RH, Skinner M. Worsening of congestive heart failure in amyloid heart disease treated by calcium channel-blocking agent. Am J Cardiol 1985; 55:1645.

90. Griffiths BE, Hughes P, Dowdle R, Stephens MR. Cardiac amyloidosis with asymmetrical septal hypertrophy and deterioration after nifedipine. Thorax 1982; 37:711–12.

91. Rubinow A, Skinner M, Cohen AS. Digoxin sensitivity in amyloid cardiomyopathy. Circulation 1981; 63:1285–8.

92. Cassidy JT. Cardiac amyloidosis: two cases with digitalis sensitivity. Ann Intern Med 1961; 55:989–94.

93. Kyle RA, Gertz MA, Greipp PR, et al. A trial of three regimens for primary amyloidosis: colchicine alone, melphalan and prednisone, and melphalan, prednisone and colchicine. N Engl J Med 1997; 336:1202–7.

94. Skinner M, Anderson J, Simms R, et al. Treatment of 100 patients with primary amyloidosis: a randomized trial of melphalan, prednisone, and colchincine versus colchicine only. Am J Med 1996; 100:290–8.

95. Parillo JE, Borer JS, Henry WC. The cardiovascular manifestations of the hypereosinophilic syndrome: prospective study of 26 patients, with review of the literature. Am J Med 1979; 67:572–82.

96. Braunwald E. Mechanism of action of calcium-channel-blocking agents. N Engl J Med 1982; 307:1618–27.

97. Teare D. Asymmetrical hypertrophy of the heart in young patients. Br Heart J 1958; 20:1–8.

98. Maron BJ, Epstein SE. Hypertrophic cardiomyopathy. Am J Cardiol 1980; 45:141–54.

99. Clark CE, Henry WL, Epstein SE. Familial prevalence and genetic transmission of idiopathic hypertrophic subaortic stenosis. N Engl J Med 1973; 289:709–14.

100. Maron BJ, Nichols PF, Pickle LW, et al. Patterns of inheritance in hypertrophic car-

diomyopathy: assessment by M-mode and two-dimensional echocardiography. Am J Cardiol 1984; 53:1087–94.

101. Brock R. Functional obstruction of the left ventricle (acquired aortic subvalvular stenosis). Guy's Hospital Report 1957; 106:221–38.

102. Braunwald E, Lambrew CT, Rockoff SD, et al. Idiopathic hypertrophic subaortic stenosis. I: A description of the disease based upon an analysis of 64 patients. Circulation 1964; 29&30(Suppl IV):3–119.

103. Swan DA, Bell B, Oakley CM, Goodwin J. Analysis of symptomatic course and prognosis and treatment of hypertrophic obstructive cardiomyopathy. Br Heart J 1971; 33:671–85.

104. Fiddler GI, Tajik AJ, Weidman WH, et al. Idiopathic hypertrophic subaortic stenosis in the young. Am J Cardiol 1978; 42:793–9.

105. Marian AJ, Roberts R. Recent advances in the molecular genetics of hypertrophic cardiomyopathy. Circulation 1995; 92:1336–47.

106. Rosenzweig A, Watkins H, Hwang D-S, et al. Preclinical diagnosis of familial hypertrophic cardiomyopathy by genetic analysis of blood lymphocytes. N Engl J Med 1991; 325:1753–60.

107. Criley JM, Lewis KB, White RI Jr, Ross RS. Pressure gradients without obstruction: a non concept of 'hypertrophic subaortic stenosis.' Circulation 1965; 32:881–7.

108. Stewart S, Mason DT, Braunwald E. Impaired rate of left ventricular filling in idiopathic subaortic stenosis and valvular aortic stenosis. Circulation 1968; 37:8–14.

109. Sanderson JE, Gibson DG, Brown DJ, Goodwin JF. Left ventricular filling in hypertrophic cardiomyopathy: an angiographic study. Br Heart J 1977; 39:661–70.

110. Hanrath P, Mathey DG, Siegert R, Bleifeld W. Left ventricular relaxation and filling pattern in different forms of left ventricular hypertrophy: an echocardiographic study. Am J Cardiol 1980; 45:15–23.

111. Shah PM, Adelman AG, Wigle ED, et al. The natural (and unnatural) history of hypertrophic obstructive cardiomyopathy. Circ Res 1974; 34&35(Suppl II):179–95.

112. Adelman AG, Wigle ED, Ranganathan N, et al. The clinical course in muscular subaortic stenosis. A retrospective and prospective study of 60

hemodynamically proved cases. Ann Intern Med 1972; 77:515–25.

113. Hardarson T, de la Calzada CS, Curiel R, Goodwin JF. Prognosis and mortality of hypertrophic obstructive cardiomyopathy. Lancet 1973; 2:1462–7.

114. Canedo MI, Frank MJ, Abdulla AM. Rhythm disturbances in hypertrophic cardiomyopathy: prevalence, relation to symptoms and management. Am J Cardiol 1980; 45:848–55.

115. Ingham RE, Rossen RM, Goodman DJ, Harrison DC. Treadmill arrhythmias in patients with idiopathic hypertrophic subaortic stenosis. Chest 1975; 68:759–64.

116. McKenna WJ, England D, Doi YL, et al. Arrhythmia in hypertrophic cardiomyopathy. I. Influence on prognosis. Br Heart J 1981; 46:168–72.

117. Maron BJ, Savage DD, Wolfson JK, Epstein SE. Prognostic significance of 24-hour ambulatory electrocardiographic monitoring in patients with hypertrophic cardiomyopathy: a prospective study. Am J Cardiol 1981; 48:252–7.

118. Harrison DC, Braunwald E, Glick G, et al. Effects of beta adrenergic blockade on the circulation, with particular reference to observations in patients with hypertrophic subaortic stenosis. Circulation 1964; 29:84–98.

119. Flamm MD, Harrison DC, Hancock EW. Muscular subaortic stenosis. Prevention of outflow obstruction with propranolol. Circulation 1968; 38:846–58.

120. Stenson RE, Flamm MD Jr, Harrison DC, Hancock EW. Hypertrophic subaortic stenosis. Clinical and hemodynamic effects of long-term propranolol therapy. Am J Cardiol 1973; 31:763–73.

121. de la Calzada CS, Ziady GM, Hardarson T, et al. Effect of acute administration of propranolol on ventricular function in hypertrophic obstructive cardiomyopathy measured by non-invasive techniques. Br Heart J 1976; 38:798–803.

122. Swanton RH, Brooksby IAB, Jenkins BS, Webb-Peploe MM. Hemodynamic studies of beta blockade in hypertrophic obstructive cardiomyopathy. Eur J Cardiol 1977; 5:327–41.

123. Speiser KW, Krayenbuehl HP. Reappraisal of the effect of acute beta-blockade on left ventricular filling dynamics in hypertrophic obstructive cardiomyopathy. Eur Heart J 1981; 2:21–9.

124. Hess OM, Grimm J, Krayenbuehl HP. Diastolic function in hypertrophic cardiomyopathy: effects of propranolol and verapamil on diastolic stiffness. Eur Heart J 1983; 4(Suppl F):47–56.

125. Kaltenbach M, Hopf R, Kober G, et al. Treatment of hypertrophic obstructive cardiomyopathy with verapamil. Br Heart J 1979; 42:35–42.

126. Rosing DR, Condit JR, Maron BJ, et al. Verapamil therapy: a new approach to the pharmacologic treatment of hypertrophic cardiomyopathy. III. Effects of long-term administration. Am J Cardiol 1981; 48:545–53.

127. Rosin DR, Idanpaan-Heikkla U, Maron BJ, et al. Use of calcium channel blocking drugs in hypertrophic cardiomyopathy. Am J Cardiol 1985; 55:185B–95B.

128. Bonow RO, Dilsizian V, Rosing DR, et al. Verapamil-induced improvement in left ventricular diastolic filling and increased exercise tolerance in patients with hypertrophic cardiomyopathy: short and long term effects. Circulation 1985; 72:853–64.

129. Rosing DR, Kent KM, Maron BJ, Epstein SE. Verapamil therapy: a new approach to the pharmacologic treatment of hypertrophic cardiomyopathy. II. Effects on exercise capacity and symptomatic status. Circulation 1979; 60: 1208–13.

130. Paulus WJ, Nellens P, Heyndrickx GR, Andries SE. Effects of long-term treatment with amiodarone on exercise hemodynamics and left ventricular relaxation in patients with hypertrophic cardiomyopathy. Circulation 1986; 74:544–4.

131. Leon MB, Rosing DR, Maron BJ, et al. Amiodarone in patients with hypertrophic cardiomyopathy and refractory cardiac symptoms: an alternative to current medical therapy. Circulation 1984; 70(Suppl II):II–18 (abst).

132. Pollick C. Muscular subaortic stenosis: hemodynamic and clinical improvement after disopyramide. N Engl J Med 1982; 307:997–9.

133. Pollick C, Kimball B, Henderson M, Wigle ED. Disopyramide in hypertrophic cardiomyopathy: I. Hemodynamic assessment after intravenous administration. Am J Cardiol 1988; 62:1248–51.

134. Pollick C. Disopyramide in hypertrophic cardiomyopathy: II. Noninvasive assessment after oral administration. Am J Cardiol 1988; 62:1252–5.

135. Spirito P, Seidman CE, McKenna WJ, Maron BH. The management of hypertrophic cardiomyopathy. N Engl J Med 1997; 336:775–85.

136. Jeanrenaud X, Goy JJ, Kappenberger L. Effects of dual-chamber pacing in hypertrophic obstructive cardiomyopathy. Lancet 1992; 339:1318–23.

137. Fananapazir L, Epstein ND, Curiel RV, et al. Long-term results of dual-chamber (DDD) pacing in obstructive hypertrophic cardiomyopathy. Evidence for progressive symptomatic and hemodynamic improvement and reduction of left ventricular hypertrophy. Circulation 1994; 90:2731–42.

138. Nishimura RA, Trusty JM, Hayes DL, et al. Dual-chamber pacing for patients with hypertophic obstructive cardiomyopathy: a prospective randomized, double-blind cross-over study. J Am Coll Cardiol 1997; 29:435–41.

139. Sigwart U. Non-surgical myocardial reduction for hypertrophic obstructive cardiomyopathy. Lancet 1995; 346:211–14.

140. Gleichman U, Seggewiss H, Faber L. Catheter treatment of hypertrophic cardiomyopathy. Dtsch Med Wochenschr 1996; 121:679–85.

141. Knight C, Kurbaan AS, Seggewiss H. Non-surgical reduction for hypertrophic obstructive cardiomyopathy: outcome in the first series of patients. Circulation 1997; 95:2075–81.

142. Morrow AG, Brockenbrough EC. Surgical treatment of idiopathic hypertrophic subaortic stenosis: technic and hemodynamic results of subaortic ventriculomyotomy. Ann Surg 1961; 154:181–9.

143. Morrow AG. Hypertrophic subaortic stenosis. J Thorac Cardiovasc Surg 1978; 76:423–30.

144. Canedo MI, Frank MJ. Therapy of hypertrophic cardiomyopathy: medical or surgical? Clinical and pathophysiologic considerations. Am J Cardiol 1981; 48:383–8.

145. Maron BJ, Merrill WH, Freier PA, et al. Long-term clinical course and symptomatic status of patients after operation for hypertrophic subaortic stenosis. Circulation 1978; 57: 1205–13.

146. McKenna W, Deanfield J, Faruqui A, et al. Prognosis in hypertrophic cardiomyopathy: role of age and clinical, electrocardiographic and hemodynamic features. Am J Cardiol 1981; 47:532–8.

147. Cecchi F, Maron BJ, Epstein SE. Long-term outcome of patients with hypertrophic cardiomyopathy successfully resuscitated after cardiac arrest. J Am Coll Cardiol 1989; 13:1283–8.

148. Spirito P, Chiarella F, Carratino L, et al. Clinical course and prognosis of hypertrophic cardiomyopathy in an outpatient population. N Engl J Med 1989; 320:749–55.

9

Heart failure in patients with chronic renal failure

Alborz Hassankhani, Neilander Sawhney and Barry H Greenberg

Introduction

Renal insufficiency is common in heart failure, occurring in 25–50% of patients with this syndrome.[1-3] The etiology of renal impairment in heart failure patients is usually multifactorial. The causes are outlined in Table 9.1 and they include:

- reduced renal blood flow or perfusion pressure due to cardiac dysfunction
- volume depletion or reduced arterial perfusion pressure as a result of treatment with diuretics and vasodilators
- intrinsic renal disease.

The coexistence of renal disease and heart failure is not entirely unexpected as hypertension, diabetes, hyperlipidemia and/or atherosclerosis increase the risk for the development of both conditions. Determination of the cause of renal insufficiency is important as the first two situations are potentially reversible, whereas the last is not.

The presence of renal insufficiency adversely affects the heart failure patient by worsening prognosis and complicating management.[1-5] The response of the kidney to a reduction in cardiac output and/or perfusion is to promote salt and water retention and to activate the renin–angiotensin–aldosterone system (RAAS) by increasing production of renin activity. Although these responses may be helpful when the hemodynamic perturbations are due to hy-

Etiology	Therapy
Inadequate cardiac output	Optimize medical therapy Consider pulmonary artery catheterization to help 'tailor' therapy Consider inotropic support
Iatrogenic (volume depletion, reduced arterial perfusion, nephrotoxic drugs, etc.)	Judicious fluid replacement Reduce diuretic and/or vasodilator dose Discontinue nephrotoxic drugs
Intrinsic renal disease	Angiotensin-converting enzyme inhibitor or angiotensin type 1 receptor blockers for patients with diabetic nephrosclerosis and other proteinuric states Supportive therapy, as above, to help maintain renal function

Table 9.1 Etiology of renal insufficiency in patients with heart failure and its therapy

povolemia secondary to dehydration or blood loss, they are deleterious when heart failure is the cause. In this setting, they further worsen the situation by increasing the load on the failing heart and by promoting deleterious cardiac remodeling. If renal insufficiency is also present, the resultant volume overload, anemia, uremia, and electrolyte disturbances contribute to the deterioration in cardiac performance. Thus, it is not surprising that renal insufficiency adversely impacts on the clinical course of heart failure patients. In a retrospective analysis of patients with left ventricular dysfunction in the SOLVD trial, even moderate degrees of renal dysfunction were associated with an increased risk for all-cause mortality, as depicted in Figure 9.1.[1,2] This association was based predominantly on increased risk of heart failure progression, which suggests that the adequacy of renal compensation may be an indicator of overall circulatory compensation in these pa-

tients. It also suggests that therapies that preserve renal function should favorably affect the clinical course of heart failure patients. This is an important consideration to keep in mind in prescribing a treatment regimen, as the complex 'cocktail' of drugs used to treat heart failure can have significant effects on renal physiology that could paradoxically adversely effect the clinical course.

The aim of this chapter is to summarize the complicated considerations that must be taken into account when managing heart failure patients with coexistent renal insufficiency. The task is made difficult by the fact that patients with renal insufficiency were usually excluded from the clinical trials that have been cited to support and justify various therapeutic ap-

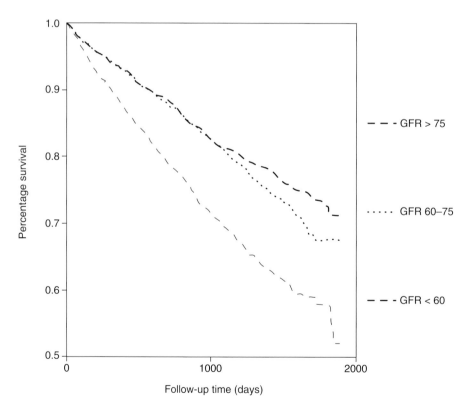

Figure 9.1   Kaplan–Meier survival analysis by level of glomerular filtration rate (GFR). Reproduced with permission from Al-Ahmad et al.[2]

proaches. To further complicate matters, even the meager insights gained from these clinical trials about the treatment of heart failure patients with renal insufficiency are limited by being based on measurement of creatinine alone as an indication of renal function. Nonetheless, important inferences regarding therapy of heart failure patients with renal insufficiency can be made from these studies. When bolstered by information about the effects of various agents on renal function and from clinical experience in heart failure patients with renal insufficiency, some rational approaches to this complicated patient group can be offered.

Angiotensin-converting enzyme inhibitors

Angiotensin-converting enzyme (ACE) inhibitors are considered to be a cornerstone of heart failure therapy.[6–10] In a meta-analysis of 7000 heart failure patients from 34 placebo-controlled trials, ACE inhibitors resulted in an overall 23% reduction in mortality, a 35% reduction in hospitalization or death, and a 20% reduction in fatal/nonfatal myocardial infarction.[11] Despite these impressive benefits, many patients with systolic left ventricular dysfunction are not given ACE inhibitors.[12] Renal insufficiency has been identified as the most common reason for failing to prescribe ACE inhibitors in heart failure patients with systolic left ventricular dysfunction.[13] Concerns about both efficacy and safety are responsible for the underutilization of ACE inhibitors in patients with renal insufficiency. A review of the available data reveals that the benefits of ACE inhibitors in patients with renal insufficiency are not nearly as well established as in patients with normal renal function, as most clinical trials excluded patients with serum creatinine concentrations above 177–221 µmol/l (2–2.5 mg/dl).

The Studies of Left Ventricular Dysfunction (SOLVD) was one of the most influential of the ACE inhibitor trials and the results of SOLVD provided evidence of ACE inhibitor benefits in patients with both symptomatic and asymptomatic left ventricular systolic dysfunction. Inferences about patients with renal insufficiency from the SOLVD database are somewhat limited by the fact that only 16% of patients had a serum creatinine above 1.5 mg/dl (133 µmol/l) on entry and only 2% had a level above 2.0 mg/dl (177 µmol/l). However, 32% of the patients had a predicted GFR (glomerular filtration rate) below 60 ml/min/1.73 m^2 and only 36% of the patients had a predicted GFR of more than 75 ml/min/1.73 m^2.[2] Although there has been no formal subgroup analysis demonstrating the beneficial effects of ACE inhibitors in patients with renal insufficiency, the majority of patients in this trial had some degree of renal insufficiency and the cohort had significant benefit from ACE inhibitors.[1,2,8]

In addition to the mortality benefit, ACE inhibitors have other potential benefits in patients with renal insufficiency and heart failure. One of the most important goals of the therapy of heart failure is to inhibit progression of left ventricular dysfunction. The effects of ramipril, an ACE inhibitor, on cardiovascular events in patients with atherosclerosis (or a predisposition to atherosclerosis based on the presence of diabetes and at least one additional risk factor) was assessed in the Heart Outcomes Prevention Evaluation (HOPE) study.[14] The results demonstrated a highly significant 22% reduction in the composite primary endpoint of cardiovascular death, myocardial infarction, or stroke. Since there were significant reductions in cardiovascular events as well as a 16% reduction in the complications of diabetes with ACE inhibitor therapy, it was not surprising that the risk of heart failure was also reduced by 23%.

The issue of whether the beneficial effects of ramipril were maintained in patients with renal insufficiency was addressed in a subsequent analysis of the HOPE patients. In this report, 980 HOPE patients with mild renal insufficiency – defined as serum creatinine of at least 1.4 mg/dl (124 µmol/l) – were compared with 8307 patients with normal renal function. The cumulative incidence of the primary outcome was higher in patients with renal insufficiency than in those without (22.2% vs 15.1%; $P < 0.001$) and it increased with serum creatinine levels. However, ramipril was associated with similar risk reduction in patients with and those without renal insufficiency (20% compared with 21%; $P > 0.2$).[15] Whether or not ACE inhibitors are associated with benefits of this magnitude in preventing cardiovascular events in patients with more severe degrees of renal impairment is not known.

There is evidence, however, that ACE inhibitors inhibit progression of renal disease, a property that is likely to be of considerable benefit to heart failure patients given the strong association between the extent of renal impairment and subsequent morbidity and mortality. ACE inhibitors are standard therapy in patients with type 1 diabetic nephropathy and other proteinuric states either with or without hypertension;[16,17] their beneficial effects are related to the reduction in proteinuria that leads to renal fibrosis.[18,19] Increases in glomerular permeability, mediated by renal injury, lead to the tubular 'escape' of intravascular proteins. Ingestion of these proteins by tubular cells initiates a proinflammatory response that ultimately leads to progressive fibrosis and renal dysfunction.[20] Angiotensin-mediated stimulation of transforming growth factor beta (TGF-β) has been identified as a final common pathway in this process.[21,22] By inhibiting production of TGF-β, ACE inhibitors attenuate proteinuria and expansion of the mesangial interstitial matrix. Results from the Collaborative Study Group Captopril Trial demonstrated a 14% reduction in serum TGF-β1 levels with ACE inhibitor therapy as opposed to an 11% increase in the placebo control group. Moreover, there was a quantitative inverse relationship between TGF-β levels at 6 months and the decline of GFR at 2 years.[23] Thus, 'to the extent that ACE-inhibitors lower the rate of urinary protein excretion, they effectively limit the progressive decline in GFR. If treatment is sufficiently prolonged, the GFR decline can be effectively halted or reversed, even in patients with remarkably severe disease'.[19]

Concerns regarding the safety of ACE inhibitors in heart failure patients with renal insufficiency are a major impediment to their use. It is not uncommon to see an increase in the serum creatinine with the initiation of ACE inhibitor therapy. This is related to a decline in glomerular hydrostatic pressure and GFR as well as a reduction in arterial perfusion pressure. This situation, however, often stabilizes with sustained therapy where a decrease in renovascular resistance overcomes the decrease in GFR and helps maintain stable renal blood flow and function. Thus, in most cases, ACE inhibitor-induced increases in creatinine do not indicate progressive structural damage to the kidney and (most importantly) they are usually *reversible* by discontinuing the drug. Thus, a 30% rise in creatinine is considered acceptable and does not warrant cessation of therapy in most patients.[24] Approximately 5% of patients develop worsening renal function with ACE inhibitor therapy; the majority can be managed by close observation and by adjustment of the diuretic dose.[25] In addition, adjustment and/or discontinuation of other agents that affect arterial pressure or renal function – e.g. nonsteroidal anti-inflammatory agents and other nephrotoxic drugs – should be considered in heart failure patients who develop worrisome increases in serum creatinine levels with ACE inhibitors. A minority of these patients may have bilateral renal artery stenosis, a condition in which there is marked sensitivity to the renal effects of the ACE inhibitors. In these cases, rapid and severe deterioration in renal function may occur, a situation that requires immediate cessation of ACE inhibitor therapy.

Based on these considerations, it is our practice to use ACE inhibitors in all heart failure patients with creatinine levels below 2.5 mg/dl (221 μmol/l) and to consider their use even in patients with creatinine levels up to 3.0 mg/dl (265 μmol/l). Increases in creatinine of up to 30% are considered acceptable in most cases, but this depends somewhat on the starting level, with more caution exerted in those patients with greater elevations at baseline. As always, ACE inhibitors are initiated at a low dose that is gradually titrated upwards. Both the initial dose and the rate of titration are modified according to the degree of renal impairment at baseline. Measurements of renal function and serum potassium levels are carried out frequently. The dose of potassium supplementation is adjusted to keep serum levels within the normal range. It is worth noting that heart failure patients with renal insufficiency are prone to developing hyperkalemia when ACE inhibitors are given. When this occurs, the dose of ACE inhibitors may need to be reduced or the drug discontinued if serum potassium levels remain at or above 5.6 mmol/l. Obviously, for patients who are intolerant of ACE inhibitors for other reasons – including angioedema, intractable cough, or symptomatic hypotension – alternative therapy with other vasodilators must be considered.

Angiotensin receptor blockers and other alternatives to therapy with angiotensin-converting enzyme inhibitors

The theoretical benefits of blockade of the RAAS at the receptor level by angiotensin type 1 receptor blockers (ARBs) include more complete prevention of the effects of angiotensin II by avoidance of the 'ACE-escape' phenomenon and the lack of undesirable ACE inhibitor effects due to inhibition of the breakdown of substances such as bradykinin. The possibility that ARBs might be less likely than ACE inhibitors to cause worsening renal function was assessed in the Evaluation of Losartan In The Elderly (ELITE) Study.[26] The ELITE population consisted of older ACE inhibitor naive patients with symptomatic heart failure due to left ventricular systolic dysfunction. The results, however, demonstrated that there was a similar 10.5% incidence of a persistent increase in serum creatinine levels by at least 0.3 mg/dl (26.5 μmol/l) in each group. Less than 2% of patients in either group had to discontinue therapy because of renal dysfunction during the 48 weeks of follow-up. Persisting increases in serum potassium levels of 0.5 mmol/l or more above baseline while on therapy was observed in 18.8% of losartan-treated patients and 22.7% of captopril-treated patients ($P = 0.069$). Although ELITE suggested that losartan might benefit survival compared to captopril, rigorous testing of this hypothesis in ELITE-2 failed to confirm this effect.[27] Thus, since ARBs have similar effects on renal function without additional clinical benefits they are reserved for use in patients who cannot tolerate ACE inhibitors secondary to side effects such as cough or angioedema. Of note, several recent trials support the use of ARBs in retarding the progression to end-stage renal disease in patients with renal insufficiency and type 2 diabetes.[28,29] However, whether ARBs have any advantage over ACE inhibitors in this regard is uncertain.

The effects of combining ACE inhibitor and ARB therapy in the treatment of heart failure patients were recently evaluated in the Valsartan in Heart Failure Trial (Val-HeFT).[30] The results demonstrated a significant reduction in the combined risk of mortality and morbidity due primarily to a 27% reduction in heart failure hospitalization. However, a higher mortality was detected in the subset of patients who were also taking beta-blockers, raising concerns about the combination of all three agents in heart failure patients. Although the combination of an ACE inhibitor with an ARB has not been evaluated in heart failure patients with renal insufficiency, we currently avoid this combination based on the potentially adverse effects on renal function and retention of potassium. In Val-HeFT 7% of patients were not on ACE inhibitors and in this sub-group valsartan significantly reduced both morbidity and mortality. Thus, ARBs are now considered the first line alternative for patients who are considered to be intolerant of ACE inhibitors.

For heart failure patients with renal insufficiency who develop dramatic worsening of renal function or who develop significant hyperkalemia with ACE inhibitor or ARB therapy, alternative therapy is an option. The combination of hydralazine and isosorbide dinitrate does not have significant nephrotoxicity and it is well suited for these patients. In the Ventricular function in Heart Failure Trial (V-HeFT-I), this combination improved survival compared with either prazosin (an α_2-agonist) or placebo.[31] However, this combination may result in

significant reductions in arterial pressure that in some patients may cause worsening renal function. Also, V-HeFT II demonstrated that enalapril significantly reduced mortality in a heart failure population compared with the hydralazine–nitrate combination.[32] Thus, we reserve this option for patients with severe impairment of renal function – e.g. creatinine levels at or above 3.0 mg/dl (265 μmol/l) – or another limiting side effect of these agents. However, if a patient with renal disease progresses to dialysis, we usually reinstitute therapy with an ACE inhibitor or an ARB at that time.

Diuretics

Loop diuretics are the most effective agents available for treating salt and water retention in the heart failure patient. Few (if any) clinical trials have assessed loop diuretic efficacy in heart failure patients, either with or without renal insufficiency. Thus, their continued use is a matter of faith and broad-based clinical experience. Perhaps the most troublesome problem regarding the use of diuretics in heart failure patients with renal insufficiency is the development of 'diuretic resistance,' a condition in which the patient responds poorly to diuretic doses that had previously been effective. When diuretic resistance occurs, contributory causes must be considered. These include the degree of renal insufficiency, presence of the nephrotic syndrome, extent of hypoalbuminemia, level of sodium and fluid intake, impaired absorption of oral diuretics secondary to the presence of gut edema, and counterregulatory mechanisms that are set in motion to restore effective circulatory volume.[33]

Most patients who develop diuretic resistance have evidence of renal insufficiency. The reason for this is that abnormal renal function impairs secretion of the diuretic into the tubular fluid, where it inhibits salt and water reabsorption. Thus, increasing the frequency of loop diuretic dosing is rarely successful in correcting the problem, as it only serves to repeatedly deliver a subtherapeutic dose of the diuretic to the tubule. This problem can be overcome, however, by increasing the dose of the loop diuretic. Heart failure patients with renal insufficiency who continue to have congestive symptoms and inadequate diuresis despite large doses of loop diuretics often respond to the addition of a thiazide diuretic to the regimen. The rationale for this approach is based on the fact that thiazides act on a site in the nephron that is distal to the region at which loop diuretics work. We frequently add 2.5–5 mg of metolazone once or twice per day to such refractory patients. In some patients with worsening heart failure and renal insufficiency, diuretic resistance is due to a reduction in cardiac output and/or arterial perfusion. In this case, intravenous inotropic support may be required to establish adequate blood flow and pressure to the kidney. In our experience this approach often restores diuretic responsiveness. Once euvolemia has been restored, the inotropic agent can be discontinued. If the patient cannot be adequately diuresed despite all these measures, dialysis may be the only recourse.[34–36]

Heart failure patients with renal insufficiency are particularly sensitive to problems associated with overdiuresis. When left ventricular filling pressure falls below the optimal level in these patients, there is a reduction in GFR and in arterial perfusion pressure that results in worsening azotemia. This often leads to the diuretics being held, with the not-unexpected consequence of worsening edema and congestion. It also may result in discontinuation or suboptimal dosing of beta-blockers and ACE inhibitors. This is unfortunate, as overdiuresis further activates the RAAS and the sympathetic nervous systems, both of which adversely affect the immediate situation and the long-term prognosis. Thus, it is particularly important to achieve the appropriate balance between an adequate diuresis and maintenance of an optimal left ventricular filling pressure; this may be difficult, as some patients require intravascular volumes above the 'normal' range to support their GFR. Often the optimal volume status for these patients can only be ascertained by trial and error in which the diuretic dose is titrated against further rises in renal function tests. When the empirical approach does not work, it may be necessary to obtain direct measurement of left ventricular filling pressures by means of a right heart catheter in order to optimize therapy. The results of direct measurement of filling pressures and cardiac output may also demonstrate that the problem is due to abnormally low cardiac output. In this instance, the temporary use of inotropic agents (as outlined above) may be required to achieve adequate diuresis without provoking worsening azotemia or hypotension.

Digoxin

Cardiac glycosides, digoxin and related compounds, are amongst the oldest modes of therapy for heart failure. Digoxin, the most commonly used compound of its class, is well tolerated and safe in most patients.[37] While withdrawal of digoxin from stable heart failure patients has been shown to increase symptoms, decrease exercise capacity, and increase heart failure-related hospitalizations, it does not adversely affect survival.[38,39] Since digoxin is cleared by the kidneys, most cases of toxicity occur in heart failure patients with renal insufficiency. Thus, in these patients, a dose reduction of 50–75% from the standard of 0.25 mg/day is required. Patients with advanced renal insufficiency are usually given 0.125 mg thrice weekly. More frequent monitoring of drug levels is usually recommended in heart failure patients with renal insufficiency. Given that patients with renal insufficiency are at increased risk of toxicity, and because there is no survival benefit with digoxin therapy, we reserve its use only for patients who remain symptomatic on standard therapy or for those who require it for rate control in atrial fibrillation. Furthermore, we maintain a low threshold for discontinuing digoxin in heart failure patients with renal insufficiency if it contributes to bradycardia that limits the use of beta-blockers.

Beta-blockers

Numerous clinical trials – involving thousands of patients – have unequivocally demonstrated clinically important benefits of beta-blocker therapy in heart failure patients.[40–44] Overall, beta-blockers reduce mortality in the range of 35%, and this benefit is additive to the 20–25% reduction already seen with the ACE inhibitors. Today, beta-blocker treatment of heart failure has become a standard of care in stable New York Heart Association (NYHA) class II–III patients. Recent evidence indicates that these agents may also benefit patients with more advanced heart failure.[44] The clinical trial database supporting the use of beta-blockers in heart failure patients is strongly skewed toward patients with normal renal function or only mild renal insufficiency. However, the presence of chronic renal insufficiency has been associated with elevated plasma catecholamine levels,[45] suggesting that beta-blockers might be even more effective in this population. Thus, it is no surprise that there is evidence from recent trials supporting the benefits of beta-blockade in heart failure patients and renal insufficiency.

In a study of 114 hemodialysis patients with NYHA class II or III, the addition of carvedilol to conventional therapy was associated with improved left ventricular function, reduction of left ventricular volumes, and marked improvement of clinical status.[46] All of the clinical indices mentioned above reached statistical significance after only 6 months of beta-blocker therapy, and the effects remained constant after 1 year of follow-up.

The primary concern of beta-blocker use in patients with renal insufficiency is knowing the metabolism of the drug chosen and its route of elimination. Atenolol, for example, is excreted by the kidney and it tends to accumulate in renal failure. It should therefore be used with caution to avoid untoward side effects. Metoprolol, on the other hand, is predominantly metabolized by the liver and there is no need for dose adjustment in renal failure. Carvedilol is a chiral compound with only the S-enantiomer possessing beta-blocking activity. The pharmacodynamics of carvedilol were recently studied in hypertensive patients with chronic renal insufficiency (GFR 30 ml/min or less). The area under the curve values were 40% and 50% higher on days 1 and 9 in renal insufficiency patients, primarily due to higher levels of the R-enantiomer. The S-isomer, however, is primarily hepatically metabolized, with less than 2% of the dose excreted renally. Thus, no changes in dosing of carvedilol are warranted in patients with moderate-to-severe renal insufficiency.[47] Bisoprolol is metabolized by the liver and excreted by the kidney at similar rates, and no dose adjustment due to renal insufficiency is considered necessary.

Spironolactone

The Randomized Aldactone Evaluation Study (RALES) reported that this competitive antagonist of the aldosterone receptor enhanced survival in heart failure patients with severe NYHA class III–IV symptoms and low left ventricular ejection fraction.[48] Spironolactone is hepatically metabolized and the serum half-life of 12–36 hours is unchanged in renal insufficiency. However, due to interference with potassium homeostasis, it has been associated with life-threatening hyperkalemia, particularly in patients with renal insufficiency and those on ACE inhibitor therapy. Spironolactone is currently not recommended when the creatinine clearance is less than 30 ml/min, or in patients with high baseline potassium levels who are already on ACE inhibitors. The usual close monitoring of serum potassium and creatinine that are part of the prudent monitoring of heart failure patients should be carried out even more vigorously if patients with mild renal insufficiency are started on spironolactone.

Management of chronic heart failure in patients on chronic dialysis

Heart failure patients on chronic dialysis pose a particular challenge to the clinician. In a multivariate analysis of 822 patients starting dialysis, severity of heart failure was an independent predicator of early mortality.[49] On the other hand, various studies have reported improvements in all indices of left ventricular function in end-stage renal disease patients after the initiation of dialysis.[50–53]

It is often assumed that a patient's volume and electrolyte status can be fine-tuned with dialysis therapy. However, rapid shifts of volume and electrolytes occurring during hemodialysis are often poorly tolerated in patients with concomitant left ventricular systolic dysfunction. Thus, dialysis-induced hypotension,

arrhythmias, and even hypoxia have all been reported.[54] Systemic hypotension usually occurs as a result of rapid removal of intravascular volume, particularly in those undergoing hemodialysis. Other confounding factors are the presence of underlying autonomic dysfunction, diastolic dysfunction, and concomitant antihypertensive drug therapy. Withholding antihypertensive medications 4–6 hours prior to initiation of dialysis helps alleviate the latter problem. Additional measures include lengthening the dialysis run, avoidance of excessive ultrafiltration, and allowing the patient to gain fluid in between dialysis runs. Use of low-dose, nonselective beta-blockers that would potentiate unopposed alpha-receptor-mediated vasoconstriction by endogenous catecholamines has also been proposed in this setting.[55]

Another problem occasionally encountered in hemodialysis patients is the development of high-output failure due to increased blood flow through an arteriovenous fistula. When this occurs, revision of the fistula and consideration of peritoneal dialysis or renal transplantation are other options to be considered. Finally, in the past, complications associated with dialysis membranes, such as complement activation, causing dialysis-induced hypoxemia (with cuproaphane membranes) and anaphylactoid reactions in patients receiving ACE inhibitors (due to polyacrylonitrile AN69 membranes),[55] were observed. These complications have been circumvented by using biocompatible membranes.

Cardiovascular consequences of renal transplantation

There is limited data to suggest that cardiac function improves in heart failure patients undergoing renal transplantation. In four patients with end-stage renal disease and NYHA class III–IV heart failure due to left ventricular systolic dysfunction, renal transplant increased ejection fraction from 43% to 69%, and relieved symptoms of heart failure.[56] All these patients, however, were younger men (age range 31–56 years) with nonischemic cardiomyopathy. Interestingly, despite adequate dialytic therapy, pre-transplant left ventricular dysfunction and heart failure symptoms persisted. This suggests the persistence of factors that adversely affect cardiac function even in face of adequate dialysis. Thus, renal transplantation in some patients with nonischemic cardiomyopathy can lead to improved cardiac performance and relief of symptoms.

Finally, some investigators have reported on their selective experience with combined heart–kidney transplant.[57] It appears that the incidence of both the heart and kidney allograft rejection is much improved when compared with single transplant cohorts. Long-term follow-up of these patients and further multicenter, randomized trials are needed to establish this as a standard of care in patients with end-stage renal and heart failure.

Summary

The presence of renal insufficiency in a heart failure patient is an ominous sign as it is associated with a worse prognosis and it may complicate therapeutic decisions. When assessing a heart failure patient with concomitant renal insufficiency, the following issues must be carefully evaluated:

- what is the baseline renal function?
- has there been a recent exacerbation of renal dysfunction? If so, is it due to reversible or irreversible causes?
- are there underlying comorbidities that adversely affect renal function that can be treated?
- is the renal insufficiency iatrogenic and can the condition be corrected?
- are there risk factors that may lead to worsening of renal or cardiac dysfunction? If so, can these risk factors be modified?
- what measures can be taken to minimize damage to the kidneys without necessarily compromising the management of the heart failure?

The principles of management of the heart failure patient with renal insufficiency include increased vigilance for the possibility that over-medication resulting in hypoperfusion and hypovolemia might worsen renal function, appropriate selection and dosing of medications, and more frequent laboratory and clinical follow-up. These considerations are summarized in Table 9.2. While clinical data about the efficacy of various therapeutic approaches in this specific population are scant, the overall poor prognosis mandates that aggressive medical therapy to both treat the heart failure and prevent further worsening of the underlying renal insufficiency is warranted.

Class of drugs	Benefit in HF demonstrated in clinical trials[a]	Benefit in HF and RI	Dose recommendation in RI and HF	Comments
ACEIs	+++	Some evidence in patients with mild RI	Start at lower dose and gradually titrate up; Close follow-up of potassium and renal function is imperative	Particularly useful in proteinuric states, diabetic nephropathy, and hypertensive nephrosclerosis
ARBs	++	ND	Same as ACEIs	No apparent advantage over ACEIs
Beta-blockers	+++	Limited information from large-scale trials/some information from small studies[46]	The same dose can be used in patients with or without RI (see comments)	Avoid atenolol and other renally metabolized agents. Carvedilol and metoprolol are metabolized primarily by the liver
Diuretics	ND[b]	ND	Higher doses in patients with RI May need to combine loop diuretics with thiazides	Cautious use in patients on ACEI/ARBs Avoid dehydration
Digoxin	++	–	Not recommended in RI	No mortality benefit in DIG trial Need dose adjustment in RI
Spironolactone	+	ND	Use with caution in patients with RI. Close follow-up of serum potassium mandatory	Patients with serum creatinine >2.5 mg/dl were excluded from the RALES trial

[a] +, Benefit clearly established in large randomized clinical trials; –, potentially harmful.
[b] ND, no data from large randomized trials.
ACEIs = angiotensin-converting enzyme inhibitors; ARBs = angiotensin type 1 receptor blockers.

Table 9.2 Impact of renal insufficiency (RI) on pharmacotherapy of heart failure (HF)

References

1. Dries DL, Exner D, Domanski MJ, et al. The prognostic implications of renal insufficiency in asymptomatic and symptomatic patients with left ventricular systolic dysfunction. J Am Coll Cardiol 2000; 35:681–9.

2. Al-Ahmad A, Rand WM, Manjunath G, et al. Reduced kidney function and anemia as risk factors for mortality in patients with left ventricular dysfunction. J Am Coll Cardiol 2001; 38:957–61.

3. Hillege HL, Gribes ARJ, de Kam PJ, et al. Renal function, neurohumoral activation, and survival in patients with chronic heart failure. Circulation 2000; 102:203–10.

4. Ruilope LM, van Veldhuisen DJ, Ritz E, Luscher TF. Renal function: the Cinderella of cardiovascular risk profile. J Am Coll Cardiol 2001; 38:1782–5.

5. Owen WF, Madore F, Brenner BM. An observational study of cardiovascular characteristics of long-term end-stage renal disease survivors. Am J Kidney Dis 1996; 28:931–6.

6. The CONSENSUS Trial Study Group. Effects of enalapril on mortality in severe congestive heart failure: results of the Cooperative Northern Scandinavian Enalapril Survival Study (CONSENSUS). New Engl J Med 1987; 316:1429–35.

7. Massie BM. All patients with left ventricular systolic dysfunction should be treated with an angiotensin-converting enzyme inhibitor: a protagonist's viewpoint. Am J Cardiol 1990; 66:439–43.

8. The SOLVD investigators. Effect of enalapril on survival in patients with reduced left ventricular ejection fractions and congestive heart failure. New Engl J Med 1991; 325:293–302.

9. Pfeffer MA, Braunwald E, Moye LA, et al. Effect of captopril on mortality and morbidity in patients with left ventricular systolic dysfunction after myocardial infarction – results of the survival and ventricular enlargement trial. New Engl J Med 1992; 327:669–77.

10. Massie B, Amidon T. Angiotensin-converting enzyme inhibitor therapy for congestive heart failure: rationale, results, and current recommendations. In: Hosenpud JD, Greenberg BH, eds, Congestive Heart Failure: pathophysiology, differential diagnosis, and comprehensive approach to therapy. New York: Springer-Verlag, 1993.

11. Garg R, Yusuf S. Overview of randomized trials of angiotensin-converting enzyme inhibitors on mortality and morbidity in patients with heart failure. J Am Med Assoc 1995; 273:1450–5.

12. Clinical Quality Improvement Network Investigators. Mortality risk and patterns of practice in 4606 acute care patients with congestive heart failure. The relative importance of age, sex, and medical therapy. Arch Intern Med 1996; 156:1669–73.

13. Bart BA, Gattis WA, Diem SJ, O'Connor CM. Reasons for underuse of angiotensin-converting enzyme inhibitors in patients with heart failure and left ventricular dysfunction. Am J Cardiol 1997; 79:1118–20.

14. The HOPE Study Investigators. Effects of angiotensin converting enzyme inhibitor, ramipril, on death from cardiovascular causes, myocardial infarction, and stroke in high-risk patients. New Engl J Med 2000; 342:145–53.

15. Mann JF, Gerstein HC, Pogue J, et al. Renal insufficiency as a predictor of cardiovascular outcomes and the impact of ramipril: the HOPE randomized trial. Ann Int Med 2001; 134:629–36.

16. Laffel LMB, McGill JB, Gans D, on behalf of the North American Microalbuminuria Study Group. The beneficial effect of angiotensin-converting enzyme inhibition with captopril on diabetic nephropathy in normotensive IDDM patients with microalbuminuria. Am J Med 1995; 99:497–504.

17. Morales A, Dennis V. Should an ACE inhibitor be stopped if signs of renal insufficiency appear? Cleveland Clin J Med 2001; 68:280–2.

18. Bart BA, Goldsmith SR. Aggravated renal dysfunction and the acute management of advanced chronic heart failure. Am Heart J 1999; 138:200–2.

19. Ruggenenti P, Remuzzi G. The role of protein traffic in the progression of renal diseases. Ann Rev Med 2000; 51:315–27.

20. Hall PM. Strategies to prevent progression of renal disease. Cleveland Clin J Med 2001; 68:143–52.

21. Wolf G, Mueller E, Stahl RA, Ziyadeh FN. Angiotensin II-induced hypertrophy of cultured murine proximal tubular cells is mediated by endogenous transforming growth factor-beta. J Clin Invest 1993; 92:1366–72.

22. Kaneto H, Morrisy J, Klahr S. Increased statement of TGF-β mRNA in the obstructed kidney of rats with unilateral ureteral ligation. Kidney Int 1993; 44:313–21.

23. Sharma K, Eltayeb BO, McGowan TA, et al. Captopril-induced reduction of serum levels of transforming growth factor beta correlates with long-term renoprotection in insulin-dependent diabetic patients. Am J Kid Dis 1999; 34:818–23.

24. Franklin SS, Smith RD. Comparison of effects of enalapril plus hydrochlorothiazide versus standard triple therapy on renal function in renovascular hypertension. Am J Med 1985; 79(Suppl 3):14–23.

25. Gottlieb SS, Weir MR. Renal effects of angiotensin-converting enzyme inhibition in congestive heart failure. Am J Cardiol 1990; 66(Suppl D):14D–20D.

26. Pitt B, Segal R, Martinez FA, et al. Randomized trial of losartan verses captopril in patients over 65 with heart failure. Lancet 1997; 349:747–57.

27. Pitt B, Poole-Wilson P, Segal R, et al. Effect of losartan compared with captopril on mortality in patients with symptomatic heart failure: randomised trial – the Losartan Heart Failure Survival Study ELITE II. Lancet 2000; 355; 1582–7.

28. Brenner BM, Cooper ME, de Zeeuw D, et al. Effects of losartan on renal and cardiovascular outcomes in patients with type 2 diabetes and nephropathy. New Engl J Med 2001; 345:861–9.

29. Lewis EJ, Hunsicker LG, Clarke WR, et al. Renoprotective effect of the angiotensin-receptor antagonist irbesartan in patients with nephropathy due to type 2 diabetes. New Engl J Med 2001; 345:851–60.

30. Cohn JN, Tognoni G. Valsartan Heart Failure Trial Investigators. A randomized trial of the angiotensin-receptor blocker valsartan in chronic heart failure. New Engl J Med 2001; 345:1667–75.

31. Cohn JN, Archibald DG, Ziesche S, et al. Effect of vasodilator therapy on mortality in chronic congestive heart failure: results of a VA cooperative study. New Engl J Med 1986; 314:1547–52.

32. Cohn JN, Johnson G, Ziesche S, et al. A comparison of enalapril with hydralazine–isosorbide dinitrate in the treatment of chronic congestive heart failure. New Engl J Med 1991; 325: 303–10.

33. Kramer BK, Schweda F, Riegger GA. Diuretic treatment and diuretic resistance in heart failure. Am J Med 1999; 106:90–6.

34. Brater DC. Diuretic therapy. New Engl J Med 1998; 339:387–95.

35. Weinfeld M, Chertow GM, Stevenson LW. Aggravated renal dysfunction during intensive therapy for advanced chronic heart failure. Am Heart J 1999; 138:285–90.

36. Marenzi G, Lauri G, Grazi M, et al. Circulatory response to fluid overload removal by extracorporeal ultrafiltration in refractory congestive heart failure. J Am Coll Cardiol 2001; 38:963–8.

37. The Digitalis Investigation Group. The effect of digoxin on mortality and morbidity in patients with heart failure. New Engl J Med 1997; 336:525–33.

38. Packer M, Gheorghiade M, Young JB, et al. Withdrawal of digoxin from patients with chronic heart failure treated with angiotensin-converting-enzyme-inhibitors. New Engl J Med 1993; 329:1–7.

39. Packer M, Bristow MR, Cohn JN, et al. The effect of carvedilol on morbidity and mortality in patients with chronic heart failure. New Engl J Med 1996; 334:1338–49.

40. Packer M, Coats AJS, Fowler MB, et al. Effect of carvedilol on survival in severe chronic heart failure. New Engl J Med 2001; 344:1651–8.

41. Swedberg K, Hjalmarson A, Waagstein F, Wallentin I. Beneficial effects of long-term beta-blockade in congestive cardiomyopathy. Br Heart J 1980; 44:117–33.

42. Waagstein F, Bristow MR, Swedberg K, et al., for the Metoprolol in Dilated Cardiomyopathy (MDC) trial study group. Beneficial effects of metoprolol in idiopathic dilated cardiomyopathy. Lancet 1993; 342:1331–46.

43. Waagstein F, Hjalmarson A, Varnauskas E, Wallentin I. Effect of chronic beta-adrenergic receptor blockade in congestive cardiomyopathy. Br Heart J 1975; 37:1022–36.

44. Braunwald E. Expanding indications for beta-blockers in heart failure. N Engl J Med 2001; 344:1711–12.

45. Ban M, Matsuno T, Ogawa K, Satake T. Plasma norepinephrine and dopamine-beta-hydroxylase

activity in chronic renal failure. Jpn Circ J 1979; 43:627–32.

46. Cice C, Ferra L, Di Benedetto A, et al. Dilated cardiomyopathy in dialysis patients – beneficial effects of carvedilol: a double-blind, placebo-controlled trial. J Am Coll Cardiol 2001; 37: 407–11.

47. Gehr TW, Tenero DM, Boyle DA, et al. The pharmacokinetics of carvedilol and its metabolites after single and multiple dose oral administration in patients with hypertension and renal insufficiency. Eur J Clin Pharmacol 1999; 55: 269–77.

48. Pitt B, Zannad F, Remme WJ, et al. The effect of spironolactone on morbidity and mortality in patients with severe heart failure. Randomized Aldactone Evaluation Study Investigators. New Engl J Med 1999; 341:709–17.

49. Barrett BJ, Parfrey PS, Morgan J, et al. Prediction of early death in end-stage renal disease patients starting dialysis. Am J Kidney Dis 1997; 29: 214–22.

50. Leenen FH, Smith DL, Khanna R. Changes in left ventricular hypertrophy and function in hypertensive patients started on continuous ambulatory peritoneal dialysis. Am Heart J 1985; 110:102–6.

51. Hung J, Harris PJ, Uren RF, et al. Uremic cardiomyopathy: effect of hemodialysis on left ventricular function in end stage renal failure. New Engl J Med 1980; 302:547–51.

52. Bornstein A, Gaasch WH, Harrington J. Assessment of the cardiac effects of hemodialysis with systolic time intervals and echocardiography. Am J Cardiol 1983; 51:332–5.

53. Nixon JV, Mitchell JH, McPhaul JJ, et al. Effect of hemodialysis in left ventricular function. Dissociation of changes in filling volume and in contractile state. J Clin Invest 1983; 71:377–84.

54. Leier CV, Boudoulas H. Renal disorders and heart disease. In: Braunwald E, ed., Heart Disease: a textbook of cardiovascular medicine. Philadelphia: WB Saunders, 1997.

55. Veressen L, Waer M, Vanrenterghen Y, Michielsen P. Angiotensin converting enzyme inhibitors and anaphylactoid reaction to high-flux membrane dialysis. Lancet 1990; 336: 1360–2.

56. Burt RK, Gupta-Burt S, Suki WN, et al. Reversal of left ventricular dysfunction after renal transplantation. Ann Int Med 1989; 111:635–40.

57. Castillo-Lugo JA, Brinker KR. An overview of combined heart and kidney transplantation. Curr Opin Cardiol 1999; 14:121–5.

10

Chronic heart failure and coronary artery disease

Cord Manhenke and Kenneth Dickstein

Epidemiology

Coronary artery disease is one of the leading health problems in the developed countries.[1] Important decreases in the incidence of myocardial infarction and coronary mortality have been achieved with aggressive risk factor modification, increasing awareness of the importance of adequate primary and secondary prophylaxis, and improvements in medical treatment options and coronary revascularization procedures.[2,3] On the other hand, an increasing burden of coronary artery disease deaths in developing countries has recently been documented.[4] Ischemic heart disease was the leading cause of death worldwide in 1990[5] and a change cannot be expected until at least 2020.[6]

The prevalence of coronary artery disease is difficult to estimate because serious ischemic heart disease may exist without clinical manifestations or symptoms. The presence of silent ischemia predicts an increased risk of coronary events and cardiac death.[7]

As a result of better survival, the prevalence and incidence of chronic heart failure due to coronary artery disease has changed over time. According to the Framingham study, there has been an increase in ischemic heart disease as the primary attributable cause of heart failure from 22% in the 1950s to 67% in the 1980s.[8] Recently, the frequency of ischemic heart disease as a cause of heart failure in the community setting in a population of 292,000 in the United Kingdom has been evaluated.[9] The crude incidence rate of heart failure was 0.9 cases per 1000 people per year. Coronary artery disease was the cause of 52% of incident heart failure in the general population under 75 years (Figure 10.1). More than 60% of the chronic heart failure that occurs in the US general population may be attributable to coronary heart disease.[10]

The most common cause of chronic heart failure due to coronary artery disease is myocardial infarction. One report from the Framingham study investigated long-term time trends in the occurrence of chronic heart failure after an initial episode of Q-wave myocardial infarction in the period 1950–1989.[11] An absence of decline in chronic heart failure incidence (Figure 10.2) has been noted. The authors argue that improvements in treatment in the 1980s may have salvaged more patients with myocardial infarctions with extensive left ventricular dysfunction, leading to an increasing pool of myocardial infarction survivors at high risk for heart failure development.

The term myocardial infarction was recently redefined as any detectable amount of myocardial cell necrosis due to coronary artery disease.[12] This new definition may influence future epidemiologic data evaluating the development and course of chronic heart failure secondary to myocardial infarction.

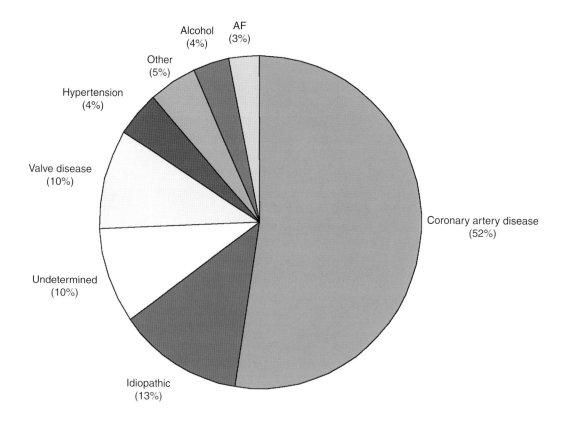

Figure 10.1   Etiology of heart failure. AF = atrial fibrillation. Reproduced with permission from Fox et al.[9]

Pathophysiology

Left ventricular dysfunction in coronary artery disease is the consequence of a dysequilibrium of myocardial oxygen demand and coronary oxygen supply, which can occur in stable/unstable angina pectoris and myocardial infarction.[13] This mismatch can be transient or persistent. In general, four major entities are responsible for left ventricular dysfunction in coronary artery disease:

- left ventricular remodeling
- apoptosis
- hibernation
- stunning.

Left ventricular remodeling and apoptosis

Myocyte necrosis leads to a reparative process in the infarct area, which also involves the border zone[14] and the remote noninfarcted myocardium. In order to counterbalance the abrupt hemodynamic changes in myocardial infarction, ventricular remodeling involves dilatation, hypertrophy, and formation of a collagen scar.

In early remodeling, within 3 hours after injury, activation of matrix metalloproteinases released by neutrophil granulocytes in the infarct area leads to degradation of extracellular matrix, mainly type I and III col-

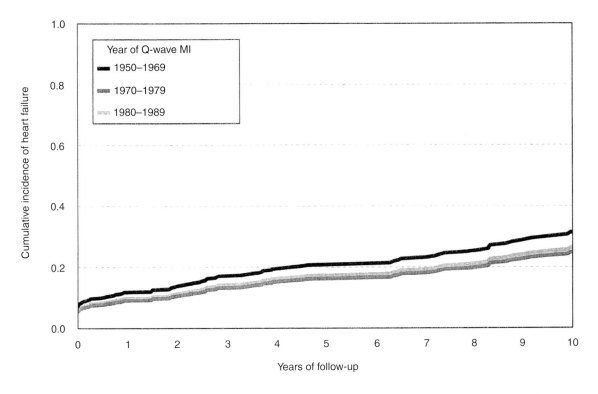

Figure 10.2 Cumulative incidence of congestive heart failure as a function of time period of initial Q-wave myocardial infarction (MI). Reproduced with permission from Guidry et al.[11]

lagen.[15] The lack of normal matrix allows myocytes that were previously bound in sarcomeres to slide apart. The result of the loss of collagen struts is local wall thinning and ventricular dilatation. There is evidence that the extent of microvascular obstruction during the early phase of reperfusion predicts left ventricular enlargement after reperfusion, independently of the infarct size.[16] The number of viable myocytes seems also to decrease in the infarct zone, possibly due to apoptosis.[17] Apoptosis is a form of regulated cell death in which external stresses or internal signals induce a cascade leading to genetically programmed cell destruction. Both an increase in wall stress and hypoxia have been shown to induce apoptosis of myocytes *in vivo*.[18,19]

According to the law of Laplace, wall stress increases with cavity dilatation, which in itself is a stimulus for volume load hypertrophy of the surviving viable myocytes, mediated by the neurohumoral system, activation of the local renin–angiotensin system, and paracrine/autocrine factors.[20] Angiotensin II seems to be an important mediator of hypertrophy in the remote infarct zone.[21] The early collagen degradation is followed by fibrinogenic tissue repair. Among others, angiotensin II is a potent stimulator of transcription of collagen type I and type III mRNA. Collagen synthesis after myocardial infarction can be seen even 90 days after injury in the infarct zone and to a lesser extent also in the remote infarct area,[22] providing the potential for extensive scar development.

Hibernation and stunning

Hibernating myocardium can be described as a matching of reduced coronary perfusion and myocardial contractility.[23] As a response to an ischemic event, non-necrotic myocytes have the ability to down-regulate contractile function and, by that, their energy demand, using their energy household to maintain cell integrity.[24] Hibernating myocardium retains its responsiveness to inotropic challenge and can be detected by noninvasive viability assessment. It has been assumed that up to 50% of patients with severely impaired left ventricular function (ejection fraction <30%) secondary to coronary artery disease have hibernating myocardium detected by positron emission tomography (PET).[25] Restoration of blood supply to the area of hibernating myocytes can lead to significant improvement of left ventricular systolic function[26] and long-term survival.[27]

In contrast to hibernation, stunning can be described as a transient mismatch between normal coronary perfusion and reduced myocardial contractility. Short-term total or subtotal obstruction of blood flow leads to a limited period of left ventricular dysfunction despite the absence of irreversible myocardial damage, followed by spontaneous recovery over time.[28] Stunning is a phenomenon that has been postulated to exist in a variety of ischemic situations, such as reperfused myocardial infarction, unstable angina, coronary artery spasm, following recovery of exercise-induced ischemia, or after coronary artery bypass surgery.[29]

It has recently been demonstrated by using dual-isotope, gated single-photon emission computed tomography (SPECT) imaging that myocardial hibernation, stunning, remodeling, and scarring often coexist in patients with ischemic cardiomyopathy. All these changes can occur together in the same vascular territory or even in the same imaging segment.[30]

Diagnostic approach

The challenge in patients with chronic heart failure and symptoms compatible with coronary artery disease is to determine whether or not the heart failure is aggravated by ischemia. Patients with a history of severe coronary artery disease and/or former coronary revascularization procedures prior to the onset of heart failure will usually be classified as having ischemic cardiomyopathy.

Erroneously, it is widely believed that symptoms typical of angina pectoris could be used to split ischemic from nonischemic cardiomyopathy. Clinical and angiographic characteristics and outcomes associated with ischemic ($n = 3113$) and nonischemic ($n = 675$) cardiomyopathy and a left ventricular ejection fraction <40% have been described.[31] Patients were classified as having ischemic cardiomyopathy by the evidence of previous myocardial infarction, former coronary intervention procedures, or significant coronary artery disease angiographically. All patients underwent coronary angiography and were followed for a median of 5.7 years. Patients with ischemic origin were generally older, more likely to be men, and had a higher incidence of risk factors. The nonischemic group tended to have more severe heart failure symptoms, a lower left ventricular ejection fraction, and a longer time period from the onset of heart failure symptoms to cardiac catheterization. In fact, 34% in the nonischemic group had typical angina pectoris symptoms but apparently normal coronary arteries at angiography. The 5-year survival was significantly lower in the ischemic cardiomyopathy group, even after adjusting for differences in baseline characteristics. The prognostic value of the extent of coronary artery disease was greater than that of the clinical diagnosis of ischemic or non-ischemic cardiomyopathy (Figure 10.3).

These mortality data are consistent with a retrospective cohort study in a hospitalized population in Sweden where ICD9 codes were used to determine the cause of cardiomyopathy.[32] Coronary artery disease was the most common cause of chronic heart failure (40%). Ischemic heart disease was an independent predictor of mortality ($P < 0.001$) in a 5-year survival analysis. In contrast, data from the SOLVD registry[33] showed no differences in mortality between ischemic and nonischemic heart failure groups, possibly because the diagnosis was based on clinical judgment alone.

Thus, when coronary artery disease is suspected in patients with chronic heart failure, in addition to a carefully obtained patient history, risk profile inquiry, clinical examination including echocardiography, and evaluation by stress electrocardiogram (ECG), coronary angiography should be performed in virtually all patients suitable for revascularization procedures when the etiology of heart failure cannot be definitely determined.

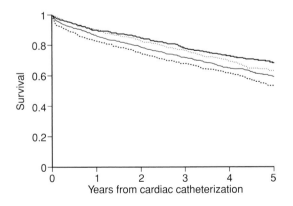

Figure 10.3 Adjusted Kaplan–Meier survival estimates for patients. CAD, coronary artery disease

Viability assessment

Detection of hibernating myocardium with the potential to revive contractility after restoration of flow is essential in order to evaluate whether or not a patient with severe left ventricular dysfunction should undergo mechanical revascularization. Careful non-invasive assessment designed to detect viable myocardium predicts which patients will improve left ventricular function and prolong survival after revascularization.[34] A number of techniques currently available are now considered.

Thallium-201

Thallium-201 (^{201}Tl) is a cation that behaves similarly to potassium. After intravenous injection at rest, about 88% of ^{201}Tl entering the coronary circulation is incorporated by normal myocardium at first pass.[35] Because of this high first-pass extraction, blood flow is an important determinant of ^{201}Tl distribution.[36] Reduction in the coronary blood flow distribution to viable myocardium leads to an initial resting defect with delayed defect resolution called rest redistribution. Myocytes with defect cell membranes are not able to incorporate ^{201}Tl. Thus, defect resolution is not seen in irreversibly damaged myocardium. Because redistribution is flow-dependent, this can be a very slow process in severely under-perfused segments. Late redistribution imaging after 18–72 hours may be required.[37] Protocols using an additional late resting injection[38] and reinjection of ^{201}Tl at rest after a preceding stress injection[39] may improve redistribution imaging. A pooled data analysis showed that the average sensitivity of ^{201}Tl rest–redistribution imaging was 90% but specificity was 54%; i.e. poor for prediction of regional recovery of left ventricular dysfunction after revascularization.[40] In this analysis, ^{201}Tl stress redistribution reinjection reached similar results, with a sensitivity and specificity of 86% and 47%, respectively.

Technetium-99m

The use of technetium-99m (^{99m}Tc) MIBI and ^{99m}Tc tetrofosmin has some theoretical advantages over ^{201}Tl in myocardial imaging. ^{99m}Tc-labeled perfusion agents with their photon energy peak of 140 keV are optimal for detection with SPECT. In addition, due to their relatively short half-life of about 6 hours, 10–15 times higher doses can be administered, leading to better image quality in a shorter time.[41] With these agents, less severe coronary artery stenoses and smaller myocardial infarctions can be successfully detected.[42] On the other hand, there is no significant redistribution of ^{99m}Tc tracers after injection. In chronic hypoperfused myocardial areas, low activity of these tracers is expected, thereby possibly underestimating viability.

Despite this theoretical background, several studies have shown that the differences between sensitivity and specificity,[43] as well as predictive values,[44] were statistically not significant when directly compared to ^{201}Tl imaging. Pooled data from 10 studies with ^{99m}Tc MIBI with or without additional use of nitroglycerin revealed a sensitivity of 83% and a specificity of 69% for detection of functional recovery after revascularization.[40] Dual isotope protocols combining ^{201}Tl and ^{99m}Tc imaging[45] may help to characterize damaged myocardium as hibernated, stunned, remodeled, or nonviable.[30]

Positron emission tomography

Scintigraphic evaluation with PET usually uses two different positron-emitting tracers: nitrogen-13 ammonia (N13) as a flow tracer to study regional myocardial perfusion and fluorine-18 fluorodeoxyglucose (^{18}FDG) used as a metabolic tracer to detect the difference between viable myocardium and scar tissue. Hibernated myocardium is characterized by enhanced uptake of ^{18}FDG despite diminished coronary flow in that region, detected by N13. Sensitivity and specificity for the prediction of improved regional function after revascularization is acceptably high: 88% and 73%, respectively.[40] Due to its high spatial resolution, the possibility for attenuation correction and high-count density images, many experts see PET as the gold standard in noninvasive assessment of viability. The major drawbacks of this technique are its high cost and limited availability. In addition, positron emission isotopes have short half-lives, requiring an on-site or nearby cyclotron.

Stress echocardiography

In stress echocardiography, regional function is enhanced by the inotropic properties of low-dose dobutamine, usually at 5–10 μg/kg/min. Drug-induced tachycardia or increase in blood pressure, subsequently leading to ischemia, occurs commonly at higher doses ranging up to 40 μ/kg/min. Stunned myocardium, which is supplied by a patent vessel will improve contraction during increasing stimulation of β_1-receptors. Hibernated myocardium supplied by a stenosed artery will, at low doses, improve contractility followed by deterioration in regional function as ischemia occurs. Necrotic tissue will obviously not respond to inotropic stimuli. Low-dose dobutamine stress echo is widely used in the assessment of myocardial viability and has gained wide clinical experience. The sensitivity and specificity for prediction of improvement in regional function after revascularization is 84% and 81%, respectively, in the hands of skilled observers.[40] Figure 10.4 summarizes the sensitivities and specificities of these classic viability assessment approaches.

A recent study tested the impact of preoperative myocardial function on prediction of

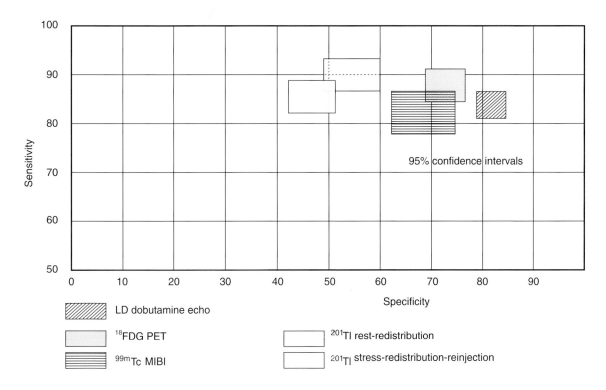

Figure 10.4 Sensitivity and specificity of various viability assessment techniques. For description of techniques, see text. Receiver operating display indicates 95% confidence intervals for each technique. The most effective modalities are located in the right upper corner. The smaller the square, the higher the accuracy of the technique. Reproduced with permission from Bax et al.[40]

global left ventricular recovery after bypass surgery in 59 patients with a mean ejection fraction of 28%.[46] Compared to PET, dipyridamole (a coronary vasodilator), and high-dose dobutamine–atropine stress, the strongest predictor of overall improvement of postoperative left ventricular function was an increase in ejection fraction with low-dose dobutamine infusion.

Stress echocardiography is inexpensive and has a widespread availability. On the other hand interpretation relies on subjective visual interpretation of wall motion,[47] while nuclear imaging allows semiquantitative analysis. Longitudinal pulsed-wave Doppler tissue velocity sampling may add quantita-

tive information for the assessment of myocardial viability and may be complementary to traditional dobutamine-stress echocardiography.[48]

Magnetic resonance imaging
Recently, contrast-enhanced magnetic resonance imaging (MRI)[49] showed promising results in the assessment of myocardial viability. In contrast to all the techniques described above, contrast-enhanced MRI can differentiate subendocardial from transmural damage. The method showed an impressive predictive accuracy, but one has to take into account that patients with only moderately depressed left ventricular function (mean ejection fraction

43%) were included. Low-dose dobutamine cine MRI also yields useful information in this setting.[50]

Treatment considerations

Risk stratification by combining clinical, hemodynamic, and angiographic parameters helps to define patients with poor long-term survival. Prognosis depends mainly on the extent of underlying coronary artery disease and left ventricular dysfunction, presence of inducible ischemia, detection of viable myocardium, comorbidity, age, and treatment strategy. The major aims of the treatment in patients with coronary artery disease and chronic heart failure are listed in Table 10.1.

Revascularization

Compared to patients with preserved left ventricular systolic function, reduced left ventricular function is associated with a higher perioperative risk and lower long-term survival in patients undergoing coronary artery bypass surgery. Low ventricular ejection fraction with or without clinical signs of heart failure is predictive of higher operative mortality rates in connection with coronary artery bypass grafting.[51] Mortality rates and incidence of low-output syndrome in patients with moderate-to-severe left ventricular

- Relief of the symptoms of coronary artery disease
- Increased exercise capacity
- Improved quality of life
- Improved long-term survival
- Prevention of deterioration and reinfarction of myocardium

Table 10.1   Major aims of treatment

systolic dysfunction undergoing coronary artery bypass grafting have declined over the last 20 years,[52] but left ventricular ejection fraction is still an independent risk factor of both short- and long-term mortality. Data from the CASS registry[53] estimated that the average operative mortality in 6630 patients undergoing coronary artery bypass grafting was 2.3%. There was a range from 1.9% in patients with an ejection fraction >50% to 6.7% in patients with an ejection fraction <19%. More recent studies documented improvement in both short- and long-term survival rates.

Progress in defining the appropriate group of patients most likely to profit from coronary artery bypass grafting, improvement in anesthetic techniques, advances in cardiac protection, more complete revascularization, and better perioperative management are most likely the main contributing factors to this encouraging trend. One study[54] including coronary artery bypass grafting procedures from 1981 to 1995 evaluated the survival rates in 156 patients with a preoperative left ventricular ejection fraction of <25%, estimated by uniplanar or biplanar left ventriculography. Thirty-eight percent had overt symptoms of chronic heart failure; the risk of in-hospital mortality was 3.8%; 1- and 5-year survival rates were 90% and 64%, respectively. These data were confirmed by a more recent study,[55] analysing early and long-term outcome in 167 patients with a mean ejection fraction of <30% determined by biplanar left ventricular angiograms before surgery. Patients underwent coronary artery bypass surgery during a period from 1991 to 1998. Early cardiac death has been estimated to be as low as 1.7%. Major nonfatal postoperative complications were reported in 24% of patients. Long-term prognosis was satisfactory, with 1- and 5-year survival of 94% and 75%, respectively.

Operative outcome is highly dependent on patient selection and surgical expertise. In addition to left ventricular dysfunction and clinical symptoms of chronic heart failure, older age, comorbid conditions, female gender, and the extent of coronary artery disease are all independent risk factors for early mortality. Multivariate correlates of long-term survival include severity of preoperative angina class, evidence of chronic heart failure, number of diseased vessels, and incomplete revascularization.[54]

Compared to medical treatment alone, myocardial revascularization has proven beneficial effects with regard to symptom relief, exercise tolerance, and long-term survival,[56] with results comparable to cardiac transplantation.[57]

Careful patient selection is crucial for achieving the beneficial effects of revascularization. It has been suggested that there is a positive correlation between the amount of dysfunctional but viable myocardium in patients with moderate-to-severe left ventricular systolic dysfunction and functional improvement as well as prognosis after successful coronary revascularization.[58]

Lack of early improvement in ejection fraction after coronary artery bypass surgery in patients with an ejection fraction <30% cannot be used to predict poorer outcome with respect to angina pectoris, heart failure symptoms, and survival.[59] It should be pointed out that the majority of studies estimating the accuracy of preoperative viability assessment in this setting had improvement of regional but not global myocardial recovery as the endpoint.[60] In concordance with the guidelines for coronary artery bypass surgery of the American College of Cardiology and the American Heart Association,[56] coronary artery bypass surgery in patients with poor left ventricular function can be recommended in the following conditions:

- significant left main coronary artery stenosis or left main artery equivalent (≥70% stenosis of the proximal left anterior descent artery and proximal left circumflex artery).
- proximal left anterior descent artery stenosis with two- or three-vessel disease.
- significant viable noncontracting revascularizable myocardium (Class IIa indication).

Referring to the European guidelines on the management of stable angina pectoris,[61] coronary artery bypass surgery is recommended in patients with stable angina and an ejection fraction <30% when there is evidence of left main coronary artery stenosis, or triple-vessel disease, particularly when the proximal left anterior descent artery is involved.

Transmyocardial laser revascularization

In highly symptomatic patients with end-stage coronary artery disease in whom, for several reasons revascularization is not feasible, larger randomized trials demonstrated that treatment with transmyocardial[62–64] (TMLR) or percutaneous transmyocardial laser revascularization[65] (PTMLR) compared to medical treatment alone increased exercise tolerance, and improved quality of life and angina symptoms. Although all these trials generally allowed inclusion of patients with markedly depressed ejection fraction of 30% or less, mean ejection fraction was above 45% in all studies. Thus, the value of TMLR or PTMLR in patients with poor left ventricular function with or without heart failure symptoms and severe angina pectoris, refractory to therapy, is still not satisfactorily evaluated. The mechanism leading to improvement has not been conclusively elucidated.

One might be concerned about the possibility of worsening contractile function by a technique that actively damages myocardial tissue. In fact, in the ATLANTIC study[62] ejection fraction worsened significantly by 3% at 3 months. While experimental data suggest deterioration of systolic function early after creation of myocardial laser channels,[66] no change in hemodynamic or left ventricular status could be found in the clinical setting with preserved ejection fraction.[67] However, there is evidence that patients with an ejection fraction <35% might have a perioperative decrease of left ventricular function requiring insertion of an intra-aortic balloon pump perioperatively. It has therefore been recommended to start intra-aortic balloon pump preoperatively in these patients.[68]

Surgical repair

As described above, remodeling of the myocardium after myocardial infarction may lead to dilation and contractile impairment of the left ventricle, possibly resulting in chronic heart failure. Surgical anterior ventricular endocardial restoration (SAVER) of normal left ventricular size and shape is based on the Dor procedure,[69] reducing ventricular size by replacing the akinetic or dyskinetic segment with an intraventricular patch. This approach has recently been evaluated in 439 patients with a mean ejection fraction of 29%.[70] In 89%, the SAVER procedure was performed immediately after coronary artery bypass surgery; mitral valve repair was performed in 22% and mitral valve replacement in 4% of patients; hospital mortality was 6.6%. Postoperative ejection fraction increased by a mean of 11% and preoperative left ventricular end systolic volume index decreased from mean 109 ml/m^2 to 69 ml/m^2 postoperatively.

Survival at 18 months was 88% in patients undergoing SAVER and coronary artery bypass surgery and, thus, is comparable to coronary artery bypass surgery alone. Long-term follow-up data beyond 18 months are not yet available. A large multicenter trial is planned to compare directly (1) the SAVER procedure combined with coronary artery bypass surgery and aggressive medical treatment with (2) coronary artery bypass surgery and medical treatment alone.[71] Only when these data are available, can one weigh up the possible benefits from the risks of this promising procedure.

Pharmacologic treatment

In most of the landmark trials for the treatment of chronic heart failure the majority of patients had ischemic cardiomyopathy. Thus, the general treatment recommendations can be applied to this group. There are, however, some special considerations one has to take into account.

Aspirin

Aspirin is widely used in patients with coronary artery disease. Pooled data analysis from about 20,000 patients revealed a 20% reduction in long-term mortality by the use of aspirin in these patients.[72]

The use of aspirin is generally recommended to all patients with chronic stable angina or those with clinical or laboratory evidence of coronary artery disease and should be continued indefinitely.[73] However, there are concerns about combining aspirin or nonsteroid anti-inflammatory drugs (NSAIDs) in general with an angiotensin-converting enzyme (ACE) inhibitor. As ACE inhibitors promote the release of vasodilatory prostaglandins by an increase in circulating bradykinin, inhibition of prostaglandin synthesis by blocking cyclooxygenase-1 could theoretically attenuate the beneficial effects of ACE inhibitors in heart failure and hypertension.[74] Several subgroup analyses have reported a negative interaction between aspirin and ACE inhibitors.[75-77] Data from SOLVD[75] showed that use of antiplatelet agents was associated with a substantial survival benefit in patients with an ejection fraction ≤35%. No influence on survival could be seen with enalapril, when given in addition to antiplatelet therapy, although a beneficial effect on the combined endpoint of death or hospital admission for heart failure could be documented. The authors point out that one of the possible mechanisms may be overlapping mechanisms of action, detracting from benefit when given together. They concluded that antiplatelet agents and ACE inhibitors may interact at multiple levels with various degrees of agonistic and antagonistic effects, depending on their relative concentration and the balance between vasodilating and vasoconstricting prostaglandins.

On the other hand, a cohort study of 11,575 patients suffering from coronary artery disease with and without heart failure showed a statistically significant absolute 8% reduction in mortality at 5 years in patients receiving aspirin combined with ACE inhibitors compared with ACE inhibition alone.[78] The benefit was substantial even after adjusting for potential confounders. Another retrospective cohort study looked at 1-year survival in a population of 1110 patients older than 65 years with evidence of coronary artery disease and chronic heart failure. These patients revealed a greater survival benefit on aspirin even after adjusting for the use of ACE inhibitors.[79]

In summary, there still is conflicting evidence concerning the efficacy of the combined use of aspirin and ACE inhibitors. Agonistic and antagonistic effects may be dose-dependent. Use of low-dose aspirin (75–100 mg/day) may have less influence on the synthesis of vasodilating prostaglandins, while still keeping its full antiplatelet efficacy,[80] and is therefore routinely recommended.

Angiotensin-converting enzyme inhibitors
There is a large body of evidence documenting the safety and efficacy of ACE inhibitors, when given to patients with reduced left ventricular function and coronary artery disease. As discussed above, angiotensin II is an important player in the complex process of postinfarction remodeling. Treatment with ACE inhibitors lowers angiotensin II levels and thus attenuates left ventricular dilatation and deterioration after acute myocardial infarction.[81,82] Other ACE inhibitor-mediated effects that may be desirable in both chronic heart failure and coronary artery disease are improvement in endothelial dysfunction,[83] reduction in sympathetic activity,[84] improvement in fibrinolytic activity by decreasing plasminogen activator inhibitor (PAI) 1 and increasing tissue plasminogen activator (t-PA),[85] and alterations of cytokine levels.[86]

The HOPE trial evaluated the effects of ramipril on 9297 patients at high risk for cardiovascular events.[87] Patients without known ejection fraction <40% and without evidence of chronic heart failure were included who had either established atherosclerotic disease or diabetes with at least one additional cardiovascular risk factor. The study was stopped prematurely at 4.5 years because of a 22% reduction in the combined primary endpoint of myocardial infarction, stroke, or death from cardiovascular disease in the ramipril group compared to placebo (P<0.001). A significant reduction in each of the individual components of the primary endpoint was also seen.

The cardioprotective effect of ACE inhibitors in patients undergoing revascularization has been addressed in two smaller trials. In the Quo Vadis trial, 149 patients undergoing coronary artery bypass surgery without traditional indications for ACE inhibitor treatment were randomized to treatment with quinapril 40 mg/day or placebo.[88] Treatment was started at least 2 weeks before coronary artery bypass surgery. At 1 year, patients receiving quinapril had an 80% reduction in ischemic events, defined as myocardial infarction, recurrence of angina pectoris, ischemic stroke, or transient ischemic attack. The APRES trial included 159 patients with a left ventricular ejection fraction between 30% and 50%, without signs of chronic heart failure following revascularization, who were randomly assigned to ramipril or placebo.[89] At a median follow-up of 33 months there was a 58% risk reduction in the combined endpoint of cardiac death, myocardial infarction, and chronic heart failure ($P = 0.031$).

The use of ACE inhibitors is fundamental in the treatment of patients with left ventricular dysfunction and clinical symptoms of chronic heart failure. The data discussed above strengthen the indication even more in patients at high risk for cardiovascular events.

Angiotensin type 1 receptor blockers
The use of angiotensin type 1 receptor blockers (ARBs), either instead of or in combination with ACE inhibitors, has some theoretical treatment advantages in patients with coronary artery disease and chronic heart failure. Due to a side-effect profile comparable with placebo, ARBs are generally well tolerated. ARBs directly block the angiotensin subtype 1 (AT-1) receptor, which mediates important effects of angiotensin II, such as peripheral vasoconstriction, growths of the left ventricle and arterial walls, and secretion of aldosterone by the adrenal cortex.[90]

The ELITE II trial was the first large study that prospectively compared the effectiveness of the ARB losartan to captopril in terms of survival and morbidity in patients with symptomatic chronic heart failure.[91]

A total of 3152 patients were randomized and titrated to either losartan 50 mg once daily or captopril 50 mg three times daily, if tolerated; 79% of patients had a history of coronary artery disease and the mean ejection fraction was 31% in both groups. Most of the patients were either in New York Heart Association (NYHA) functional class II (52%) or III (43%). Median follow-up was 1.5 years. No statistically significant differences in the predefined endpoints could be observed.

The Val-HeFT (Valsartan Heart Failure Trial) study investigated whether the addition of the ARB valsartan in patients considered optimally treated for chronic heart failure reduces mortality and morbidity; 5010 patients were randomized in a double-blind, placebo-controlled, parallel group study design. Inclusion criteria were chronic heart failure with NYHA functional class II–IV symptoms and an ejection fraction below 40%, and 2 weeks of pharmacologic treatment stability. Coronary artery disease was the primary cause of chronic heart failure in about 60% of patients. At baseline, about 93% of patients included were on an ACE inhibitor and approximately 35% were on beta-blocker therapy.

Overall, in a mean observation period of 23 months, the addition of valsartan significantly reduced the combined endpoint of mortality and morbidity with relative risk reduction of 13.2% compared with placebo ($P = 0.009$), mainly by a 24% reduction in hospitalization for heart failure ($P < 0.001$). Mortality was similar in both treatment groups.

Subgroup analysis revealed that the addition of valsartan in patients with ischemic etiology of heart failure did not lead to a significant reduction in the combined endpoint. Patients treated with both a beta-blocker and an ACE inhibitor at baseline (32%) had worse outcome in terms of morbidity and mortality when valsartan was added. As this study was not designed to look at this patient population in particular, these findings should be interpreted with caution.

In summary, the value of ARBs either alone or in combination with ACE inhibitors for treatment of chronic heart failure due to coronary artery disease is currently under investigation. In patients who are intolerant to ACE inhibitors the use of an ARB is recommended.

Spironolactone

The RALES study showed that addition of the aldosterone receptor blocker spironolactone at doses of 12.5–50 mg significantly improved survival and reduced hospitalization for worsening of heart failure and angina symptoms in patients with severe chronic heart failure and a mean ejection fraction of about 25%.[92] Of 1663 patients in the study, about 55% had chronic heart failure due to coronary artery disease. Treatment with spironolactone was equally effective in patients with heart failure of ischemic or nonischemic etiology.

Endogenous aldosterone may play an important role in the remodeling process. Recent results indicate that treatment with spironolactone improves left ventricular volume and mass and reduced plasma procollagen type III aminoterminal peptide levels, a biochemical marker of myocardial fibrosis, in patients with nonischemic cardiomyopathy.[93] The prognostic significance of serological markers of extracellular matrix turnover has been investigated in a substudy of the RALES trial.[94,95] Blood samples from 261 patients were obtained at baseline. Blood samples after 6 months could be taken in only 151 patients. The etiology of heart failure was heterogenic, with only 35% of patients having cardiomyopathy of ischemic origin.

In a multivariate analysis, serum procollagen type III aminoterminal peptide levels, at baseline, were significantly higher in patients

with ischemic heart disease (5.2 µg/ml for ischemic vs 4.7 µg/ml for nonischemic heart disease). The study demonstrated that serum markers of collagen synthesis decreased in the spironolactone group, whereas markers of collagen degradation did not change, indicating a reduction in the extracellular matrix turnover rate. Serum procollagen type III aminoterminal peptide levels of ≥3.85 µg/ml had prognostic significance with negative correlation to survival and hospitalization-free survival due to chronic heart failure in the placebo group but not in the spironolactone group. The role of aldosterone receptor blockers in the remodeling process in ischemic cardiomyopathy is investigated by ongoing research.

Beta-blockers

Beta-blockers have become part of standard treatment for patients with chronic heart failure. The question whether the efficacy of beta-blockers is influenced by the cause of heart failure has been addressed in one meta-analysis.[96] Data from 21 trials with 5849 patients, including the Cardiac Insufficiency Bisoprolol Study II (CIBIS-II),[97] but not the Metoprolol CR/XL Randomized Intervention Trial in Congestive Heart Failure (MERIT-HF)[98] and Carvedilol Prospective Randomized Cumulative Survival Study (COPERNICUS),[99] were analysed. The overall mortality benefit from treatment with beta-blockers was similar in patients with chronic heart failure due to coronary artery disease and nonischemic heart failure.

The MERIT-HF included 3991 patients with chronic heart failure in NYHA functional class II–IV with an ejection fraction of 40% or less; the patients were randomized to metoprolol CR/XL or placebo. Medication was titrated to a target dose of 200 mg once daily if tolerated. About 65% of patients in both groups had chronic heart failure due to coronary artery disease. The study was stopped prematurely at a mean follow-up of 1 year due to a highly significant 34% relative risk reduction in mortality, which was the primary endpoint, in the metoprolol group. Subgroup analysis showed a statistically significant survival benefit of patients with ischemic chronic heart failure, when treated with metoprolol CR/XL compared with placebo.

The COPERNICUS trial included 2289 patients with chronic heart failure in NYHA functional class IV without clinical signs of heart failure decompensation, severe hypotension, or renal insufficiency at inclusion. Mean ejection fraction was about 20%. The patients were randomized to either carvedilol, titrated to a target dose of 25 mg twice daily, if tolerated, or placebo. Coronary artery disease was the cause of chronic heart failure in more than 65% of patients included. This study also was stopped prematurely, at a mean follow-up of 10.4 months, due to a 35% decrease in the risk of death in the carvedilol group.

In addition, beta-blockers have been outlined as the first-line treatment for angina pectoris.[100] Occurrence of both conditions – i.e. chronic heart failure and coronary artery disease – strengthens the indication for treatment.

Calcium channel blockers

The use of calcium channel blockers is generally not recommended in patients with left ventricular systolic dysfunction or chronic heart failure. Nifedipine,[101] verapamil,[102] diltiazem,[103] and nisoldipine[104] have shown disappointing results with clinical deterioration in this group of patients. Felodipine and amlodipine seem to have no overall influence on mortality or hospitalization in patients with chronic heart failure;[105,106] however, these two drugs may be safely used in patients requiring additional treatment for angina pectoris or hypertension.

Nitrates

Administration of sublingual nitroglycerin is the favored treatment for acute episodes of angina pectoris. Long-acting nitroglycerin preparations have beneficial effects on symptoms of coronary artery disease but their role in treatment of chronic heart failure is more unclear. One study indicates that nitrates as an adjunct to treatment with ACE inhibitors may improve exercise tolerance and left ventricular size and systolic function.[107] Long-acting nitrate preparations can be safely used as additional treatment in patients with coronary artery disease and chronic heart failure remaining symptomatic on therapy with beta-blockers, or in those intolerant to beta-blocker therapy.

Statins

HMG-CoA-reductase inhibitors (statins) are established as effective in the primary and secondary prophylaxis of coronary artery disease. Statins have properties that go far beyond lipid lowering. Plaque stabilization,[108] reversal of endothelial dysfunction,[109] and antioxidative properties[110] are only some of the plausible additional effects of these agents.

Conclusion

Coronary artery disease is currently the major cause of left ventricular dysfunction and chronic heart failure. Specific considerations regarding assessment and treatment are essential in the optimal management of this large and heterogeneous population. It is essential to decide whether coronary artery disease represents only the underlying cause of chronic heart failure or is an active player that determines the cause and prognosis in this disease. Symptoms suggestive of angina pectoris should be carefully evaluated. When satisfactory pharmacologic therapy is not possible, revascularization should be considered, especially when there is evidence of myocardial viability. Improvements in prognosis after coronary artery bypass surgery are highly correlated to careful selection of those patients most likely to profit from this procedure. Ongoing research will provide answers regarding the role of novel pharmacologic agents, newer methods for assessing myocardial viability, and more sophisticated revascularization techniques.

References

1. Lopez AD. Assessing the burden of mortality from cardiovascular disease. World Health Stat Q 1993; 46:91–6.

2. Sans S, Kesteloot H, Kromhout D. The burden of cardiovascular diseases mortality in Europe. Task Force of the European Society of Cardiology on Cardiovascular Mortality and Morbidity Statistics in Europe. Eur Heart J 1997; 18:1231–48.

3. Rosamond WD, Chambless LE, Folsom AR, et al. Trends in the incidence of myocardial infarction and in mortality due to coronary heart disease, 1987 to 1994. N Engl J Med 1998; 339:861–7.

4. Reddy KS, Yusuf S. Emerging epidemic of cardiovascular disease in developing countries. Circulation 1998; 97:596–601.

5. Murray CJL, Lopez AD. Mortality by cause of eight regions of the world: global burden of disease study. Lancet 1997; 349:1269–76.

6. Murray CJL, Lopez AD. Alternative projection of mortality and disability by cause 1990–2020: global burden of disease study. Lancet 1997; 349:1498–504.

7. Deedwania PC, Carbajal EV. Silent myocardial ischemia – a clinical perspective. Arch Intern Med 1991; 151:2373–82.

8. Kannel WB, Ho K, Thom K. Changing epidemiological features of cardiac failure. Eur Heart J 1994; 72 (Suppl):S3–9.

9. Fox KF, Cowie MR, Wood DA, et al. Coronary artery disease as the cause of incident heart failure in the population. Eur Heart J 2001; 22:221–36.

10. He J, Ogden LG, Bazzano LA, et al. Risk factors for congestive heart failure in US men and women. NHANES I epidemiologic follow-up study. Arch Int Med 2001; 161:1996–2002.

11. Guidry UC, Evans JC, Larson MG, et al. Temporal trends in event rates after Q-wave myocardial infarction. The Framingham study. Circulation 1999; 100:2054–9.

12. The Joint European Society of Cardiology/ American College of Cardiology Committee. Myocardial infarction redefined. Eur Heart J 2000; 2:1502–13.

13. Opie LH. The ever expanding spectrum of ischemic left ventricular dysfunction. Cardiovasc Drugs Ther 1994; 8(Suppl 2):297.

14. Melillo G, Lima JAC, Judd RM, et al. Intrinsic myocyte dysfunction and tyrosine kinase pathway activation underlie the impaired wall thickening of adjacent regions during postinfarct left ventricular remodeling. Circulation 1996; 93:1447–58.

15. Li YY, McTiernan CF, Feldman AM. Interplay of matrix metalloproteinases, tissue inhibitors of metalloproteinases and their regulators in cardiac matrix remodelling. Circ Res 2000; 46:214–24.

16. Gerber BL, Rochitte CE, Melin JA, et al. Microvascular obstruction and left ventricular remodeling early after acute myocardial infarction. Circulation 2000; 101:2734–41.

17. Kajstura J, Cheng W, Reiss K, et al. Apoptotic and necrotic myocyte cell death are independent contributing variables of infarct size in rats. Lab Invest 1996; 74:86–107.

18. Cheng W, Li B, Kajstura J, et al. Stretch-induced programmed myocyte cell death. J Clin Invest 1995; 96:2247–59.

19. Tanaka M, Ito H, Adachi S, et al. Hypoxia induces apoptosis with enhanced expression of Fas antigen messenger RNA in cultured neonatal rat cardiomyocytes. Circ Res 1994; 75: 426–33.

20. St John Sutton MG, Sharpe N. Left ventricular remodeling after myocardial infarction. Pathophysiology and therapy. Circulation 2000; 101:2981–8.

21. Lindpainter K, Lu W, Neidermejer N, et al. Selective activation of cardiac angiotensinogen gene expression in post ventricular remodeling in the rate. J Mol Cell Cardiol 1993; 25: 133–43.

22. Cleutjens JPM, Verluyten MJA, Smits JFM, Daemen MJAP. Collagen remodeling after myocardial infarction in the rat heart. Am J Pathol 1995; 147:325–38.

23. Ross J. Myocardial perfusion–contraction matching. Implications for coronary heart disease and hibernation. Circulation 1991; 83: 1076–83.

24. Schulz R, Heusch G. Hibernating myocardium. Heart 2000; 84:587–94.

25. Al-Mohammad A, Mahy IR, Norton MY, et al. Prevalence of hibernating myocardium in patients with severely impaired left ventricles. Heart 1998; 80:559–64.

26. Elefteriades JA, Tolis G Jr, Levi E, et al. Coronary artery bypass grafting in severe left ventricular dysfunction: excellent survival and improved EF and functional state. J Am Coll Cardiol 1993; 22:1411–17.

27. Pasquet A, Robert A, D'Hont AM, et al. Prognostic value of myocardial ischemia and viability in patients with chronic left ventricular ischemic dysfunction. Circulation 1999; 100:141–8.

28. Braunwald E, Kloner RA. The stunned myocardium: prolonged, postischemic ventricular dysfunction. Circulation 1982; 66:1146–9.

29. Gerber BL, Wijns W, Vanoeverschelde JLJ, et al. Myocardial perfusion and oxygen consumption in reperfused noninfarcted dysfunctional myocardium after unstable angina. Direct evidence for myocardial stunning in humans. J Am Coll Cardiol 1999; 34:1939–46.

30. Narula J, Dawson MS, Singh BK, et al. Noninvasive characterization of stunned, hibernating, remodelled and nonviable myocardium in ischemic cardiomyopathy. J Am Coll Cardiol 2000; 63:1913–19.

31. Bart BA, Shaw LK, McCants CB, et al. Clinical deteminants of mortality in patients with angiographically diagnosed ischemic or nonischemic cardiomyopathy. J Am Coll Cardiol 1997; 30:1002–8.

32. Andersson B, Waagstein F. Spectrum and outcome of congestive heart failure in a hospitalized population. Am Heart J 1993; 126:632–40.

33. SOLVD Investigators. Effect of enalapril on survival in patients with reduced left ventricular ejection fractions and congestive heart failure. N Engl J Med 1991; 325:293–302.

34. Bax JJ, Poldermans D, Elhendy A, et al. Improvement of left ventricular ejection fraction, heart failure symptoms and prognosis after revascularization in patients with chronic coronary artery disease and viable myocardium detected by dobutamine stress echocardiography. J Am Coll Cardiol 1999; 34:163–9.

35. Weich HF, Strauss HW, Pitt B. The extraction of thallium-201 by the myocardium. Circulation 1977; 56:188–91.

36. Nielsen AP, Morris KG, Murdock R, et al. Linear relationship between the distribution of thallium-201 and blood flow in ischemic and nonischemic myocardium during exercise. Circulation 1980; 61:797–801.

37. Yang LD, Berman DS, Kiat H, et al. The frequency of late reversibility in SPECT thallium-201 stress-redistribution studies. J Am Coll Cardiol 1990; 15:334–40.

38. Ragosta M, Beller GA, Watson DD, et al. Quantitative planar rest–redistribution ^{201}Tl imaging in detection of myocardial viability and prediction of improvement in left ventricular function after coronary bypass surgery in patients with severely depressed left ventricular function. Circulation 1993; 87:1630–41.

39. Rocco TP, Dilsizian V, McKusick KA, et al. Comparison of thallium redistribution with rest 'reinjection' imaging for the detection of viable myocardium. Am J Cardiol 1990; 66:158–63.

40. Bax JJ, Wijns W, Cornel JH, et al. Accuracy of currently available techniques for prediction of functional recovery after revascularization in

patients with left ventricular dysfunction due to chronic coronary artery disease: comparison of pooled data. J Am Coll Cardiol 1997; 30:1451–60.

41. Marcus Cardiac Imaging: a Companion to Braunwald's Heart Disease, 2nd edn. Philadelphia: WB Saunders, Company, 1996: 1004.

42. Cuocolo A, Soricelli A, Nicolai E, et al. Technetium-99m-tetrofosmin regional myocardial uptake at rest: relation to severity of coronary artery stenosis in previous myocardial infarction. J Nucl Med 1995; 36:907–13.

43. Marzullo P, Parodi O, Reisenhofer B, et al. Value of rest thallium-201/technetium-99m sestamibi scans and dobutamine echocardiography for detecting myocardial viability. Am J Cardiol 1993; 71:166–72.

44. Udelson JE, Coleman PS, Metherall J, et al. Predicting recovery of severe regional ventricular dysfunction. Comparison of resting scintigraphy with ^{201}Tl and 99mTc-sestamibi. Circulation 1994; 89:2552–61.

45. Iskandrian AE, Acio E. Methodology of a novel myocardial viability protocol. J Nucl Cardiol 1998; 5:206–9.

46. Pasquet A, Lauer MS, Williams MJ, et al. Prediction of global left ventricular function after bypass surgery in patients with severe left ventricular dysfunction. Impact of pre-operative myocardial function, perfusion, and metabolism. Eur Heart J 2000; 21:124–36.

47. Hoffmann R, Lethen H, Marwick T, et al. Analysis of interinstitutional observer agreement in the interpretation of dobutamine stress echocardiogram. J Am Coll Cardiol 1996; 27:330–6.

48. Rambaldi R, Poldermans D, Bax JJ, et al. Doppler tissue velocity sampling improves diagnostic accuracy during dobutamine stress echocardiography for the assessment of viable myocardium in patients with severe left ventricular dysfunction. Eur Heart J 2000; 21:1091–8.

49. Kim RJ, Wu E, Rafael A, et al. The use of contrast-enhanced magnetic resonance imaging to identify reversible myocardial dysfunction. N Engl J Med 2000; 343:1445–53.

50. Baer FM, Voth E, Schneider CA, et al. Comparison of low-dose dobutamine–gradient echo magnetic resonance imaging and positron emission tomography with [^{18}F] fluorodeoxyglucose in patients with chronic artery disease: a functional and morphological approach to the detection of residual myocardial viability. Circulation 1995; 91:1006–15.

51. Baker DW, Jones R, Hodges J, et al. Management of heart failure. III: The role of revascularization in the treatment of patients with moderate to severe left ventricular systolic dysfunction. JAMA 1994; 272:1528–34.

52. Yau TM, Fedak PW, Weisel RD, et al. Predictors of operative risk for coronary bypass operations in patients with left ventricular dysfunction. J Thorac Cardiovasc Surg 1999; 118:1006–13.

53. Kennedy JW, Kaiser GC, Fisher LD, et al. Clinical and angiographic predictors of operative mortality from the collaborative study in coronary artery surgery (CASS). Circulation 1981; 63:793–802.

54. Tachiotis GD, Weintraub WS, Johnston TS, et al. Coronary artery bypass grafting in patients with advanced left ventricular dysfunction. Ann Thorac Surg 1998; 66:1632–9.

55. Luciani GB, Montalbano G, Casali G, Mazzuco A. Predicting long-term functional results after myocardial revascularization in ischemic cardiomyopathy. J Thorac Cardiovasc Surg 2000; 120:478–89.

56. Eagle KA, Guyton RA, Davidoff R, et al. ACC/AHA Guidelines for Coronary Artery Bypass Surgery. A Report of the American College of Cardiology/American Heart Association Task Force on Practice guidelines (Committee to Revise the 1991 guidelines for Coronary Artery Bypass graft Surgery). J Am Coll Cardiol 1999; 34:1262–347.

57. Tjan TD, Kondruweit M, Scheld HH, et al. The bad ventricle–revascularization versus transplantation. Thorac Cardiovasc Surg 2000; 48:9–14.

58. Meluzin J, Cerny J, Frelich M, et al. Prognostic value of the amount of dysfunctional but viable myocardium in revascularized patients with coronary artery disease and left ventricular dysfunction. J Am Coll Cardiol 1998; 32:912–20.

59. Samady H, Elefteriades JA, Brian G, et al. Failure to improve left ventricular function after coronary revascularization for ischemic cardiomyopathy is not associated with worse outcome. Circulation 1999; 100:1298–304.

60. Stahle E. Patients with ischemic heart disease and severe left ventricular dysfunction – who

should not be revascularized? Eur Heart J 2000; 21:101–3.

61. Task Force of the European Society of Cardiology. Management of stable angina pectoris. Eur Heart J 1997; 18:394–413.

62. Burkhoff D, Schmidt S, Schulman SP, et al. for the ATLANTIC investigators. Transmyocardial laser revascularization compared with continued medical therapy for the treatment of refractory angina pectoris: a prospective randomised trial. Lancet 1999; 354:885–90.

63. Allen KB, Dowling RD, Fudge TL, et al. Comparison of transmyocardial revascularization with medical therapy in patients with refractory angina. N Engl J Med 1999; 341:1029–36.

64. Frazier OH, March RJ, Horvath KA, for the Transmyocardial Carbon Dioxide Laser Revascularization Group. Transmyocardial revascularization with a carbon dioxide laser in patients with end-stage coronary artery disease. N Engl J Med 1999; 341:1021–8.

65. Oesterle SN, Sanborn TA, Ali N, et al. Percutaneous transmyocardial laser revascularization for severe angina: the PACIFIC randomised trial. Lancet 2000; 356:1705–10.

66. Hughes CG, Shah AS, Yin B, et al. Early postoperative changes in regional systolic and diastolic left ventricular function after transmyocardial laser revascularization: a comparison of holmium:YAG and CO_2 lasers. J Am Coll Cardiol 2000; 35:1022–30.

67. Dixon SR, Schreiber TL, Rabah M, et al. Immediate effect of percutaneous myocardial laser revascularization on hemodynamics and left ventricular systolic function in angina pectoris. Am J Cardiol 2001; 87:516–19.

68. Lutter G, Saurbier B, Nitzsche E, et al. Transmyocardial laser revascularization (TMLR) in patients with unstable angina and low ejection fraction. Eur J Cardiothorac Surg 1998; 13:21–6.

69. Dor V, Saab M, Coste P, et al. Left ventricular aneurysm: a new surgical approach. Thorac Cardiovasc Surg 1989; 37:11–19.

70. Athanasuleas CL, Stanley AWH Jr, Buckberg GD, et al. Surgical anterior ventricular endocardial restoration (SAVER) in the dilated remodeled ventricle after anterior myocardial infarction. J Am Coll Cardiol 2001; 37:1198–209.

71. Jones RH. Is it time for a randomized trial of surgical treatment of ischemic heart failure? J Am Coll Cardiol 2001; 37:1210–13.

72. Antiplatelet Trialist's Collaboration: Collaborative overview of randomised trials of antiplatelet therapy I: Prevention of death, myocardial infarction, and stroke by prolonged antiplatelet therapy in various categories of patients. BMJ 1994; 308:81–106.

73. Cairns JA, Theroux P, Louis HD, et al. Antithrombotic agents in coronary artery disease. Chest 1998; 114:611S.

74. Houston MC. Nonsteroidal anti-inflammatory drugs and antihypertensives. Am J Med 1991; 90:42S–7S.

75. Al-Khadra AS, Salem DN, Rand WM, et al. Antiplatelet agents and survival: a cohort analysis from the Study of Left Ventricular Dysfunction (SOLVD) trial. J Am Coll Cardiol 1998; 31:419–25.

76. Nguyen KN, Aursnes I, Kjekshus J. Interaction between enalapril and aspirin on mortality after acute myocardial infarction: subgroup analysis of the Cooperative New Scandinavian Enalapril Survival Study II (CONSENSUS II). Am J Cardiol 1997; 79:115–19.

77. Peterson JG, Laur MS, Young JB, et al. Evidence for an adverse interaction between ACE inhibitors and aspirin following myocardial infarction: the GUSTO-I trial. J Am Coll Cardiol 1998; 31(Suppl A):96A.

78. Leor J, Reicher-Reiss H, Goldbourt U, et al. Aspirin and mortality in patients treated with angiotensin-converting enzyme inhibitors. A cohort study of 11,575 patients with coronary artery disease. J Am Coll Cardiol 1999; 33:1920–5.

79. Krumholz HM, Chen YT, Radford MJ. Aspirin and the treatment of heart failure in the elderly. Arch Intern Med 2001; 161:577–82.

80. Guazzi MD, Compodonico J, Celeste F, et al. Antihypertensive efficacy of angiotensin converting enzyme inhibition and aspirin counteraction. Clin Pharmacol Ther 1998; 63:79–86.

81. Bonarjee V, Carstensen S, Caidahl K, et al. Attenuation of left ventricular dilatation after myocardial infarction by early initiation of enalapril therapy. Am J Cardiol 1993; 72:1004–9.

82. Konstam M, Kronenberg M, Rousseau M, et al. Effects of the angiotensin-converting enzyme in-

hibitor enalapril on the long-term progression of left ventricular dilatation in patients with asymptomatic systolic dysfunction. Circulation 1993; 88:2277–83.

83. Hornig B, Arakawa N, Haussmann D, Drexler H. Differential effects of quinaprilat and enalaprilat on endothelial function of conduit arteries in patients with chronic heart failure. Circulation 1998; 98:2842–8.

84. Patten RD, Kronenberg MW, Benedict CR, et al. Acute and long-term effects of the angiotensin converting enzyme inhibitor, enalapril, on adrenergic activity and sensitivity during exercise in patients with left ventricular dysfunction. Am Heart J 1997; 134:37–43.

85. Vaughan DE. Endothelial function, fibrinolysis, and angiotensin converting enzyme inhibition. Clin Cardiol 1997; 20(Suppl 2):II-34–7.

86. Gullestad L, Aukrust P, Ueland T, et al. Effect of high- versus low-dose angiotensin converting enzyme inhibition on cytokine levels in chronic heart failure. J Am Coll Cardiol 1999; 34:2061–7.

87. The Heart Outcomes Prevention Evaluation Study Investigators. Effects of an angiotensin converting enzyme inhibitor, ramipril, on cardiovascular events in high-risk patients. N Engl J Med 2000; 342:145–53.

88. Oosterga M, Voors A, Veeger N, et al. Quo Vadis (effects of Quinapril On Vascular ACE and Determinants of Ischemia). Circulation 1998; 98(Suppl I):I-636.

89. Kjoller-Hansen L, Steffensen R, Grande P. The Angiotensin-converting Enzyme Inhibition Post Revascularization Study (APRES). J Am Coll Cardiol 2000; 35:881–8.

90. Goodfriend TL, Elliott ME, Catt KJ. Angiotensin receptors and their antagonists. N Engl J Med 1996; 334:1649–54.

91. Pitt B, Poole-Wilson PA, Segal R, et al. Effect of losartan compared with captopril on mortality in patients with symptomatic heart failure: randomised trial – the Losartan Heart Failure Survival Study ELITE II. Lancet 2000; 355:1582–7.

92. Pitt B, Zannad F, Remme WJ, et al. for the Randomized Aldactone Evaluation Study Investigators. The effect of spironolactone on morbidity and mortality in patients with severe heart failure. N Engl J Med 1999; 341:709–17.

93. Tsutamoto T, Wada A, Maeda K, et al. Effect of spironolactone on plasma brain natriuretic peptide and left ventricular remodeling in patients with congestive heart failure. J Am Coll Cardiol 2001; 37:1228–33.

94. Zannad F, Dousset B, Alla F. Treatment of congestive heart failure: interfering the aldosterone–cardiac extracellular matrix relationship. Hypertension 2001; 38:1227–32.

95. Zannad F, Alla F, Dousset B, et al. Limitation of extracellular matrix turnover may contribute to survival benefit of spironolactone therapy in patients with congestive heart failure: insights from the Randomized Aldactone Evaluation Study (RALES). Circulation 2000; 102:2700–6. [Erratum, Circulation 2001; 103:476.]

96. Bonet S, Agusti A, Arnau JM, et al. β-adrenergic blocking agents in heart failure. Benefits of vasodilating and nonvasodilating agents according to patients characteristics: a meta analysis of clinical trials. Arch Intern Med 2000; 160:621–7.

97. CIBIS-II Investigators and Committees. The Cardiac Insufficiency Bisoprolol Study II (CIBIS-II): a randomised trial. Lancet 1999; 353:9–13.

98. MERIT-HF Study Group. Effect of Metoprolol CR/XL in chronic heart failure: Metoprolol CR/XL Randomised Intervention Trial in Congestive Heart Failure (MERIT-HF). Lancet 1999; 353:2001–7.

99. The Carvedilol Prospective Randomized Cumulative Survival Study Group. Effect of carvedilol on survival in severe chronic heart failure. N Engl J Med 2001; 344:1651–8.

100. Gibbons RJ, Chatterjee K, Daley J, et al. ACC/AHA/ACP-ASIM guidelines for the management of patients with chronic stable angina: a report of the American College of Cardiology/American Heart Association Task Force on Practice Guidelines (Committee on Management of Patients with Chronic Stable Angina). J Am Coll Cardiol 1999; 33:2092–197.

101. Elkayam U, Amin J, Mehra A, et al. A prospective randomized, double-blind, crossover study to compare the efficacy and safety of chronic nifedipine therapy with that of isosorbide dinitrate and their combination in the treatment of congestive heart failure. Circulation 1990; 82:1954–61.

102. Mohindra SK, Udeani OG. Long acting verapamil and heart failure. JAMA 1989; 261:994.

103. The Multicenter Diltiazem Postinfarction Trial Research Group. The effect of diltiazem on mortality and reinfarction after myocardial infarction. N Engl J Med 1988; 319:385–92.

104. Barjon JN, Rouleau JL, Bichet D, et al. Chronic renal and neurohumeral effects of the calcium entry blocker nisoldipine in patients with congestive heart failure. J Coll Cardiol 1987; 9:622–30.

105. Cohn JN, Ziesche S, Smith R, et al. Effect of the calcium antagonist felodipine as supplementary vasodilator therapy in patients with chronic heart failure treated with enalapril: V-HEFT III Vasodilator-Heart Failure Trial (V-HEFT) study group. Circulation 1997; 96:856–63.

106. Packer M, O'Connor CM, Ghali JK, et al. Effect of amlodipine on morbidity and mortality in severe chronic heart failure. Prospective Randomized Amlodipine Survival Study. N Engl J Med 1996; 335:1107–14.

107. Elkayam U, Johnson JV, Shotan A. Double-blind, placebo-controlled study to evaluate the effect of organic nitrates in patients with chronic heart failure treated with angiotensin converting enzyme inhibition. Circulation 1999; 99:2652–7.

108. Williams JK, Sukhova GK, Herrington DM, Libby P. Pravastatin has cholesterol-lowering independent effects on the artery wall of atherosclerotic monkeys. J Am Coll Cardiol 1998; 31:684–91.

109. Treasure CB, Klein JL, Weintraub W, et al. Beneficial effects of cholesterol lowering on the coronary endothelium in patients with coronary artery disease. N Engl J Med 1995; 332:481–7.

110. Girona J, La Ville AE, Sola R, et al. Simvastatin decreases aldehyde production derived from lipoprotein oxidation. Am J Cardiol 1999; 83:846–51.

11

Heart failure and valvular disease

Helen Oxenham and Norman Sharpe

Introduction

Primary valvular heart disease is an uncommon cause of heart failure in the general population, accounting for only 7% of patients with new presentation heart failure in the community[1] and approximately 4% of patients included in heart failure clinical trials.[2] However, it is an important condition to diagnose because effective remedial intervention can significantly alter outcome.

Data from longitudinal studies such as the Framingham study show that the incidence of heart failure secondary to rheumatic heart disease has fallen steadily over the past 30 years so that it now accounts for heart failure in only 2% of men and 3% of women in Western countries.[3] However, rheumatic heart disease still represents an important cause of heart failure in India and other developing nations.[4]

Valvular dysfunction places a hemodynamic burden on the left or right ventricle, or both, which can be compensated for initially with little, if any, associated symptoms. However, myocardial dysfunction and congestive heart failure develop eventually[5] with the degree of left ventricular dysfunction prognostically important.[6]

Three questions should be considered when assessing any patient who presents with heart failure and valvular disease:

1. *Severity of valve disease.* Is the valve disease severe enough to cause morbidity and mortality for which intervention would be beneficial?
2. *Coexisting diseases.* What other conditions contribute to the clinical picture? Coronary artery disease increases surgical mortality and morbidity, may contribute to left ventricular dysfunction, and affects long-term outcomes.
3. *Treatment.* What is the best surgical or medical therapy to minimize morbidity and mortality?

Assessment of valvular heart disease

Echocardiography has replaced cardiac catheterization as the definitive method for diagnosis and assessment of valvular heart disease. It is noninvasive, portable, accurate, and easily reproducible.[7]

Cardiac catheterization provides supportive information and may be needed for the following:[8]

- identification of coexisting coronary artery disease in patients with ischemic symptoms, males 35 years of age or older, postmenopausal females, or patients with multiple coronary risk factors
- determination of the pressure gradient across stenotic aortic or mitral valves
- assessment of mitral or aortic regurgitation with ventriculography or aortography

• determination of pulmonary artery pressure and other hemodynamic variables.

Use of echocardiography in valvular heart disease[7]

• Definition of the primary valve lesion.
• Determination of the severity of the valve lesion.
• Evaluation of cardiac chamber size and left ventricular function.
• Detection of abnormalities secondary to the primary lesion.
• Establishment of baseline data for serial follow-up or re-evaluation after intervention.

The four major acquired left-sided valve lesions are discussed further:

• aortic stenosis
• aortic regurgitation
• mitral stenosis
• mitral regurgitation.

Aortic stenosis

The diagnosis of aortic stenosis (AS) in patients presenting with heart failure is important for two reasons:

• treatment with valve replacement significantly improves symptoms and outcome
• this group of patients otherwise have an extremely poor prognosis.

Epidemiology

AS is a disease of the elderly, caused mainly by degenerative changes: 3% of persons aged 75–86 years were found to have critical AS in the Helsinki aging study.[9] Since 1930, there has been a decline in AS due to rheumatic heart disease so that congenital bicuspid valve currently accounts for most cases of AS in people younger than 70 years.

Pathophysiology

Diastolic dysfunction, systolic dysfunction, or both, can cause heart failure in patients with AS. Diastolic dysfunction occurs as a result of a restriction to left ventricular filling secondary to left ventricular hypertrophy with increased wall thickness and collagen content. Systolic impairment develops as a result of excess afterload, decreased contractility, or a combination of these factors.[5] Aortic valve replacement allows an increase in ejection fraction as the relief of obstruction to outflow reduces ventricular afterload and can provide marked symptomatic relief.

Prognosis

Symptoms indicating severe or critical AS typically include dyspnea, angina, and syncope. Dyspnea, which implies underlying left ventricular dysfunction, is the presenting symptom in 38% of patients[10] and is the most common initial symptom in the elderly.[11] Sudden death is rare in the absence of previous symptoms (3–5%) but rises dramatically to 15–20% per year after symptoms develop[12] so that up to 75% of patients die within 3 years of their initial manifestation unless the aortic valve is replaced.[5] Patients who develop or present with congestive heart failure as a consequence of severe AS have significantly reduced survival. In a study by Horskotte and Loogen[12] all patients with AS and heart failure had died within 29 months of developing heart failure.

Independent predictors of survival in patients with untreated AS[12]

- Valve gradient.
- Pulmonary artery systolic pressure.
- Coronary artery disease severity.
- Congestive heart failure score.
- Raised left ventricular filling pressures at cardiac catheterization.

Diagnosis

The diagnosis and grading of aortic stenosis is usually made using echocardiography. Doppler echo assessment of velocity change across the aortic valve using the modified Bernouilli equation and calculation of the aortic valve area using the continuity equation have been shown to provide accurate, reproducible estimates of the severity of aortic valve disease. A pre- to post-valve peak Doppler velocity ratio of >1:4 or an aortic valve area, of <1.0 cm^2 indicates severe stenosis.

Evaluation of aortic stenosis in patients with left ventricular dysfunction

Severe AS and significant left ventricular dysfunction often coexist in the elderly. Whereas the assessment of AS in patients with normal left ventricular function is usually straightforward, patients with significantly impaired function and relatively low transvalvular gradients pose a serious diagnostic challenge.[13] Aortic valve areas calculated using either Doppler or the Gorlin formula are flow-dependent and the true anatomic valve area may be underestimated when there is low cardiac output. Dobutamine stress echo can be used to identify patients with low-gradient 'severe' aortic stenosis by evaluating

their hemodynamic response to dobutamine infusion.

Dobutamine stress echo to evaluate the severity of aortic stenosis

Low-dose dobutamine is infused and titrated at 10-min intervals up to a maximum dose of 20 mg/kg/min. Results obtained from Doppler hemodynamic assessment and 2D echo during the study allow patients to be placed in one of three groups (Table 11.1).[14]

Patients who achieve an aortic valve area >1.0 cm^2 during dobutamine infusion do not have severe AS.[13]

Medical therapies

Except for prophylaxis against endocarditis, there is no proven medical therapy for AS. Studies in small numbers of patients with severe heart failure and mild-to-moderate AS have shown that afterload reduction using hydralazine or prazosin appears to improve cardiac performance by lowering systemic vascular resistance, despite a reduction in aortic valve area.[15] However, these drugs are contraindicated in patients with severe stenosis in whom potential harmful effects are predicted when using afterload reduction.

Surgical treatment

Balloon aortic valvuloplasty

Valvuloplasty was initially proposed for use in the elderly as an alternative to valve replacement, but initial enthusiasm decreased after significant periprocedural morbidity and disappointing long-term outcome was documented. Procedural morbidity is high, with a 10–30% complication rate, and 30-day mortality is 14%.[10,16] Serious complications such as death, stroke, aortic rupture, and aortic regurgi-

Group	Results obtained from dobutamine stress echo	Interpretation of findings	Treatment
1	>20% increase in wall motion score (preserved contractile function) and AVA increase of >0.3 cm^2 or AVA >1.0 cm^2 and no substantial change in transvalvular gradient	Left ventricular dysfunction is unrelated to (relatively mild) aortic valve disease	Conservative. This group does not benefit from AVR
2	>20% increase in wall motion score (preserved contractile function) and <0.3 cm^2 increase in AVA and increase in pressure gradient (A baseline AVA of <0.6 cm^2 nearly always indicates severe AS[13])	Severe (fixed) aortic valve disease. Significant stenosis with recoverable LV function	This group does well with surgery
3	No increase in stroke volume with dobutamine (patients without contractile reserve)	Severity of AS cannot be determined	This group has a very poor prognosis. It is unclear how best to treat them

AS = aortic stenosis; AVA = aortic valve area; AVR = aortic valve replacement; LV = left ventricular.

Table 11.1 Dobutamine stress echo in aortic stenosis[14]

tation occur in 25% of patients with New York Heart Association (NYHA) class III or IV heart failure[5,17] and there is a restenosis rate of 75% at 6 months.[16] Long-term event-free and actuarial survival after valvuloplasty is dismal and resembles the natural history of untreated aortic stenosis. There is a 94% probability of death, valve replacement, or repeat valvuloplasty within 3 years of the initial procedure.[5] Patient age and left ventricular ejection fraction (LVEF) best predict survival.[18]

Although absolute increases in valve area are in the order of 0.2–0.4 cm^2, peak-to-peak gradient is generally reduced by 50% immediately after the procedure.[19] Valvuloplasty

may thus acutely improve cardiac hemodynamics and palliate symptoms sufficiently to produce dramatic short-term clinical recovery.[16,18] However, substantial residual outflow obstruction frequently remains and acceptable long-term results generally require valve replacement.[10,20]

Indications for the use of balloon aortic valvuloplasty in patients with severe AS and heart failure

1. As a bridge to valve replacement if immediate surgery is inadvisable.[21] Valvuloplasty is highly successful in converting patients with cardiogenic shock and medically

refractory pulmonary edema caused by critical AS to a better surgical risk.[10]

2. In selected patients with AS in whom another condition precludes valve replacement.
3. When other major surgery is proposed for underlying disease with an uncertain prognosis.[22]
4. Pregnancy.

Valve replacement following valvuloplasty

In a nonrandomized, retrospective review, Lieberman et al. showed that actuarial survival in patients undergoing valve replacement after valvuloplasty was excellent and superior to repeat valvuloplasty or medications alone.[23] There was low perioperative mortality and excellent palliation of symptoms. Survival 1 year after valvuloplasty was 52% in patients treated with valvuloplasty alone compared with 95% in patients treated with valvuloplasty and subsequent valve replacement. Survival 3 years after valve replacement was 75% compared with 13% or 20% 3 years after initial or repeat valvuloplasty, respectively.[23] These data confirm the effectiveness of using valvuloplasty as a bridge to surgery in a select group of patients with severe AS.[16]

Aortic valve replacement

Unless there are exceptional circumstances, surgery is always indicated for severe AS and age is not a contraindication to surgery even when advanced heart failure is present. The presence of left ventricular impairment solely due to AS is an indication for urgent surgery.[21] Substantial improvement has been shown following valve replacement in patients with long-standing disease and ejection fractions below 20%. Irreversible left ventricular dysfunction may occur due to myocardial damage from coexisting coronary artery disease or when significant afterload mismatch was present for more than 3–6 months before aortic valve replacement.[24]

Aortic regurgitation

Pathophysiology

Chronic aortic regurgitation (AR) causes:

- volume overload
- increased afterload
- increased end-systolic wall stress.

In an attempt to normalize wall stress, there is left ventricular hypertrophy and left ventricular dilatation, which may progress to left ventricular systolic dysfunction.

Symptoms

An insidious deterioration of ventricular function may occur without clinical signs[25] and symptoms may not appear until left ventricular dysfunction is well advanced.[5] Symptoms are usually those of left-sided heart failure and herald the transition from a compensated to a decompensated state.

Asymptomatic patients

The prognosis of asymptomatic patients with normal left ventricular size and function is excellent.[26] The risk of death is less than 0.5% per year and the risk of death or aortic valve replacement is between 4% and 5% per year.[27,28] However, there is compelling evidence that AR should be corrected before the onset of left ventricular damage because an increase in left ventricular end-systolic dimension dramatically decreases survival even in asymptomatic patients.[25] When the end-systolic dimension is greater than 50 mm, the risk of heart failure or the need for valve replacement is 20% and more than 25% when the end-systolic dimension is greater than 55 mm.[29]

Symptomatic patients

Within 10 years of diagnosis, patients with severe, chronic AR have a 75% chance of death or valve replacement and an 83% risk of a cardiac event.[30] Even mild heart failure symptoms increase mortality and surgery is indicated in all patients with NYHA class II symptoms or more, if these are attributable to severe AR. Higher risk is also associated with:

• severe symptoms, even if transient and responding to treatment
• ejection fraction <55%
• atrial fibrillation.

Exercise testing can identify under-reporting of symptoms and an abnormal left ventricular response to exercise may be useful in evaluating early depression of left ventricular function. The value of exercise data in addition to resting measures of left ventricular size and function is unknown.[8]

Diagnosis

Echocardiography is the most useful modality to identify and quantify AR as well as left ventricular size and function. Aortography can add important information regarding regurgitant volume and left ventricular end-diastolic pressure. Magnetic resonance imaging is a developing imaging technique that can be used to assess regurgitant volume in addition to left ventricular volumes and mass.[31]

Medical treatment

Bradycardia will increase aortic regurgitant flow, but pacing-induced tachycardia offers little if any benefit as therapy for patients with AR.

Vasodilators reduce both aortic and left ventricular diastolic pressure and as a result, the transvalvular pressure gradient is unaltered and regurgitant volume is unchanged.[32] However, small, nonrandomized studies using hydralazine, nifedipine, enalapril, or quinapril have observed significant reductions in ventricular volumes and regurgitant fraction, with or without an increase in ejection fraction. In a larger trial comparing digoxin with nifedipine, Scognamiglio et al.[33] showed that nifedipine can delay the need for surgery by 2 or 3 years in asymptomatic patients with severe aortic regurgitation and normal left ventricular function. No patient had symptoms or signs of congestive heart failure but patients with the most significant left ventricular chamber dilatation benefited most from treatment with vasodilator therapy. Vasodilators have also been shown to favorably affect left ventricular remodeling and to delay surgery but have not been shown to improve survival of patients with severe AR.[30] There is some concern over the potential masking of left ventricular dysfunction when angiotensin-converting enzyme (ACE) inhibitors are used in patients with AR, as left ventricular dysfunction precedes the development of symptoms in these patients.[33] Vasodilators should, therefore, be reserved for patients who do not have an indication for surgery. When they are used, the vasodilator dose needs to be adjusted in order to achieve a decrease in arterial pressure[8] and these patients should be closely monitored to identify changes in left ventricular size or function (Table 11.2).

Patients with clear indications for surgery should not be treated with vasodilator therapy in the hope of postponing aortic valve replacement except when surgery is not possible.

Acute aortic regurgitation

Although vasodilators such as nitroprusside are useful in the short term, treatment with aortic

Severity of aortic regurgitation	Symptoms attributed to AR	LV systolic function	LV dimensions	Management
Mild	None	Normal (>55% or FS >0.27)	Normal	Nil
Moderate/severe	None	Normal	Normal or minimal LV enlargement, up to LVEDD 70 mm	Medical (vasodilator therapy) with close follow-up
Moderate/severe	None	Normal or LVEF approaching 50%	LVEDD >70 mm or LVESD >55 mm or LVESV >55 ml/m²	AVR
Moderate/severe	None	LV systolic dysfunction		AVR
Moderate/severe	NYHA II or more	Normal	Normal	AVR
Moderate/severe	NYHA II or more	LV systolic dysfunction		AVR
Severe	Severe symptoms	Significant impairment of LV systolic function		Medical treatment pre-AVR

AR = aortic regurgitation; AVR = aortic value replacement; FS = fractional shortening; LV = left ventricle; LVEDD = left ventricular end-diastolic diameter; LVEF = left ventricular ejection fraction; LVESD = left ventricular end-systolic diameter; LVESV = left ventricular end-systolic volume; NYHA = New York Heart Association.

Table 11.2 Guidelines for the treatment of chronic aortic regurgitation[25]

valve replacement is recommended for all cases of acute aortic regurgitation and pulmonary edema.[8]

Surgical treatment

Aortic valve replacement
In the majority of patients with chronic severe AR, valve replacement has been shown to substantially reduce left ventricular dilatation, improve systolic function, and reduce cardiovascular mortality.[27] Aortic valve replacement carries an operative mortality of 2.4–4.9% or less in the absence of coronary artery disease.[34] Good surgical results can be expected, even in patients with left ventricular

dysfunction, if the duration of left ventricular dysfunction is less than 14 months.[27] However, patients with NYHA class III or class IV symptoms have higher surgical and long-term mortality in the setting of severe AR.[35] It is important to identify left ventricular dysfunction early in order to achieve maximum benefit from valve replacement (Table 11.3).[36]

Choice of valve replacement
The choice of aortic valve replacement depends largely on patient factors. Bioprosthetic aortic valves do not require long-term anticoagulation[37] but are less durable than mechanical valves and have an expected life of 10–15 years,

Outcome	LVEF <35% ($n = 43$)	LVEF 35–50% ($n = 134$)	LVEF >50% ($n = 273$)	P value
Operative mortality	14%	7%	4%	$P < 0.04$
10-year survival	$41 \pm 9\%$	56 ± 5	70 ± 3	$P < 0.0001$
10 year incidence of heart failure	25%	17%	9%	$P < 0.003$
Postoperative EF increase	$+4.9 \pm 2.5\%$	$+4 \pm 1.2\%$	-2.3 ± 0.8	

EF = ejection fraction; LVEF = left ventricular ejection fraction.

Table 11.3 Outcomes following aortic valve replacement in patients with severe aortic regurgitation and markedly reduced ejection fraction[36]

although this may be longer in people over 65 years. Two large, randomized trials comparing bioprosthetic and mechanical aortic valves showed an increased risk of reoperation but reduced risk of bleeding with bioprosthetic valves, and overall patient survival was significantly better with a mechanical aortic valve replacement.[38,39]

Despite improvements in left ventricular function and size following valve replacement, patients with prosthetic valves still have significant 10-year mortality and morbidity.[40,41] Guidelines recommend the use of mechanical aortic prostheses in patients younger than 65 or those in whom coexisting conditions exist for which anticoagulation is necessary.[8] Bioprosthetic valves should be used in the elderly or those with a significant contraindication to anticoagulation.

Mitral stenosis

Epidemiology

Mitral stenosis (MS) is almost always due to rheumatic deformity and scarring of the mitral apparatus. It is therefore now rare in Western countries, except in the elderly,[42] but still remains common in developing nations.[43]

Symptoms

Patients with MS usually have symptoms typical of left-sided heart failure. These stem from increased left atrial pressure and reduced cardiac output due to obstruction of filling of the left ventricle. Left ventricular systolic function is often normal but right heart failure develops secondary to pulmonary vasoconstriction:[5] 60% of asymptomatic patients remain symptom-free after 10 years, whereas only 60% of patients with NYHA II symptoms survive after 10 years.

Diagnosis

Echocardiography is central to the diagnosis of MS. Assessment of severity uses pressure half time and mitral valve area calculated from Doppler transmitral flow velocities during diastole and planimetry. Features suggestive of suitability for percutaneous balloon valvuloplasty (PBV) should be identified.

The Wilkins score is an echo index that takes into account:

- mobility of mitral valve leaflets
- leaflet thickness
- degree of subvalvular abnormality

- severity and location of calcification.

A value from 0 to 4 is assigned to each of the above categories and these values are added together to give a final 'score'. Scores of eight or less predict a good response to PBV.[44] This scoring system is still widely used, although it is less useful in certain situations, such as in the elderly, where commissural calcification seems to have a significant impact on procedural success.[42]

Other important features to identify prior to mechanical intervention include:[7]

- left atrial size and presence of thrombus
- presence and severity of mitral regurgitation
- left ventricular size and function
- associated lesions
- pulmonary artery systolic pressure.

Exercise Doppler echocardiography is a clinically established tool for assessing the functional significance of MS.[13] If discrepancies exist between the clinical picture and resting mitral valve area, the capability of performing 10 min of exercise on a standard treadmill rules out severe disease.

Treatment

- No medical therapies for MS have been shown to improve survival.
- Digoxin and diuretics can be used effectively for symptoms of congestion and heart rate control.
- Beta-blockers and calcium channel blockers can help palliate rapid atrial arrhythmias.
- MS is effectively treated using PBV, open surgical commissurotomy or mitral valve replacement.

Percutaneous balloon valvuloplasty

Indications for surgery or percutaneous balloon valvuloplasty:

- cardiac symptoms plus at least moderate MS (valve area ≤ 1.5 cm^2)
- pulmonary hypertension with moderate to severe MS.

PBV increases valve area by commissural splitting, fracture of calcium and leaflets, and partial valve disruption. Valve area increases typically from approximately 1 cm^2 to 1.8–2.0 cm^2 but may increase by only 50% in the elderly.[45] A successful procedure is defined as:

- mitral valve area increase >50%
- final valve area >1.5 cm^2
- mitral regurgitation $\leq$ grade 2.

This procedure has low hospital mortality (1–3%), morbidity, and 30-day mortality in selected individuals.[20] The rate of serious complications such as cerebrovascular accident or cardiac tamponade is 1–2%. Five-year event-free survival is greater than 70%[46] and there is a 30% rate of restenosis during the first 10 years. Thus, all patients with symptomatic MS should be actively considered for PBV.[21]

PBV is considered the treatment of choice for patients with MS if the valve is pliable and uncalcified.[47] The 5-year event-free survival of 84% after PBV is similar to that expected after surgical commissurotomy[48] and survival can be predicted by:

- mitral valve Wilkins echo score <8
- left ventricular end-diastolic pressure less than or equal to 10 mmHg
- baseline NYHA functional class II or III[49]

Although the symptom-free period is shorter than after mitral valve replacement, the procedure is cheaper with less morbidity and can be used to delay valve replacement for at least a few years. It should be used to treat MS in patients with a high risk of hemodynamic complications such as during pregnancy or where there is pulmonary hypertension. PBV has also been shown to significantly reduce the incidence of thromboembolism. It should therefore also be used in patients with few or no symptoms who have significant thromboembolic risk if they also have favorable anatomy.[50]

Patients with calcified mitral valves have been shown to achieve good immediate results following PBV but deterioration of these initial benefits occurs over time. Predictors of late deterioration include increasing age, atrial fibrillation, left ventricular systolic dysfunction, NYHA class III or IV, and markers suggestive of increased valve rigidity. PBV is thus best reserved for people with favorable characteristics[47] or for patients in whom surgical intervention is not possible.[42] Although PBV and surgical commissurotomy have comparable initial results and low rates of restenosis, open surgical commissurotomy will continue to be useful for patients with severe subvalvular disease, calcification, or left atrial thrombus.

Mitral valve replacement

No randomized comparisons have been made between valve replacement surgery and PBV in patients who are not well suited by echocardiographic criteria for PBV.[10] Valve replacement has operative mortality rates of 10–15% in the elderly but the risk increases with left ventricular dysfunction, pulmonary hypertension, advanced age, and other comorbidities.

Mitral regurgitation

Severe mitral regurgitation (MR) is most commonly caused by mitral valve prolapse. It causes progressive left ventricular remodeling, which results in increased left atrial and ventricular sizes. LVEF can be maintained in the 'normal' range despite significantly impaired left ventricular function and many patients remain asymptomatic until irreversible left ventricular dysfunction has already occurred. If one waits to operate until LVEF falls below normal, it may be too late for surgery to improve left ventricular size. Early identification of MR is therefore critical.[43]

The natural history of chronic severe MR depends upon the underlying disease process. The prognosis of patients with severe MR treated conservatively is poor[26] and NYHA class III or IV symptoms confer an annual mortality of 34% compared with 4% in patients with class I or II symptoms. The prognosis of patients treated with valve repair or replacement depends upon LVEF: if LVEF is less than 50%, survival is poor; however, survival is almost equivalent to that of the normal population if LVEF is greater than 60%.[51]

Diagnosis

Transesophageal echocardiography is useful in all patients in whom surgery is contemplated. It helps to:

- identify the mechanism of MR
- clarify the severity of MR.

Medical treatment

Despite the widespread use of ACE inhibitors in patients with congestive heart failure, hemodynamic and volumetric data on the effects of these agents in chronic MR are relatively sparse and the results conflicting.[32]

There is currently no apparent benefit from using vasodilators long term for mitral regurgitation, especially in asymptomatic patients. There have been no long-term studies showing that vasodilators delay surgery, improve survival, or improve outcome. However, patients with markedly elevated systolic left ventricular pressure such as severe hypertension or aortic stenosis may have a dramatic reduction in MR with vasodilator therapy.[52]

Concerns about vasodilator treatment in chronic mitral regurgitation

Vasodilator therapy may:

* mask the development of left ventricular dysfunction
* worsen MR in some patients.

Rheumatic valves often have fixed orifices that are unlikely to change with load manipulation, so that regurgitant volume may increase after nitrate administration.[32] Alternatively, reducing left ventricular size in a patient with mitral valve prolapse may increase the regurgitant orifice, and therefore increase MR. Vasodilator therapy should therefore generally be avoided unless MR is due to dilated cardiomyopathy.

Indications for surgery in severe chronic mitral regurgitation

* Symptoms attributed to severe MR (even NYHA class II).
* Asymptomatic, with left ventricular end-systolic diameter ≥45 mm.
* Asymptomatic, with left ventricular ejection fraction ≤60%.

Patients with right ventricular ejection fraction <30% are at especially high risk. Surgery is likely to improve symptoms and prevent further deterioration of left ventricular function even in patients with severely depressed left ventricular function.[27]

Surgical treatment

Mitral regurgitation can be treated with:

* valve repair
* mitral valve replacement, with preservation of the mitral apparatus
* mitral valve repair, with removal of the mitral apparatus.

Mitral valve repair

Successful mitral valve repair improves symptoms and preserves left ventricular function.[53] It is feasible in up to 70% referred for surgery and should be carried out rather than mitral valve replacement wherever possible.[54] This is the procedure of choice in patients with MR caused by degenerative disease and is most successful when MR is due to localized prolapse of part of the posterior leaflet but has also been used for rheumatic mitral valves.[55]

Repair is associated with low operative mortality and morbidity and excellent late survival. Retrospective, nonrandomized comparisons report 10-year survival rates after valve repair of 88% compared with 73% after mitral valve replacement. Predictors of survival include age, NYHA class, atrial fibrillation, coronary artery disease, LVEF, and left ventricular end-systolic volume.[56,57] LVEF fraction increases by approximately 4% in patients with preoperative left ventricular dysfunction. However, 16% of patients require reoperation within 10 years of the initial procedure and the chances of reoperation increase with increased complexity of the initial operation.[58]

Advantages of valve repair over valve replacement[7]

* Lower perioperative mortality rates.[52]
* Less prosthetic material used.

- Reduced need for anticoagulation.

- Lower incidence of infective endocarditis.

- Preservation of left ventricular function through retention of mitral subvalvular apparatus.

- Better late outcome than mitral valve replacement.[52]

Disadvantages

- Greater technical demands.

- Long-term durability less well-defined than for prosthetic valves.

- Not applicable to all patients.[5]

Patient selection

- Moderate distortion of valvular anatomy but pliable anterior leaflet and chordae.

- Mild disease with low Wilkins echo scores.

- Absence of aortic or tricuspid disease.

- Mixed mitral stenosis/mitral regurgitation have an increased risk of reoperation or failure.

Valve repair is highly operator-dependent, and operative mortality and long-term success are related to the experience and expertise of the surgeon and operating center. Centers operating on large numbers of patients have shown equivalent results when comparing anterior and posterior valve prolapse repair; however, smaller centers still favor anterior leaflet repair.

Mitral valve replacement

The most significant predictor of persistent left ventricular enlargement following mitral valve replacement, in patients with MR or mixed mitral stenosis and MR, is a large end-systolic volume preoperatively. Therefore, surgery should be considered before the ejection fraction decreases to < 0.5, end-systolic volume

index is greater than 50 ml/m^2, or pulmonary hypertension develops.[57]

Should valve replacement prove necessary, as much of the subvalvular apparatus as possible should be conserved to maintain left ventricular geometry and function. Division of all the chordae tendinae is accompanied by a significant reduction in left ventricular E_{max};[37] however, postoperative left ventricular function and survival improves when the apparatus is preserved.

Choice of valve replacement

Mechanical mitral valve replacements are associated with significantly lower rates of reoperation due to valve failure but a higher risk of bleeding. In two large, randomized trials comparing bioprosthetic with mechanical mitral valve replacements, actuarial patient survival was not significantly different after prolonged follow-up.[38,39]

Mechanical mitral valve replacements should be used when there are coexisting reasons for anticoagulation. Bioprostheses can be used in patients over 70 years of age.

Conclusions

- Primary valvular disease is an uncommon but treatable cause of heart failure. Heart failure secondary to severe aortic stenosis has an extremely poor prognosis but aortic valve replacement results in significant improvements in symptoms and survival.

- Aortic valvuloplasty does not improve long-term survival, carries significant periprocedural mortality and morbidity, and should only be used as a bridge to aortic valve replacement or as palliation in severely ill patients.

- Dobutamine stress echo evaluates the severity of aortic stenosis in patients with impaired left ventricular systolic function and low transvalvular gradients.

- Aortic valve replacement should not be postponed by the use of vasodilators in patients with severe aortic regurgitation and clear indications for aortic valve replacement.

- Primary balloon valvuloplasty is the treatment of choice in patients with mitral stenosis and suitable valve anatomy.

- There is no apparent benefit from using vasodilators in patients with mitral regurgitation secondary to valve disease.

- Mitral valve repair should be carried out whenever possible rather than mitral valve replacement in patients with severe mitral regurgitation.

- Mechanical prosthetic valves should be used in young patients and in those where anticoagulation is required for a coexisting condition.

References

1. Cowie MR, Wood DA, Coats AJ, et al. Incidence and aetiology of heart failure; a population-based study. Eur Heart J 1999; 20:421–8.
2. Teerlink JR, Goldhaber SZ, Pfeffer MA. An overview of contemporary etiologies of congestive heart failure. Am Heart J 1991; 121(6 Pt 1):1852–3.
3. Massie B, Shah N. Evolving trends in the epidemiologic factors of heart failure: rationale for preventive strategies and comprehensive disease management. Am Heart J 1997; 133:703–12.
4. Lip GY, Gibbs CR, Beevers DG. ABC of heart failure: aetiology. BMJ 2000; 320:104–7.
5. Carabello BA, Crawford FA Jr. Valvular heart disease N Engl J Med 1997; 337:32–41 [published erratum appears in N Engl J Med 1997 Aug 14; 337:507].
6. Wilkins GT. Valvular heart disease: putting guidelines into practice. BMJ 1997; 314: 1428–9.
7. Currie PJ. Valvular heart disease. A correctable cause of congestive heart failure. Postgrad Med 1991; 89:123–6, 131–6.
8. Bonow RO, Carabello B, de Leon AC Jr, et al. Guidelines for the management of patients with valvular heart disease: executive summary. A report of the American College of Cardiology/American Heart Association Task Force on Practice Guidelines (Committee on Management of Patients with Valvular Heart Disease). Circulation 1998; 98:1949–84.
9. Mangion JR, Tighe DA. Aortic valvular disease in adults. A potentially lethal clinical problem. Postgrad Med 1995; 98:127–35, 140.
10. Marzo K, Prigent FM, Steingart RM. Interventional therapy in heart failure management. Clin Geriatr Med 2000; 16:549–66.
11. Otto CM, Burwash IG, Legget ME, et al. Prospective study of asymptomatic valvular aortic stenosis. Clinical, echocardiographic, and exercise predictors of outcome. Circulation 1997; 95: 2262–70.
12. Horstkotte D, Loogen F. The natural history of aortic valve stenosis. Eur Heart J 1988; 9(Suppl E):57–64.
13. Schwammenthal E, Vered Z, Rabinowitz B, et al. Stress echocardiography beyond coronary artery disease. Eur Heart J 1997; 18(Suppl D):D130–7.
14. deFilippi CR, Willett DL, Brickner ME, et al. Usefulness of dobutamine echocardiography in distinguishing severe from nonsevere valvular aortic stenosis in patients with depressed left ventricular function and low transvalvular gradients. Am J Cardiol 1995; 75:191–4.
15. Greenberg BH, Massie BM. Beneficial effects of afterload reduction therapy in patients with con-

gestive heart failure and moderate aortic stenosis. Circulation 1980; 61:1212–16.

16. Smedira NG, Ports TA, Merrick SH, Rankin JS. Balloon aortic valvuloplasty as a bridge to aortic valve replacement in critically ill patients. Ann Thorac Surg 1993; 55:914–16.

17. Kastrup J, Wennevold A, Thuesen L, et al. Short- and long-term survival after aortic balloon valvuloplasty for calcified aortic stenosis in 137 elderly patients. Danish Med Bull 1994; 41:362–5.

18. Lieberman EB, Bashore TM, Hermiller JB, et al. Balloon aortic valvuloplasty in adults: failure of procedure to improve long-term survival. J Am Coll Cardiol 1995; 26:1522–8.

19. Anonymous. Percutaneous balloon aortic valvuloplasty. Acute and 30-day follow-up results in 674 patients from the NHLBI Balloon Valvuloplasty Registry. Circulation 1991; 84:2383–97.

20. Anonymous. Complications and mortality of percutaneous balloon mitral commissurotomy. A report from the National Heart, Lung, and Blood Institute Balloon Valvuloplasty Registry. Circulation 1992; 85:2014–24.

21. Prendergast BD, Banning AP, Hall RJ. Valvular heart disease: recommendations for investigation and management. Summary of guidelines produced by a working group of the British Cardiac Society and the Research Unit of the Royal College of Physicians. J Roy Coll Phys London 1996; 30:309–15.

22. Park R, Schmidt DH, Shalev Y, Bajwa TK. Percutaneous balloon aortic valvuloplasty in high-risk elderly patients. Wisconsin Med J 1995; 94:537–41.

23. Lieberman EB, Wilson JS, Harrison JK, et al. Aortic valve replacement in adults after balloon aortic valvuloplasty. Circulation 1994; 90(5 Pt 2): II205–8.

24. Rahimtoola SH. Severe aortic stenosis with low systolic gradient: the good and bad news [editorial; comment]. Circulation 2000; 101:1892–4.

25. Gaasch WH, Sundaram M, Meyer TE. Managing asymptomatic patients with chronic aortic regurgitation. Chest 1997; 111:1702–9.

26. Grayburn PA. Vasodilator therapy for chronic aortic and mitral regurgitation. Am J Med Sci 2000; 320:202–8.

27. Bonow RO, Dodd JT, Maron BJ, et al. Long-term serial changes in left ventricular function and reversal of ventricular dilatation after valve replacement for chronic aortic regurgitation. Circulation 1988; 78(5 Pt 1):1108–20.

28. Siemienczuk D, Greenberg B, Morris C, et al. Chronic aortic insufficiency: factors associated with progression to aortic valve replacement. Ann Intern Med 1989; 110:587–92.

29. Henry WL, Bonow RO, Borer JS, et al. Observations on the optimum time for operative intervention for aortic regurgitation. I. Evaluation of the results of aortic valve replacement in symptomatic patients. Circulation 1980; 61:471–83.

30. Dujardin KS, Enriquez-Sarano M, Schaff HV, et al. Mortality and morbidity of aortic regurgitation in clinical practice. A long-term follow-up study. Circulation 1999; 99:1851–7.

31. Sondergaard L, Aldershvile J, Hildebrandt P, et al. Vasodilatation with felodipine in chronic asymptomatic aortic regurgitation. Am Heart J 2000; 139:667–74.

32. Levine HJ, Gaasch WH. Vasoactive drugs in chronic regurgitant lesions of the mitral and aortic valves. J Am Coll Cardiol 1996; 28:1083–91.

33. Scognamiglio R, Rahimtoola SH, Fasoli G, et al. Nifedipine in asymptomatic patients with severe aortic regurgitation and normal left ventricular function. N Engl J Med 1994; 331:689–94.

34. Khan S, Chaux A, Matloff J, et al. The St. Jude Medical valve. Experience with 1,000 cases. J Thorac Cardiovasc Surg 1994; 108:1010–19; discussion 1019–20.

35. Klodas E, Enriquez-Sarano M, Tajik AJ, et al. Optimizing timing of surgical correction in patients with severe aortic regurgitation: role of symptoms. J Am Coll Cardiol 1997; 30:746–52.

36. Chaliki H, Mohty D, Averinos J, et al. Outcomes following aortic valve replacement in patients with severe aortic regurgitation and markedly reduced ejection fraction. J Am Coll Cardiol 2001; 37(Suppl A):486A.

37. Westaby S. Non-transplant surgery for heart failure. Heart 2000; 83:603–10.

38. Hammermeister K, Sethi G, Henderson W, et al. A comparison of outcomes in men 11 years after heart-valve replacement with a mechanical valve or bioprosthesis. N Engl J Med 1993; 328:1289–96.

39. Bloomfield P, Wheatley D, Prescott R, Miller H. Twelve-year comparison of a Bjork–Shiley mechanical heart valve with porcine bioprostheses. N Engl J Med 1991; 324:573–9.

40. Braunwald E. Aortic valve replacement: an update at the turn of the millennium. Eur Heart J 2000; 21:1032–3.

41. Kvidal P, Bergstrom R, Malm T, Stahle E. Long-term follow-up of morbidity and mortality after aortic valve replacement with a mechanical valve prosthesis. Eur Heart J 2000; 21:1099–111.

42. Sutaria N, Elder AT, Shaw TR. Long term outcome of percutaneous mitral balloon valvotomy in patients aged 70 and over . Heart 2000; 83:433–8.

43. Harris KM, Robiolio P. Valvular heart disease. Identifying and managing mitral and aortic lesions. Postgrad Med 1999; 106:113–14, 117–20, 125 passim.

44. Wilkins GT, Weyman AE, Abascal VM, et al. Percutaneous balloon dilatation of the mitral valve: an analysis of echocardiographic variables related to outcome and the mechanism of dilatation. Br Heart J 1988; 60:299–308.

45. Hildick-Smith DJ, Shapiro LM. Balloon mitral valvuloplasty in the elderly. Heart 2000; 83:374–5.

46. Tuzcu EM, Block PC, Griffin BP, et al. Immediate and long-term outcome of percutaneous mitral valvotomy in patients 65 years and older. Circulation 1992; 85:963–71.

47. Iung B, Garbarz E, Doutrelant L, et al. Late results of percutaneous mitral commissurotomy for calcific mitral stenosis. Am J Cardiol 2000; 85:1308–14.

48. Reyes VP, Raju BS, Wynne J, et al. Percutaneous balloon valvuloplasty compared with open surgical commissurotomy for mitral stenosis. N Engl J Med 1994; 331:961–7.

49. Cohen DJ, Kuntz RE, Gordon SP, et al. Predictors of long-term outcome after percutaneous balloon mitral valvuloplasty. New Engl J Med 1992; 327:1329–35.

50. Vahanian A, Michel PL, Cormier B, et al. Results of percutaneous mitral commissurotomy in 200 patients. Am J Cardiol 1989; 63:847–52.

51. Enriquez-Sarano M, Tajik AJ, Schaff HV, et al. Echocardiographic prediction of survival after surgical correction of organic mitral regurgitation. Circulation 1994; 90:830–7.

52. Hochreiter C, Niles N, Devereux RB, et al. Mitral regurgitation: relationship of noninvasive descriptors of right and left ventricular performance to clinical and hemodynamic findings and to prognosis in medically and surgically treated patients. Circulation 1986; 73:900–12.

53. Enriquez-Sarano M, Orszulak TA, Schaff HV, et al. Mitral regurgitation: a new clinical perspective. Mayo Clin Proc 1997; 72:1034–43.

54. Lee EM, Shapiro LM, Wells FC. Superiority of mitral valve repair in surgery for degenerative mitral regurgitation. Eur Heart J 1997; 18:655–63.

55. Yau TM, El-Ghoneimi YA, Armstrong S, et al. Mitral valve repair and replacement for rheumatic disease. J Thorac Cardiovasc Surg 2000; 119:53–60.

56. Enriquez-Sarano M, Schaff HV, Orszulak TA, et al. Congestive heart failure after surgical correction of mitral regurgitation. A long-term study. Circulation 1995; 92:2496–503.

57. Crawford MH, Souchek J, Oprian CA, et al. Determinants of survival and left ventricular performance after mitral valve replacement. Department of Veterans Affairs Cooperative Study on Valvular Heart Disease. Circulation 1990; 81:1173–81.

58. Ling LH, Enriquez-Sarano M, Seward JB, et al. Clinical outcome of mitral regurgitation due to flail leaflet. N Engl J Med 1996; 335:1417–23.

12

Heart failure and arrhythmia
Irina Savelieva and A John Camm

Introduction: mortality and cardiac arrhythmias in heart failure

The syndrome of chronic heart failure has a multifactorial etiology and involves multiple mechanisms of pathogenesis operating at different stages as the disease progresses. The annual mortality rate associated with this condition is high, ranging from 5–15% in mild heart failure to 20–50% in moderate-to-severe heart failure and often exceeding 50% in patients with advanced disease.[1] Sudden death is responsible for about half of all cardiac deaths in patients with heart failure. From a recent report from MERIT-HF (Metoprolol CR/XL Randomized Intervention Trial in Congestive Heart Failure) study, the relative prevalence of sudden death in patients with NYHA (New York Heart Association) class II, III, and IV heart failure was 64%, 59%, and 33%, respectively.[2] Nonsustained ventricular tachycardia and atrial fibrillation are common findings in heart failure and are generally associated with more severe left ventricular dysfunction and increased mortality. However, the prognostic significance of these arrhythmias remains largely unproven, suggesting a complex interplay between mechanisms of arrhythmogenesis and the progression of circulatory failure. Empirical antiarrhythmic therapy aimed at suppression of the arrhythmia is, therefore, often ineffective for improvement of prognosis and may have an increased risk of proarrhythmia and worsening heart failure. The utility of conventional risk factors is limited in heart failure patients, and strategies need to be devised to identify those who would benefit most from antiarrhythmic therapy.

Ventricular arrhythmias in heart failure

Prevalence and prognosis

Ventricular arrhythmias are almost ubiquitous in heart failure, ranging from 10–25% in patients with NYHA class I and II up to 50–80% in patients with NYHA class III or IV heart failure.[3-6]

Many (but not all) studies have shown that the presence of frequent ventricular ectopic activity and nonsustained ventricular tachycardia is associated with an increased all-cause mortality and sudden death in patients with heart failure.[4,5,7,8] In the GESICA (Gruppo de Estudio de la Sobrevida en la Insuficiencia Cardiaca en Argentina) study of 516 patients (80% NYHA class III or IV), those with nonsustained ventricular tachycardia had a nearly 3-fold increased risk for sudden death compared with those without this arrhythmia.[4] The presence of nonsustained ventricular tachycardia was also associated with an increased 2-year all-cause mortality (50.5% vs 30.9%). However, in the CHF-STAT (Congestive Heart Failure – Survival Trial of Antiarrhythmic Therapy) study involving 667 patients with an ejection fraction ≤40%, and ≥10 ventricular premature beats per hour, the presence of nonsustained ventricular tachycardia (80% of patients) was associated with sudden death in univariate analysis, but lost its predictive power in multivariate models.[5] Furthermore, in patients with moderate-to-severe heart failure, the presence of ventricular arrhythmias on 24-hour Holter electrocardiogram (ECG) recording does not specifically predict sudden death. Although in the Vasodilator in Heart Failure Trial II (V-HeFT II), the occurrence of sudden death was higher in patients with ventricular ectopic activity on Holter ECG than in those without arrhythmias (15.9% vs 10.3%), the presence of ventricular arrhythmias was an independent predictor for total mortality (44.2% vs 24.9%) but not for sudden death after adjustment for other univariate predictors.[9] In 1080 patients with NYHA III or IV class symptoms, studied in the PROMISE (Prospective Randomized Milrinone Survival Evaluation) trial, the presence and the number of episodes of nonsustained ventricular tachycardia carried a 1.12 (95% CI 1.07–1.17) relative risk for all-cause mortality and 1.16 (95% CI 1.09–1.24) for sudden death, but did not discriminate between patients who died suddenly or from progressive heart failure.[6] Finally, in the ATLAS (Assessment of Treatment with Lisinopril and Survival) study of 3164 patients with heart failure ventricular tachycardia preceded heart failure death in 9.4% of cases compared with 7.3% of cases of sudden cardiac death.[10] Therefore, there is uncertainty whether the presence of ventricular ectopic activity is an independent determinant for

sudden death or merely related to the extent of myocardial dysfunction and the severity of heart failure. It is likely that the frequency and complexity of ventricular arrhythmias more closely relate to the progression of heart failure and all-cause mortality than sudden arrhythmic death. There are data suggesting that ventricular arrhythmias appear to be more specific predictors of sudden death in patients with less severe heart failure, whereas in patients with advanced heart failure, other mechanisms, such as bradycardia and electromechanical dissociation, may be responsible for cardiac arrest.[8,11]

'Antiarrhythmic effects' of angiotensin-converting enzyme inhibitors

Role of neurohormonal activation and stretch in arrhythmogenesis

Increased neurohormonal activity is nearly omnipresent in patients with heart failure and appears to contribute independently to progression of the disease and mortality. In the SOLVD (Studies Of Left Ventricular Dysfunction) and SAVE (Survival And Ventricular Enlargement) studies, patients with even clinically asymptomatic left ventricular dysfunction who died or developed severe heart failure had markedly and persistently elevated levels of plasma neurohormones, including norepinephrine, aldosterone, and atrial natriuretic peptide.[12,13]

There are a number of ways by which neurohumoral imbalance may contribute to arrhythmogenesis in heart failure, including progression of myocardial dysfunction, facilitation of myocardial hypertrophy and fibrosis, and promotion of electrophysiologic instability. Angiotensin II promotes interstitial myocardial fibrosis, which may create a substrate for re-entrant tachyarrhythmias. Myocardial hypertrophy in heart failure is invariably associated with prolonged repolarization and early afterdepolarizations that may initiate triggered activity. Excessive adrenergic stimulation can increase inward calcium currents, potentiating delayed afterdepolarizations and enhanced automaticity.

The stretch-mediated pathophysiologic mechanism of arrhythmogenesis is responsible for a significant proportion of atrial and ventricular arrhythmias in heart failure. The presence of various types of stretch-specific channels, which may generate both inward and outward currents, has been identified in cardiac myocytes, including nonselective calcium/sodium and potassium ion channels and selective potassium or chloride ion channels.[14,15] Activation of an inward current (i_{SA}) and inactivation of an outward current (i_{SI}) favor the development of triggered activity arising from delayed and early afterdepolarizations. Finally, stretch has been shown to further stimulate the synthesis of angiotensin II, which can induce myocyte hypertrophy and contributes to electrophysiologic instability by direct effects on membrane currents.

Effects of angiotensin-converting enzymes inhibitors on ventricular arrhythmias and sudden death

The beneficial effects of angiotensin-converting enzymes (ACE) inhibitors on survival in heart failure have been consistently shown in a large number of trials in patients with overt heart failure[16–19] and less severe or clinically asymptomatic left ventricular systolic dysfunction[10–23] (Table 12.1). A combined analysis of data from 32 studies in over 7000 patients with heart failure and a recent meta-analysis of 15 trials in over 15,000 patients with myocardial infarction have uniformly shown that treatment with ACE inhibitors significantly reduced all-cause mortality (by 23% and 17%, respectively).[24] There was a trend toward reduction in sudden death in patients with heart failure, including the CONSENSUS and SOLVD populations, and a 20% decrease in risk for sudden death in patients with myocardial infarction, including TRACE, AIRE, and SAVE populations with clinical or asymptomatic left ventricular systolic dysfunction. In the V-HeFT I and II studies, the suppression of nonsustained ventricular tachycardia by 27% in patients treated with enalapril compared with the hydralazine–isosorbide dinitrate group was associated with a 52% reduction in sudden death at 1 year.[25] Furthermore, treatment with enalapril prevented the occurrence of new ventricular tachycardia by 54%. Recently, the Task Force on Sudden Cardiac Death of the European Society of Cardiology classified the results of clinical trials on survival benefits of ACE inhibition as a high level of evidence and put ACE inhibitors, along with beta-blockers and aldosterone receptor blockers as class I recommended drugs for primary prevention of sudden death in myocardial infarction and heart failure among the agents without electrophysiologic properties.[26]

The beneficial effect of ACE inhibitors on mortality appears to be due to other mechanisms rather than merely modification of ventricular remodeling, prevention of ischemia, and improvement of mechanical ventricular function. These include alleviation of wall stress, modulation of refractoriness, interference with ion currents, modification of cardiac autonomic status, and stabilization of electrolyte balance. However, in other studies, such as CONSENSUS and SOLVD, ACE inhibitors reduced total mortality but did not

ACEI	Study	No. of patients	Patient characteristics	Follow-up	Effect on arrhythmias	Effect on sudden death	Risk reduction for all-cause mortality
Enalapril: Initial dose 2.5 mg Treatment dose 5–20 mg; up to 40 mg in CONSENSUS	CONSENSUS[17] SOLVD Px[19]	253 4228	HF NYHA IV Asymptomatic ventricular dysfunction, EF ≤0.35	188 days >3 years	– No effects on VA in a substudy	– 4.6% ACEI vs 5.0% placebo (*P* = 0.10); 10% reduction in death due to arrhythmias	27% 8%
	SOLVD Rx[20]	2568	Symptomatic HF, >3 years EF ≤0.35	>3 years	–	8.2% ACEI vs 8.8% placebo; 10% risk reduction (*P* >0.25)	16%
	V-HeFT II[25]	804	HF NYHA I–III, EF ≤0.45, CTR >0.55	2.5 years	Suppression of NSVT by 27% and prevention of new VA by 54%	52% risk reduction ACEI vs hydralazine	Mortality 32.7% ACEI vs 38.2% hydralazine (*P* = 0.016)
Cantopril: Initial dose 12.5 mg Treatment dose 50–100 mg; up to 400 mg in Hy-C	SAVE[23]	2231	MI 3–16 days, asymptomatic ventricular dysfunction, EF ≤0.40	42 months	Suppression of VA in a Holter substudy	9.4% ACEI vs 11.2% placebo	19%
	Hy-C[18]	117	HF NYHA III–IV	8 ± 7 months	–	5% ACEI vs 37% hydralazine	Mortality 19% ACEI; 49% hydralazine
Ramipril: Initial dose 1.25–2.5 mg Treatment dose 5–10 mg	AIRE[22]	2006	MI 3–10 days, clinical HF	15 months	Severe SVA leading to death occurred in 11 patients on ACEI vs 37 patients on placebo	30% risk reduction	27%

Continued

Table 12.1 Clinical evidence of effects of angiotensin-converting enzyme inhibitors on arrhythmias and sudden death in patients with left ventricular dysfunction

| Trandolapril: Initial dose 1 mg Treatment dose 2–4 mg | TRACE[21] | 1749 | MI 2–6 days, NYHA I, II (59% symptomatic), EF ≤0.35 | 24–50 months | 55% risk reduction for AF | 24% risk reduction; reduction in arrhythmia cause of death (24 patients on ACEI vs 36 patients on placebo) | 22% |
| Lisinopril: Initial dose 2.5 mg Treatment dose 2.5–5 mg (low) 32.5–35 mg (high) | ATLAS[16] | 3164 | HF NYHA II–IV, EF ≤0.30, other risk factors | 46 months | – | – | 8% with a high dose Mortality 44.1% if antiarrhythmics present vs 43.6% if no antiarrhythmics |

ACEI = angiotensin-convering enzyme inhibitor; AF = atrial fibrillation; CTR = cardiothoracic ratio; EF = ejection fraction; HF = heart failure; MI = myocardial infarction; NSVT = nonsustained ventricular tachycardia; NYHA = New York Heart Association; SVA = supraventricular arrhythmia; VA = ventricular arrhythmia.

Table 12.1 *Continued*

suppress ventricular arrhythmias and did not prevent sudden death, although less ventricular ectopy was noted in Holter substudies.[27,28] This discrepancy may be explained, in part, by different interpretation of mode of death and definitions of sudden death used in these studies as it has been proved for SOLVD and V-HeFT trials. Agreement in classification of mode of death in the V-HeFT population by V-HeFT and SOLVD investigators was achieved for only half the cases. In some studies, death from cardiac arrest following significant worsening heart failure was qualified as death from progressive pump failure. In the V-HeFT studies, the beneficial effects of an ACE inhibitor on ventricular arrhythmias were seen over hydralazine and isosorbide dinitrate but were not evaluated against placebo. Pharmacologic differences between the different types of ACE inhibitors and a higher proportion of patients taking beta-blockers in later studies may account for the difference in the effects of ACE inhibitors on sudden death.

Beta-blockers

Rationale for beta-blocker therapy in heart failure

Although raised circulating catecholamines and increased cardiac adrenergic drive are aimed to compensate for decreased cardiac output at early stages of heart failure, they ultimately lead to exacerbation of myocardial dysfunction, directly correlating with disease progression and mortality. Cardiotoxic effects of catecholamines can be mediated through both beta- and alpha$_1$-adrenoreceptors, which are constitutively activated in heart failure and have been shown to promote myocardial hypertrophy. Excessive sympathetic stimulation

and shift in the cardiac myocyte adrenergic receptor profile result in augmentation of excitability due to delayed afterdepolarizations and triggered activity.[29,30]

Effects of beta-blockers on sudden death

In a meta-analysis of 22 trials in 10,135 patients with heart failure, treatment with beta-blockers confers a significant survival benefit by reducing the risk of death by 35%.[31] Although this reduction in mortality rates was primarily due to the prevention of death from worsening heart failure, the results of large trials have suggested that the beneficial survival effects of beta-blockade are not limited to the prevention of progression of heart failure but may result from the reduction in sudden cardiac death (Table 12.2).[2,32–40]

The MERIT-HF[2] and CIBIS II[38] (Cardiac Insufficiency Bisoprolol Study II) using selective beta$_1$-blockers, metoprolol and bisoprolol, enrolled over 6600 patients with clinically significant heart failure and showed nearly identical results: the risk of all-cause death was reduced by 34% in both studies, which was largely attributable to the reduction in risk of sudden death (41% and 52%, respectively). In two recently completed studies in patients with advanced heart failure and a left ventricular ejection fraction <25% (COPERNICUS: Carvedilol Prospective Randomized Cumulative Survival) and in patients with myocardial infarction and left ventricular dysfunction (CAPRICORN: Carvedilol Post-Infarct Survival Control in Left Ventricular Dysfunction), treatment with carvedilol was associated with a 24% and 26% reduction in risk for sudden death, respectively.[39,40]

However, another study of the efficacy of beta-blocker therapy with bucindolol 50–100

Beta-blocker	Study	No. of patients	Patient characteristics	Follow-up	Risk reduction for all-cause mortality	Risk reduction for sudden death
Propranolol: 180 mg	BHAT-CHF[37]	710	MI 5–21 days, clinical HF	25 months	27%	47%
Metoprolol: Initial dose 10 mg Target dose 100–150 mg (mean 108 mg)	MDC[34]	383	EF <0.40	12–18 months	34%	–
Metoprolol CR/XL: Initial dose 12.5–25 mg Target dose 200 mg (mean 159 mg)	MERIT-HF[2]	3991	NYHA II–IV, EF ≤0.40	1 year	34%	41%
Bisoprolol: Initial dose 1.25 mg Target dose 5 mg, 10 mg in CIBIS II	CIBIS I[32]	641	NYHA III, IV EF <0.40	22.8 months	20%	21%
	CIBIS II[38]	2647	NYHA III, IV EF ≤0.35	1.3 years	34%	52%
Carvedilol 12.5–50 mg	MOCHA[33]	345	6-min walk 15–450 m, EF ≤0.35	6 months	73%	–
Carvedilol: 50 mg	ANZ[35]	415	Stable HF, EF <0.45	19 months	25%	9%
Carvedilol: 50–100 mg	US Carvedilol[36]	1094	NYHA II–IV EF ≤0.35	6–12 months	65%	–
Carvedilol: Initial dose 6.25 mg Titration dose biweekly 12.5–25 mg Target dose 50 mg	COPERNICUS[39]	2289	NYHA III, IV EF ≤0.25	10.4 months	30%	24%
Carvedilol: Target dose 50 mg	CAPRICORN[40]	1959	± NYHA, EF ≤0.40, MI 3–21 days	1.3 years	23%	26%

Continued

Table 12.2 Clinical evidence of effects of beta-blockers on ventricular arrhythmias and sudden death in patients with left ventricular dysfunction

Bucindolol: Initial dose 6 mg Titration dose 12.5, 25, 50 mg Target dose 100 mg; 200 mg if weight ≥75 kg	BEST[41]	2708	NYHA III (92%), IV	2 years	Annual mortality 15% on bucindolol vs 17% on placebo; 10% risk reduction (P = 0.10)	14% risk reduction for cardiovascular death (P = 0.04), 12% risk reduction for sudden death (P = 0.21)

Table 12.2 *Continued*

mg twice daily in 2708 patients with NYHA class III and IV heart failure, Beta-blocker Evaluation of Survival Trial (BEST), did not show any benefit in terms of all-cause mortality or sudden death.[41] Like carvedilol, bucindolol is a third-generation nonselective beta-blocker with mild vasodilating action. However, compared with carvedilol, the alpha$_1$-blocking properties of bucindolol are significantly weaker (beta$_1$/alpha$_1$ selectivity is 2.4 vs 66) and the beta$_2$-blocking effects are stronger (beta$_1$/beta$_2$ selectivity is 7.3 vs 1.4), making it an exclusively sympatholytic agent. In the BEST study, bucindolol decreased systemic norepinephrine levels by 19%. It is possible that irreversible loss of adrenergic support to the failing heart caused by sympatholytic effects of bucindolol and insufficient vasodilating action, which potentially counteracts the initial decrease in cardiac output, may attenuate benefits of bucindolol in patients with severely depressed ventricular function early in the course of therapy. Furthermore, the myocardial alpha$_1$-receptors have been implicated in hypertrophy and remodeling.

Presently, only bisoprolol, carvedilol, and metoprolol have been recommended by the Task Force for the Diagnosis and Treatment of Chronic Heart Failure of the European Society of Cardiology for treatment of patients with heart failure.[42] The effects of different types of beta-blockers on the risk of death and hospitalizations during a 3-year follow-up will be compared in the Carvedilol or Metoprolol European Trial (COMET) in more than 3000 patients with NYHA II to IV heart failure due to ischemic or nonischemic cardiomyopathy. Nebivolol, a third-generation beta-blocking agent with a nearly 300-fold affinity to beta$_1$-adrenoreceptors, without alpha$_1$-blocking properties, is now under investigation (SENIORS).

Suppression of ventricular arrhythmias

Although an antiarrhythmic effect of beta-blockade is generally accepted, there is uncertainty as to whether these agents reduced sudden death in patients with heart failure by preventing ventricular arrhythmias. In the BHAT study, propranolol suppressed ventricular ectopic activity and prevented sudden cardiac death in post myocardial infarction patients.[43] In the CIBIS I study of 641 patients with NYHA class III heart failure (95%), there was a significantly lower incidence of ventricular tachycardia or ventricular fibrillation in the bisoprolol group compared with placebo (5 vs 14 events).[32] Carvedilol has been shown to suppress all forms of ventricular ectopic activity in patients with idiopathic and ischemic heart failure and complex ventricular arrhythmias.[44] However, in the Spanish Study on Sudden Death (SSSD) of 368 post myocardial infarction patients with an ejection fraction of 20–45% and at least 3 ventricular premature beats per hour, the decline in ventricular ectopic activity on Holter in patients receiving metoprolol did not differ from spontaneous variations in the untreated group.[45]

There may be several explanations for this discrepancy. First, ventricular arrhythmias detected during Holter monitoring may not predict sudden death and, second, sudden death may not be a primary electrical event but a result of myocardial infarction, aortic rupture, or pulmonary and systemic embolism, or may be due to bradyarrhythmias and electromechanical dissociation. Autopsy data from the ATLAS study have shown that sudden death in a significant proportion of patients with ischemic heart failure was due to acute coronary event.[46]

Use of diuretics and arrhythmic death

Electrolyte imbalance due to hyperaldosteronism and diuretic therapy resulting in hypokalemia and hypomagnesemia may increase susceptibility to ventricular arrhythmias.[47] Hypokalemia favors both enhanced automaticity and the development of afterdepolarizations by means of prolonging the rapid phase of ventricular repolarization. In addition to sodium retention and potassium depletion and increased vascular resistance, aldosterone promotes heart failure by stimulating myocardial and vascular fibrosis, causing direct vascular damage, leading to excessive sympathetic stimulation and baroreceptor dysfunction, suggesting that aldosterone antagonists may have a substantial cardioprotective action.

A retrospective analysis of 6797 SOLVD participants revealed that the use of nonpotassium-sparing diuretics was associated with a nearly 2-fold increase in the risk of arrhythmic death in univariate analysis and remained significantly increased (1.33) after adjustment for other risk factors.[48] In a small series of 42 patients with moderate-to-severe heart failure, the addition of spironolactone to an ACE inhibitor and a loop diuretic in a random, placebo-controlled fashion resulted in a significant reduction in the number of ventricular ectopic beats during Holter monitoring compared with placebo.[49] Finally, in the Randomized Aldactone Evaluation Study (RALES), spironolactone reduced the risk for all-cause death by 30% compared with placebo in 1663 patients with severe heart failure who were treated with an ACE inhibitor, a loop diuretic and digoxin.[50] This reduction in total mortality was attributed to a lower risk of both deaths from progressive heart failure (36%) and sudden cardiac death (29%).

Specific antiarrhythmic therapy for ventricular arrhythmias in heart failure

Adverse effects of class I antiarrhythmic drugs

The use of antiarrhythmic drugs is known to carry a particular risk of life-threatening proarrhythmia in the setting of heart failure. The results of CAST (Cardiac Arrhythmia Suppression Trials) revealed that although class I antiarrhythmic agents effectively suppressed ventricular ectopic activity in post myocardial infarction patients, one-third of whom had an a ejection fraction less than 40% and about a half had a history of clinical heart failure, all-cause mortality and sudden death rates were increased by 2.64-fold and 3.6-fold, respectively.[51,52] In the first Stroke Prevention Atrial Fibrillation (SPAF) study, the nonrandomized use of class I antiarrhythmic agents, such as quinidine and procainamide, in patients with heart failure and atrial fibrillation, was associated with a 5.8-fold increase in risk for cardiac death.[53] Furthermore, the propafenone arm of the Cardiac Arrest Study Hamburg (CASH), in which patients were randomized to antiarrhythmic drug therapy (propafenone, metoprolol, amiodarone) or an implantable cardioverter–defibrillator (ICD), was stopped prematurely after a mean follow-up of 11.3 months. The reason was a 61% higher all-cause mortality rate, as well as arrhythmic or sudden death rates, in the drug treatment arm.[54] Data from the Multicenter UnSustained Tachycardia Trial (MUSTT) showed a trend toward worse survival in patients with coronary heart disease, an ejection fraction 40% or less and asymptomatic, nonsustained ventricular tachycardia assigned to electrophysiologically guided propafenone compared with no antiarrhythmic therapy.[55] As a result it is now generally agreed that class I drugs should be avoided in the management of heart failure patients.

Sotalol

In the ESVEM (Electrophysiology Study Versus Electrocardiographic Monitoring) study of patients with sustained ventricular tachyarrhythmias or resuscitated cardiac arrest, inducible sustained ventricular tachycardia and a mean ejection fraction of 31–34%, treatment with d,l-sotalol significantly reduced arrhythmia recurrence and was associated with a lower all-cause mortality compared with class I antiarrhythmic drugs.[56] A trend toward lower recurrence rates was also observed in a subgroup of patients with an ejection fraction less than 25% and severe heart failure. However, this study was designed to compare the predictive accuracy of two techniques for long-term therapy of sustained ventricular tachyarrhythmias and was not powered to assess survival benefits.

The Survival With Oral D-sotalol (SWORD) was a trial of a pure class III antiarrhythmic drug, d-sotalol, for prophylactic use in patients with a recent myocardial infarction and symptomatic or asymptomatic left ventricular dysfunction (an ejection fraction 40% or less) or remote myocardial infarction and clinical heart failure. The study was terminated prematurely because of an increased mortality rate associated with treatment with d-sotalol (5.5% compared with 3.1% in the placebo group), resulting in a 1.65-fold increased risk, primarily due to sudden or arrhythmic death.[57] It has been suggested that in patients with impaired myocardial perfusion secondary to coronary heart disease, d-sotalol may prolong action potential duration in a nonuniform fashion, thus promoting dispersion of

refractoriness, which may predispose to an increased risk of arrhythmias.[58] Based on these data, the Task Force on Sudden Cardiac Death of the European Society of Cardiology did not recommend sotalol for the prevention of sudden death in patients with left ventricular dysfunction.[26]

Amiodarone

Effects on survival and mode of death

Amiodarone is presently the only approved antiarrhythmic drug that has a beneficial effect on survival, largely due to the prevention of sudden/arrhythmic death in patients with left ventricular systolic dysfunction. Although adopted as a class III antiarrhythmic drug due to its blocking effects on the delayed potassium rectifying current, resulting in the prolongation of action potential duration, amiodarone exerts multichannel action by inhibiting sodium and calcium currents, adding to its antiarrhythmic effect. Amiodarone has additional benefits in the presence of heart failure by virtue of its antiadrenergic and sympatholytic effects. It has been shown to noncompetitively block alpha- and beta-adrenoreceptors and to decrease the cardiac norepinephrine spillover rate.

The two largest amiodarone trials in patients with acute or recent myocardial infarction with an ejection fraction less than 40% (EMIAT) or with frequent ventricular arrhythmias as the main inclusion criterion (CAMIAT) both reported substantial and statistically significant reductions in the risk of arrhythmic death or resuscitated cardiac arrest, but a neutral effect on overall mortality or death from progressive heart failure (Table 12.3).[59,60] The other two large trials, GESICA and CHF-STAT, have specifically addressed the issue of the efficacy of amiodarone in patients with overt heart failure, including those with idiopathic dilated

Dose of amiodarone	Study	No. of patients	Patient characteristics	Follow-up	Effect on arrhythmias	Effect on sudden death	Effect on all-cause mortality
Loading dose 600 mg for 2 weeks Maintenance dose 300 mg	GESICA[61]	516	CHF NYHA II–IV, EF ≤0.35, CTR >0.55, LVED ≥3.2 cm/m², NSVT >10 beats excluded	2 years	Persistence of NSVT was associated with an increased all-cause mortality (RR = 1.75) and sudden death (RR = 2.77)	27% risk reduction	28% risk reduction; 23% risk reduction from HF
Loading dose 800 mg for 2 weeks Maintenance dose 400 mg for 50 weeks, then 200 mg	CHF-STAT[62]	674	CHF NYHA II–IV, EF ≤0.40, CTR >0.50, LVED >5.5 cm/m², VPC ≥10/hour	2 years	Decrease in the number of patients with NSVT from 77% to 33% at 3 months; reduction in the number of VPC from 254±370 to 44±145/hour	15% on amiodarone vs 19% on placebo (ns)	No effect; 44% reduction in hospitalizations and cardiac death in nonischemic HF
Loading dose 10 mg/kg for 2 weeks Maintenance dose 400 mg (300 mg if <60 kg or >75 years) If arrhythmias suppressed, 200–300 mg daily for 4 months, then 200 mg 5–7 days per week	CAMIAT[60]	1202	MI (6–45 days), VPC ≥10/hour or NSVT, 24% clinical CHF	2 years	Suppression of the arrhythmia in 84% on amiodarone vs 35% on placebo at 4 months, in 86% vs 39% at 8 months	38.2% risk reduction for VF+arrhythmic death), 29.3% risk reduction for arrhythmic death only (*P* = 0.097)	18.3% risk reduction (ns)

Continued

Table 12.3 Clinical evidence of efficacy of amiodarone for prevention of sudden death in patients with left ventricular dysfunction

EMIAT[59]	1486	MI (>5 days), EF ≤0.40, 40% NSVT	Loading dose 800 mg for 2 weeks Maintenance dose 400 mg for 14 weeks, then 200 mg	2 years	Persistence of the arrhythmia was associated with an increased all-cause mortality (20% vs 10%)	35% risk reduction	13.9% on amiodarone vs 13.7% on placebo
Meta-analysis[63]	6500	Includes patients with MI and CHF	—	—	—	29%	13%

CHF = congestive heart failure; CTR = cardiothoracic ratio; EF = ejection fraction; HF = heart failure; LVED = left ventricular end-diastolic dimension; MI = myocardial infarction; ns = not significant; NSVT = nonsustained ventricular tachycardia; NYHA = New York Heart Association; RR = relative risk; VF = ventricular fibrillation; VPC = ventricular premature complex.

Table 12.3   *Continued*

cardiomyopathy. The GESICA study has shown that low-dose amiodarone reduced total mortality by 28%, sudden death by 27%, and death from progressive pump failure by 23%.[61] Consistent with antiadrenergic and especially sympatholytic properties of amiodarone, the subgroup analysis revealed that patients with baseline heart rate more than 90 beats/min conferred most benefit from treatment. However, in the CHF-STAT study of 674 patients with NYHA class II–IV heart failure, amiodarone did not affect sudden death or total mortality, although it showed that treatment with amiodarone resulted in a statistically significant increase in left ventricular ejection fraction.[62] The difference between these two trials may be attributable to the different proportion of patients with ischemic heart failure: 31% in GESICA and 71% in CHF-STAT, which is suggestive of the more beneficial affect of amiodarone on the reduction of risk for sudden death in nonischemic heart failure.

A recent meta-analysis of 13 trials (6500 patients) of amiodarone, 5 of which involved patients with heart failure, has shown a neutral or positive effect on total mortality (a 13% reduction), which was of borderline statistical significance, and a 29% reduction in risk for sudden death.[63]

Suppression of ventricular arrhythmias
The ability of amiodarone to suppress ventricular ectopic activity has been demonstrated in several studies. In the CAMIAT study, amiodarone almost completely abolished frequent or repetitive asymptomatic ventricular premature beats in 84% compared with only 35% in the placebo group.[60] In the CHF-STAT study, after 3 months of therapy, the proportion of patients with nonsustained ventricular tachycardia decreased from 77% to 33%.[62] Although a significant suppression of ventricular ectopy by amiodarone was observed in

CAMIAT, there were insufficient outcome data to assess whether such a suppression predicted a reduction in the risk of sudden death and cardiac arrest. In the GESICA study, amiodarone reduced sudden death by 27% but it did not modify the risk of sudden death in the subgroups with and without nonsustained ventricular tachycardia.[4] The CHF-STAT has shown that suppression of asymptomatic ventricular ectopic activity does not confer any benefit in terms of reducing arrhythmia-related death.

Furthermore, a recent meta-analysis of three secondary prevention ICD trials has revealed substantial limitations of survival benefits with amiodarone compared with an ICD: risk of arrhythmic death was increased by 50% with amiodarone as was risk for all-cause mortality (28%).[64] Most importantly, patients with a left ventricular ejection fraction of 35% or less and patients with at least NYHA class III heart failure were at higher risk with amiodarone vs an ICD. This was not seen among those with more preserved ventricular systolic function. These data suggest that the treatment of heart failure itself is more likely to prevent sudden death. Pure antiarrhythmic agents are not, therefore, recommended for prophylactic use or for routine treatment of asymptomatic, nonsustained ventricular arrhythmias in patients with heart failure.

Amiodarone and beta-blockers: interaction
In addition to its noncompetitive blockade of alpha- and beta-adrenoreceptors, amiodarone can induce a significant decrease in the number of beta-receptors and can inhibit the coupling of beta-receptors with the regulatory unit of adenylate cyclase. Therefore, the combination of amiodarone and beta-blockers may be beneficial. The favorable interaction between amiodarone and beta-blockers, resulting in a significant reduction in cardiac mor-

tality and arrhythmic death, has been shown in a recent meta-analysis of CAMIAT and EMIAT.[65] Post hoc analyses from these trials indicated that patients receiving amiodarone and a beta-blocker had a substantially lower risk of death (30–72%) compared with patients receiving amiodarone alone. Although all-cause mortality was lower in patients receiving a combination of these agents, it did not reach statistical significance. Although a similar analysis of data from the Antiarrhythmics Versus Implantable Defibrillator Trial (AVID) did not show any substantial benefit of adding beta-blockers to amiodarone, beta-blockade was independently associated with improved survival in patients who were not treated with specific antiarrhythmic therapy.[66]

Dofetilide and azimilide

The ability of dofetilide to suppress the induction of sustained ventricular tachycardia in the acute test and to prevent recurrence of the arrhythmia during long-term treatment has been found to be similar to that of sotalol, but was associated with better tolerability and a lower likelihood of withdrawal.[67] In 174 patients with an ICD, randomly assigned to receive either dofetilide (500 μg twice daily) or placebo, dofetilide increased the median time to first all-cause ICD shock by 33% and first appropriate shock by 27%, but did not modify total appropriate ICD therapy episodes, including shocks and antitachycardia pacing.[68] The effects of dofetilide on arrhythmia and mortality in patients with left ventricular dysfunction have been evaluated in a large prospective study, the Danish Investigations of Arrhythmia and Mortality on Dofetilide in Congestive Heart Failure (DIAMOND-CHF). The study enrolled 1518 patients with NYHA class II or III within the

preceding month and an ejection fraction of 35% or less who were randomly assigned to either dofetilide 500 μg twice daily or placebo.[69] After 18 months of follow-up, the overall mortality rates were similar in the dofetilide and the placebo groups (41% vs 42%) as were cardiac (33% in either arm) and arrhythmic death rates (20% in either arm).

Recently, another new class III antiarrhythmic agent, azimilide, which exerts both I_{Kr} and I_{Ks} channel blocking effects, has been shown to significantly reduce the number of appropriate shocks by 44% in 172 patients with ICD, life-threatening ventricular arrhythmias, NYHA class II or III heart failure, and a mean ejection fraction of 31%, who were randomized to three dose regimens of azimilide (35 mg, 75 mg, 125 mg daily) or placebo.[70]

Implantable cardioverter–defibrillator therapy for ventricular tachyarrhythmias

Although there was a concern that ICD therapy might be of limited efficacy in patients with severe left ventricular dysfunction because of the competing risk of death from progressive heart failure or bradyarrhythmias and electromechanical dissociation, the results of the three large prospective secondary prevention trials (AVID, CIDS, and CASH) have reported that an ICD is superior to empiric amiodarone, guided sotalol, or empiric metoprolol, with respect to overall survival (Table 12.4).[71–73] The meta-analysis of AVID, CIDS and CASH in patients with life threatening ventricular tachyarrhythmias has revealed a 28% decrease in the risk of total mortality and a 50% decrease in arrhythmic death with an ICD versus amiodarone, which was predominantly attributed to a better survival of patients with an ejection fraction of 35% or less, whereas in patients with more preserved

Study	Prevention	No. of patients	Patient characteristics	Follow-up	Antiarrhythmic therapy	Risk reduction for all-cause mortality	Risk reduction for sudden death
MADIT[74]	Primary	196	Post-MI, NSVT, inducible VT, EF ≤0.35 (mean EF = 0.26), 65% NYHA II–III	27 months	74% empiric amiodarone	54%	–
MADIT II[76]	Primary	1232	Post-MI, EF ≤0.30 (mean EF = 0.23), NYHA I–III	20 months	Not prespecified but ~12% amiodarone	31%	Arrhythmic mortality: 3.6% ICD, 9.4% conventional Rx
MUSTT[75]	Primary	704	NSVT, inducible VT, EF ≤0.40 (mean EF = 0.30), 64% NYHA II–III	39 months	Guided/empiric class I, sotalol, amiodarone	60% vs guided therapy; 55% vs no therapy	76% vs guided therapy; 73% vs no therapy
CABG Patch[77]	Primary	900	CAD, EF <0.36 (mean EF = 0.27), abnormal SAECG, elective CABG	32 months	Not prespecified; ~30% on antiarrhythmic therapy at 1 year	No difference	45%
AVID[71]	Secondary	1016	VT/VF, EF <0.40 (mean EF = 0.32), 48% NYHA I	1.5 years	Empiric amiodarone; guided sotalol	39%	57%
CIDS[72]	Secondary	656	Cardiac arrest, sustained VT ≥150 beats/min; EF ≤0.35 (mean EF = 0.34), 51% NYHA I–IV, 83% CAD	3 years	Empiric amiodarone	19.7% (ns)	32.8% (ns)
CASH[73]	Secondary	288	Cardiac arrest, 76% NYHA II,III, mean EF = 0.45	57 months	Empiric amiodarone, metoprolol[a]	23%	58%

Continued

Table 12.4 Clinical evidence of efficacy of ICD for primary and secondary prevention of sudden death in patients with left ventricular dysfunction

Trial	Prevention	N	Inclusion criteria	Follow-up	Control arm	Outcomes	
AMIOVIRT[78]	Primary	102	DCM, EF <0.35, 85% NYHS II–III, asymptomatic NSVT	20.1 months	Empiric amiodarone	Mortality at 1 year: 12% ICD, 11% amiodarone; at 2 years: 15% ICD, 21% amiodarone	–
CAT[79]	Primary	104	DCM ≤9 months, EF ≤0.30 (mean EF = 0.24), NYHA II–III	22.8 months	Not prespecified	Mortality at 1 year: 8% ICD, 3.7% conventional Rx; at 6 years: 27% ICD, 32% conventional Rx	None at 1 year

CABG = coronary artery bypass graft; DCM = dilated cardiomyopathy; EF = ejection fraction; ICD = implantable cardioverter–defibrillator; MI = myocardial infarction; NYHA = New York Heart Association; NSVT = nonsustained ventricular tachycardia; Rx = therapy; SAECG = signal-averaged electrocardiogram; VF = ventricular fibrillation; VT = ventricular tachycardia.
[a] Assignment to propafenone was discontinued because of a high all-cause mortality on the interim analysis.

Table 12.4 *Continued*

ventricular function ICD did not confer added benefit compared with amiodarone.[64]

The MADIT (Multicenter Automatic Defibrillator Implantation Trial) study has identified a high-risk group of patients without a history of cardiac arrest or sustained ventricular tachyarrhythmias in whom ICD therapy may confer greater survival benefit compared with conventional medical therapy. These are patients with prior myocardial infarction, a left ventricular ejection fraction of 35% or less, nonsustained ventricular tachycardia, and inducible, nonsuppressible sustained ventricular tachycardia during electrophysiologic testing.[74] In the MUSTT (Multicenter Unsustained Tachycardia Trial) study, 704 patients with a left ventricular ejection fraction of 40% or less, nonsustained ventricular tachycardia on Holter and inducible ventricular tachycardia during programmed ventricular stimulation, ICD therapy was associated with a 60% reduction in total mortality and a 76% reduction in arrhythmic death compared with antiarrhythmic drug therapy.[75] The results of a recently completed MADIT II study have shown that ICD therapy confers survival benefit in post myocardial infarction patients with advanced left ventricular dysfunction (left ventricular ejection fraction of 30% or less), in the absence of electrophysiologic testing to induce the arrhythmia.[76] Although in the CABG Patch study ICD therapy did not modify all-cause mortality in patients with left ventricular dysfunction and an abnormal signal-averaged ECG who underwent elective coronary bypass surgery, it reduced the arrhythmic death rate by 45%.[77]

However, primary prevention ICD trials in patients with nonischemic dilated cardiomyopathy did not show any survival benefit of an ICD compared with amiodarone (AMIOVIRT) or conventional therapy (CAT). In the Amiodarone versus Implantable Cardioverter–Defibrillator Randomized Trial (AMIOVIRT) of 102 patients with a left ventricular ejection fraction of 35% or less and asymptomatic nonsustained ventricular tachycardia, the 4-year survival rate was 85% for the amiodarone group and 79% for the ICD group.[78] The Cardiomyopathy Trial (CAT) in patients with recently diagnosed dilated cardiomyopathy, a left ventricular ejection fraction of 30% or less and without a history of ventricular tachyarrhythmias, was stopped prematurely because it failed to show an expected 6% difference in 1-year survival in favor of ICD versus no antiarrhythmic treatment.[79] Total mortality at 1 year of 5.6% was much less than an expected total mortality of 30%. Cumulative survival after 4 years of follow-up was 80% in the control group vs 86% in the ICD group.

There are now several ongoing primary prevention trials designed to evaluate the survival benefit of ICD therapy over best conventional heart failure treatment in patients with severe left ventricular dysfunction. The Sudden Cardiac Death in Heart Failure Trial (SCD-HeFT) will randomize 2500 patients with NYHA class II or III heart failure and left ventricular ejection fraction 35% or less to ICD and best conventional therapy, amiodarone and best conventional therapy, or best conventional therapy and placebo.[80] The primary endpoint is overall mortality during 2–2.5 years of follow-up.

The Beta-blocker Strategy plus Implantable Cardioverter–Defibrillator (BEST–ICD) study will test the hypothesis that electrophysiologically guided therapy and implantation of an ICD in patients with inducible ventricular tachycardia will improve survival compared with the conventional strategy.[81] All 1200 patients with a recent myocardial infarction and a left ventricular ejection fraction 35% or less and more than one of the additional risk factors, such as at least 10 ventricular premature beats per hour, decreased heart rate variability, and the presence of late potentials, will receive metoprolol and will be followed up for 2 years. The primary endpoint is overall mortality.

Atrial fibrillation in heart failure

Prevalence and prognosis

Heart failure is often associated with atrial fibrillation. Data from large clinical trials of heart failure have shown that the prevalence of atrial fibrillation in patients with mild-to-moderate heart failure is in the range of 10–20%, increasing to 50% in those with severe heart failure.[16,17,82,83] A recent European Heart Failure survey reported that 45% of 10,464 heart failure patients presented with atrial fibrillation. The onset of atrial fibrillation in patients with heart failure is often associated with overt heart failure decompensation, worsening NYHA functional class, a decrease in peak exercise oxygen consumption, a reduction in cardiac index, and an increase in valve regurgitation, implying that atrial fibrillation may be the cause and not just a marker of more severe left ventricular dysfunction. Data from the Digitalis Investigation Group (DIG) trial of 7788 patients with heart failure have shown that the presence of supraventricular tachyarrhythmias (predominantly atrial fibrillation) was associated with a nearly 2.5-fold increased risk for all-cause mortality and a 3-fold risk of worsening heart failure during 4.5 years of follow-up.[82] Atrial fibrillation conferred a 1.34-fold risk for all-cause mortality in over 6500 patients from the SOLVD Treatment and Prevention trials, largely explained by an increased risk of death from progressive pump failure, supporting the hypothesis that atrial fibrillation is implicated in progression of left ventricular dysfunction.[83] The authors concluded that the increased proportion of patients with atrial fibrillation among those with nonischemic heart failure or heart failure of unknown etiology might suggest that some of the SOLVD patients had tachycardia-induced cardiomyopathy.

However, the adverse effects of atrial fibrillation on prognosis in heart failure has not been uniformly confirmed in large clinical trials. Crijns et al.[84] found that atrial fibrillation increased the risk of death by 1.4 as a single variable but after adjustment for age, ejection fraction, NYHA class, renal function, and blood pressure, the presence of the arrhythmia was no longer related to mortality (risk ratio 0.86). In the V-HeFT-I and II studies, which included patients with less advanced heart failure (mean left ventricular ejection fraction 30%, NYHA class II and III), cumulative mortality at 2 years for patients with atrial fibrillation and patients in sinus rhythm was 34% and 30% in V-HeFT I, and 20% and 21% in V-HeFT-II.[85]

Angiotensin-converting enzyme inhibitors

In heart failure, conventional treatment aimed at unloading of the atria may prevent or delay the development of atrial fibrillation. ACE inhibition has been shown to decrease susceptibility to atrial arrhythmias in the presence of heart failure by lowering atrial pressure, reducing mitral regurgitation, and preventing left atrial enlargement. ACE inhibitors may provide additional benefit by reducing direct electrophysiologic effects of angiotensin II on the atria and by lessening the extent of fibrosis within the atrial myocardium. In the TRACE study, significantly fewer patients in the trandolapril group developed atrial fibrillation during 2–4 years of follow-up compared with the placebo group (2.8% vs 5.3%), resulting in a 55% risk reduction of development of the arrhythmia.[86] In two recently presented studies, pre-treatment with an ACE inhibitor or an angiotensin type 1 receptor blocker (ARB) appeared to facilitate electrical or pharmacologic cardioversion of atrial fibrillation and tended to reduce the recurrence rate.[87,88]

Beta-blockers

In patients with atrial fibrillation, beta-blockers have been mainly used for rate control, usually as adjuvant therapy to digoxin. Recently, metoprolol CR/XL at a dose of up to 200 mg has been shown to reduce recurrence of the arrhythmia after cardioversion in 397 patients with persistent atrial fibrillation 66% of whom were in NYHA class II and 34% in class III.[89] In the metoprolol group, 48.7% of patients relapsed into atrial fibrillation during 3 months of follow-up compared with 59.9% of patients assigned to placebo. Among those who had atrial fibrillation recurrence, the ventricular rate response was significantly slower in the active drug group. In the CAPRICORN study, therapy with carvedilol reduced risk of the development of atrial fibrillation or flutter by nearly two-thirds.[90] The preliminary data from the COPERNICUS study have suggested that in the subgroup of patients with atrial fibrillation carvedilol was associated with a better survival compared with placebo, although this effect was less pronounced than in patients with sinus rhythm. However, the subgroup analysis of CIBIS II data has shown that bisoprolol reduced all-cause mortality in patients with sinus rhythm (relative risk 0.58) but not in patients presenting with atrial fibrillation (relative risk 1.16).[91]

Digoxin

In patients with permanent atrial fibrillation or in whom attempts to maintain sinus rhythm have been ineffective over the long term, digoxin may be used to control the ventricular rate response because of its effects on prolongation of atrioventricular nodal conduction and refractoriness through vagal stimulation and by its direct effects on the atrioventricular node. Digoxin may also increase the amount of concealed conduction in the atrioventricular node by increasing the rate at which atria discharge, resulting in a further decrease in the ventricular rate. However, vagomimetic and direct effects of digoxin may be counteracted by the increased sympathetic tone, especially in patients with heart failure, limiting the ability of digoxin to control the ventricular rate on exertion. Although it has been argued that digoxin may promote conversion of atrial fibrillation as a result of its acute hemodymanic effects and the consequent reduction in left atrial pressure and volume, digoxin is usually ineffective for termination of atrial fibrillation.[92] Moreover, the drug has been shown to facilitate atrial fibrillation due to its cholinergic effects, which may cause a nonuniform reduction in conduction velocity and effective refractory periods of the atria, and to delay the reversal of remodeling after the restoration of sinus rhythm.[93] Finally, in the DIG study, treatment with digoxin did not prevent the development of atrial fibrillation.[82]

Because of the limited effects of digoxin on heart rate during exercise, concomitant use of multiple drugs may be necessary to provide an adequate ventricular rate response, among which beta-blockers should be used as first choice in combination with digoxin because of their overall favorable effects in patients with heart failure. Calcium antagonists with inhibitory effects on atrioventricular conduction, such as verapamil and diltiazem, do not have any survival benefit and may cause worsening heart failure due to negative inotropic effects.

Rate vs rhythm control for atrial fibrillation

Evidence for a close relationship between the occurrence of atrial fibrillation and increased morbidity and mortality comes from large heart failure trials[10,81,82,87,94] and suggests that restoration and maintenance of sinus rhythm may be beneficial. The success rate of electrical cardioversion in 246 patients with predominantly mild heart failure has been reported to be 70%.[95] However, in some studies, serial electrical cardioversion did not prevent heart failure in patients with persistent atrial fibrillation and did not confer additional benefit with regard to peak oxygen consumption, heart dimensions, or neurohumoral status in a small series of patients with heart failure.[84]

There is no direct evidence for superiority of rhythm control over the rate control strategy in terms of improving survival and preventing thromboembolic events, especially in patients with heart failure. In two prospective studies comparing strategies of rhythm vs rate control in patients with persistent or permanent atrial fibrillation who did not necessarily have heart failure, the PIAF (Pharmacological Intervention in Atrial Fibrillation)[96] and STAF (Strategies of Treatment in Atrial Fibrillation),[97] both strategies yielded similar clinical results. In the STAF study there was no difference in 1-year mortality and morbidity among 200 patients with atrial fibrillation of more than 4 weeks' duration and left ventricular ejection fraction of 45% or less who were randomized to cardioversion and antiarrhythmic therapy (primarily amiodarone) or rate control and anticoagulation. Only 40% of patients remained at sinus rhythm at 1 year and 26% at 2 years,

despite repeat cardioversion and use of up to four antiarrhythmic agents to maintain sinus rhythm. Of note, although there were similar numbers of primary endpoints (death, cardiovascular events or systemic embolism) in the rhythm control and the rate control groups (9 and 10, respectively), 18 of these occurred while patients were in atrial fibrillation. In the PIAF study, the rhythm control strategy resulted in better exercise capacity but did not significantly improve symptoms or quality of life and was associated with an increased number of hospitalizations for repeat cardioversion or adverse drug effects.

Data from the recently completed AFFIRM (Atrial Fibrillation Follow-up Investigation of Rhythm Management) study of over 4000 atrial fibrillation patients aged 65 years or older with at least one risk factor for stroke have shown no difference in the primary end point of all-cause mortality as well as quality of life and functional status between the two strategies during a 3.5-year follow-up.[98] The results of the RACE (Rate Control versus Electrical Cardioversion) study of 522 patients with persistent atrial fibrillation assigned to the aggressive rhythm control strategy consisting of serial cardioversions and antiarrhythmic drugs or the rate control strategy, have also shown no difference in the primary composite endpoint of cardiovascular death, hospitalizations for heart failure, thromboembolic events, major bleedings, pacemaker implantation, and adverse effects of antiarrhythmic drug therapy between the two strategies (22.6% vs 17.2%).[99] Both studies have provided evidence that anticoagulation is essential for high-risk patients treated with either strategy.

However, in patients with rheumatic heart disease, the rhythm control strategy with amiodarone resulted in an improvement in exercise capacity, NYHA class heart failure and quality of life compared with rate control, with no difference in hemorrhagic complications, thromboembolic events, and hospital admissions.[100] Finally, the ongoing AF-CHF study is powered to detect a 25% reduction in mortality with rhythm control (electrical cardioversion, amiodarone, dofetilide, or sotalol) compared with rate control (beta-blockers and digoxin) in 1450 patients with NYHA class II–IV heart failure and an ejection fraction of 35% or less.

Rate control may be appropriate in patients with heart failure and mildly symptomatic atrial fibrillation of long duration, with a low probability of effective maintenance of sinus rhythm and in whom the risk/benefit ratio from using specific antiarrhythmic agents is shifted toward increased risk. Since enhanced adrenergic stimulation in the setting of heart failure may facilitate atrioventricular conduction and favor progression of cardiomyopathy, agents with a depressant effect on atrioventricular conduction, such as digoxin, beta-blockers, and amiodarone may benefit heart failure patients. Rhythm control is preferable in patients with heart failure and recent onset atrial fibrillation, symptomatic atrial fibrillation and relatively preserved left ventricular function, and a patient is likely to benefit from a significant improvement in quality of life from this strategy.

Amiodarone

The Canadian Trial of Atrial Fibrillation (CTAF) has shown that amiodarone 200 mg/day was nearly twice as effective as the commonly used antiarrhythmic agents sotalol and propafenone in the prevention of atrial fibrillation, reducing the risk of atrial fibrillation recurrence by 57%.[101] Data from the CHF-STAT substudy showed that amiodarone was effective for conversion of atrial fibrilla-

tion to sinus rhythm and for control of the ventricular rate response in patients with overt heart failure.[102] In this study, patients who received amiodarone had a higher rate of conversion to sinus rhythm (31.3% vs 7.7%) and were twice as less likely to develop new atrial fibrillation compared with placebo (4% vs 8%). Amiodarone also produced a sustained and significant slowing of the mean and maximum ventricular responses in the range of 16–20% and 14–22%, respectively. Furthermore, there was a significantly lower mortality rate in patients with atrial fibrillation at baseline who subsequently converted to sinus rhythm on amiodarone compared with those who remained in atrial fibrillation. However, low-risk patients with better preserved left ventricular function probably converted on amiodarone more often.

Dofetilide and azimilide

Two large prospective studies, DIAMOND-CHF and SAFIRE-D, have recently evaluated the effects of dofetilide on the conversion rate and maintenance of sinus rhythm in patients with atrial fibrillation. In DIAMOND-CHF, treatment with dofetilide 500 µg twice daily was associated with a greater rate of spontaneous conversion to sinus rhythm (44% vs 14%) and a greater probability of remaining in sinus rhythm at 1 year compared with placebo (79% vs 42%) in 1518 patients with symptomatic heart failure and an ejection fraction of 35% or less.[69] Furthermore, in the treated group there was a significant reduction in the development of new atrial fibrillation (1.98% vs 6.55%). Although dofetilide had an overall neutral effect on survival, restoration and maintenance of sinus rhythm, which occurred more often with dofetilide, was associated with a 56% reduction in mortality.

In the SAFIRE-D study of 325 patients with persistent atrial fibrillation and/or atrial flutter, 73% of whom had structural heart disease and 69% were in NYHA class II and III heart failure 58% of patients receiving the maximum dose of dofetilide (500 µg twice daily) remained in sinus rhythm after 1 year of follow-up, compared with 25% in the placebo group.[103] Dofetilide may, therefore, be used as an alternative to amiodarone for maintaining sinus rhythm.

Azimilide, at a dose of 100 mg and 125 mg daily, has been shown to significantly prolong the time to first symptomatic arrhythmia recurrence compared with placebo (the hazard ratio 1.58, CI 1.24–2.16) in 384 patients with a history of atrial fibrillation or atrial flutter, 77% of whom had structural heart disease and 18% had chronic heart failure.[104] Meta-analysis of four randomized controlled studies of the effectiveness of a range of azimilide doses in 1380 patients with atrial fibrillation has shown that each of the two highest doses (100mg and 125 mg/daily) significantly prolonged the time to recurrence of atrial fibrillation and/or atrial flutter with the hazard ratios of 1.34 and 1.32, respectively.[105] Patients with a history of coronary artery disease or chronic heart failure had a significantly greater treatment effect from azimilide than those with other underlying cardiovascular pathologies (hazard ratio 1.49–1.86).

In the ALIVE (AzimiLide post Infarct surVival Evaluation Trial) of over 3000 patients with a recent (5–21 days) myocardial infarction and left ventricular dysfunction, azimilide at a dose of 100 mg daily produced a neutral effect on all-cause mortality, including patients at high risk (an ejection fraction less than 20% and depressed heart rate variability).[110] Fewer patients who started the trial in sinus rhythm developed atrial fibrillation or flutter on azimilide compared with placebo

(0.49% vs 1.15%; $P = 0.04$), and there was a tendency to higher pharmacologic conversion rates in the azimilide arm than in the placebo arm (26.8% vs 10.8%), although this difference did not reach statistical significance ($P = 0.076$). The results of the three largest trials of class III antiarrhythmic drugs for treatment of atrial fibrillation in patients with left ventricular dysfunction and heart failure – CHF-STAT, DIAMOND-MI/CHF, and ALIVE – are summarized in Table 12.5.[102,103,106,107]

'Ablate and pace' strategy

Radiofrequency ablation of the atrioventricular node followed by implantation of a permanent pacemaker, the 'ablate and pace' strategy, is now an established treatment in patients with highly symptomatic, drug-refractory atrial fibrillation, when a poorly controlled sustained rapid ventricular rate response is likely to induce or aggravate myocardial dysfunction.[108] Interruption of rapid atrioventricular conduction during atrial fibrillation was associated with a noticeable hemodynamic improvement: an increase in left ventricular ejection fraction and a decrease in left ventricular volumes, improvement in symptoms and quality of life during a 14.3-month follow-up.[109] Although an overall increase in an ejection fraction was modest (from 32% to 42%), some patients improved their left ventricular systolic function by up to 24 points over 4 weeks, suggesting a tachycardia-mediated cardiomyopathy.

In another study, 66 patients with heart failure and permanent atrial fibrillation were randomized to receive either drug therapy for rate control or ablation and implantation of VVIR pacemaker and were followed up for 12 months.[110] Patients treated with 'ablate and pace' strategy had a significant improvement in symptoms, especially palpitations and

Study	Results		
	CHF-STAT	DIAMOND-MI/CHF	ALIVE
Number of patients	667	3028	3381
Underlying cardiac pathology	NYHA II–IV, EF ≤0.40, approx. 60% IHD; approx. 50% MI	57% NYHA III–IV, EF ≤0.35, approx. 80% IHD	MI (5–21 days); EF = 15–35%
Study drug	Amiodarone 200 mg	Dofetilide 500 μcg	Azimilide 100 mg
Atrial fibrillation	103 (15%)	506 (16.7%)	93 (2.75%)
Cardioverted to sinus rhythm			
Placebo efficacy	4/52 (7.7%)	86/257 (33.5%)[a]	4/37 (10.8%)
Drug efficacy	16/51 (31.3%)	148/249 (59.4%)[a]	15/56 (26.8%)
Placebo extracted efficacy	23.6	25.9	16
Mortality, odds ratio	0.99	1.01	0.95

EF = ejection fraction; IHD = ischemic heart disease; MI = myocardial infarction; NYHA = New York Heart Association
[a] Electrical + pharmacologic cardioversion.

Table 12.5 Amiodarone, dofetilide, and azimilide in patients with heart failure and atrial fibrillation

exertional dyspnea. However, there was no difference in the improvement in cardiac performance and global quality of life. 'Ablate and pace' strategy also did not prevent the progression of heart failure. However, nearly one-third of patients initially randomized to drug therapy crossed over to ablation and pacemaker implantation because of worsening symptoms.

Atrial preventive and antitachycardia pacing

Atrial pacing, including dual-site and biatrial pacing, has been successfully used to prevent the arrhythmia by modifying the substrate and, possibly, improving atrial hemodynamics and alleviating atrial stretch in patients with atrial fibrillation.[111] Atrial preventive pacing therapies incorporated in new implantable dual-chamber ICDs and pacemakers can potentially prevent recurrence of atrial fibrilla-

tion and reduce atrial fibrillation burden in patients with or without bradycardia indications for pacing.

Data from implantable devices have also shown that atrial fibrillation often starts with regular atrial activity consistent with an atrial tachycardia, supporting the possibility that prompt antitachycardia pacing – including burst pacing, ramp pacing and high-frequency (50 Hz) burst pacing – may terminate an arrhythmic episode and prevent progression to atrial fibrillation.[112] In a recent study, 537 patients had a dual-chamber ICD Jewel AF implanted for ventricular arrhythmias.[113] Seventy-nine percent were in NYHA class II or III heart failure (mean ejection fraction less than 35%) and 74% had concomitant atrial fibrillation or flutter. Burst and ramp pacing terminated 48% of episodes of atrial tachyarrhythmias. Of note, the degree of left ventricular dysfunction did not predict outcome of antitachycardia therapy.

The concept of 'hybrid therapy,' based on the combination of several different therapeutic strategies, suggests that painless antitachycardia pacing therapy, integrated with an atrial defibrillator and preventive atrial pacing modes, may be valuable in the subsets of patients with depressed left ventricular function and atrial and ventricular tachyarrhythmias.

Bradyarrhythmias in heart failure

Prevalence and prognosis

Bradyarrhythmias, asystole, or electromechanical dissociation may account for about 25% of sudden cardiac death in the general population and this proportion increases in patients with advanced heart failure.[11,114] In a series of 216 patients with severe heart failure and a mean ejection fraction of 18%, awaiting heart transplantation, 20 of whom died suddenly in hospital, bradyarrhythmias accounted for nearly two-thirds of sudden cardiac deaths.[11] In another series of 48 patients hospitalized for worsening heart failure 20 had severe bradycardia or electromechanical dissociation at the time of cardiac arrest.[114] In this study, patients with bradyarrhythmias as a cause of cardiac arrest generally were in a higher NYHA class heart failure, tolerated lower doses of ACE inhibitors, needed intravenous inotropic drugs more often, and were less frequently successfully resuscitated than patients with ventricular tachyarrhythmias. In the AIRE (Acute Infarction Ramipril Efficacy) study of over 2000 patients with myocardial infarction and clinical evidence of heart failure, in-hospital cardiac arrest occurred in 101 cases, 64 of which were associated with electromechanical dissociation, asystole, or bradycardia.[115]

Pacing for bradycardia in heart failure

Except for conventional bradycardia indications for cardiac pacing, such as sinus node disease and high-degree atrioventricular block, one may expect a higher incidence of iatrogenic bradycardia because of extended use of beta-blockers, which may require pacing. Although high resting heart rate has been consistently shown to be associated with adverse outcome in patients with heart failure,[116] excessive bradycardia may produce deleterious effects by inadequate cardiac output or by increasing left ventricular diastolic pressure. The randomized THEOPACE study included 117 elderly patients with symptomatic sick sinus syndrome.[117] Uncorrected bradycardia of less than 50 beats/min was associated with a higher incidence of the development of overt heart failure in the control group (17%) compared with patients who received theophylline or had a pacemaker implanted (3% in either group).

Atrioventricular synchronous pacing has been shown to be associated with lower morbidity and mortality rates compared with ventricular pacing in patients with heart failure and sinus node dysfunction (the cumulative survival rates at 5 years are 75% vs 57%) or atrioventricular block (survival rates at 5 years are 69% vs 47%).[118,119] In the Danish study of 225 patients with sick sinus syndrome, atrial-based pacing prevented worsening heart failure and reduced the risk of death from heart failure by 59% compared with ventricular-based pacing during a 5.5-year follow-up.[120] Of note, in this series of patients, there was no difference in the degree of left ventricular dysfunction between atrial and ventricular-paced groups after a shorter follow-up of 3.3 years, suggesting that ventricular pacing may produce delayed effects on the myocardium.

The mechanisms by which ventricular pacing may cause myocardial dysfunction are not completely understood. Asymmetric thickness of the left ventricular wall resulting from asynchronous electric activation, disarray of myocardial fibers, and changes in myocardial perfusion leading to functional ischemia have been observed in clinical and experimental series with chronic ventricular pacing. Retrograde conduction during ventricular pacing has been reported to be associated with the pacemaker syndrome and the development of heart failure. Loss of atrioventricular synchrony may lead to valvular regurgitation and atrial contraction against closed atrioventricular valves, resulting in atrial stretch and atrial enlargement that may promote the occurrence of atrial arrhythmias. Optimization of atrioventricular mechanical synchrony and ventricular diastolic filling period and reduction in valvular regurgitation with dual-chamber pacing may contribute to the hemodynamic improvement in patients with heart failure.

Two recent prospective studies, the Pacemaker Selection in the Elderly (PASE)[121] and the Canadian Trial of Physiologic Pacing (CTOPP),[122] did not show benefit of physiologic pacing on overall mortality. However, CTOPP reported an 18% reduction in the risk of all atrial fibrillation episodes in patients who were randomized to physiologic pacing compared with those in the ventricular pacing group. A subgroup analysis from the PASE study of 407 patients, 65 years or older, 70% of whom had NYHA class I or II heart failure, has been performed. It revealed that DDDR pacing in patients with sinus node dysfunction was associated with a trend toward lower incidence of atrial fibrillation, death, stroke and hospitalizations for heart failure compared with VVIR pacing. In a recently completed study, MOST (MOde Selection Trial), 2100 patients with sinus node dysfunction with or without atrioventricular block were randomized to DDDR or VVIR pacing.[123] DDDR pacing significantly delayed the progression to atrial fibrillation (risk reduction 21%), especially in patients without a history of atrial arrhythmias prior to the pacemaker implant (risk reduction 50%), and was associated with a better NYHA class heart failure (1.1 vs 1.5) compared with VVIR pacing.

Resynchronization pacing

The rationale for resynchronization therapy in heart failure using left ventricular or biventricular pacing is based on several factors:

- the high (about 30%) prevalence of intra- and interventricular conduction delay due to loss of cardiomyocyte integrity
- post myocardial infarction remodeling and bundle branch block, resulting in mechanical asynergy
- contraction–relaxation disturbances
- a reduction in diastolic filling time and peak rate of left ventricular filling pressure
- prolonged duration of mitral and/or tricuspid regurgitation.[124,125]

The subgroup analysis of the MUltisite STimulation In Cardiomyopathies (MUSTIC) Study have shown similar benefits of resynchronization therapy for patients in sinus rhythm and for those with permanent atrial fibrillation. At 12 months of follow-up, an increase in the 6-min walk distance was 20% in the sinus rhythm group and 17% in the atrial fibrillation group. The peak VO2 uptake increased by 11% and 9% respectively, and NYHA class improved by 25% and 27% respectively. Left ventricular ejection fraction increased (5% and 4%) and quality of life improved in both groups.[126] The acute hemodynamic effects of left ventricular and biventricular pacing, resulting in a decrease in pulmonary capillary wedge pressure and V-wave amplitude and an increase in systolic blood pressure, were comparable in patients with sinus rhythm and atrial fibrillation.[127] This suggests that restoration of atrioventricular synchrony may not be the only mechanism by which atrio-biventricular pacing can realize its beneficial hemodynamic effects. Finally, upgrading to biventricular pacing after long-term right ventricular pacing in patients with heart failure and atrioventricular nodal ablation for atrial fibrillation results in an 81% reduction in hospitalizations, a 24% improvement in NYHA class heart failure, and a 33% improvement in quality of life at 6 months of follow up.[128]

Effects of resynchronization pacing on ventricular arrhythmias

The Ventak CHF study included 32 patients (78% NYHA class III–IV heart failure) with dual-chamber biventricular ICD, who were randomly assigned to VVI pacing at 40 beats/min or VDD pacing for 3 months and then crossed over to the other pacing mode.[129] At least one episode of arrhythmia requiring device therapy (antitachycardia pacing or shock) occurred in 13 patients. During support pacing, 11 patients had an event compared with only 5 patients during biventricular pacing. In two small series of patients, biventricular pacing has been shown to suppress ventricular ectopic activity[130] and render ventricular tachycardia noninducible during electrophysiologic study in 7 out of 9 patients with sustained arrhythmia.[131]

The preliminary results of the Multicenter InSync Randomized Clinical Evaluation (MIRACLE) study of 636 patients with NYHA class II ($n = 215$) or III/IV ($n = 421$) heart failure assigned to resynchronization therapy or no pacing have shown a significantly lower incidence of spontaneous ventricular tachycardia or fibrillation during the pacing phase compared with the control phase (0.21 vs 0.42 episodes/month) at 6 months of follow-up.

There are several potential mechanisms by which biventricular pacing may exert an antiarrhythmic effect. First, it may pre-excite a larger ventricular mass, resulting in earlier repolarization and a decrease in conduction delays. A ventricular premature beat is, therefore, less likely to encounter areas with partial refractoriness and initiate re-entry. Second, biventricular pacing may reduce bradycardia-dependent dispersion of refractoriness and prevent pause-induced tachyarrhythmias. Third, biventricular pacing has been shown to decrease plasma norepinephrine levels, therefore counterbalancing arrhythmogenic effects of adrenergic stimulation.[132,133] Finally, an improvement in ventricular function due to the restoration of ventricular mechanical synchrony, the reduction in valvular regurgitation, and an increase in ventricular diastolic filling time with resynchronization pacing may reduce the vulnerability to ventricular tachyarrhythmias.

Conclusions

Despite advances in pharmacologic and non-pharmacologic management, heart failure is associated with a 5–50% annual mortality, depending on the severity of left ventricular dysfunction. Nearly half of all cardiac deaths in patients with heart failure are sudden and presumably arrhythmic. Both tachy- and bradyarrhythmias may be involved and rhythm disturbances may be secondary to hemodynamic collapse due to progressive circulatory failure. Heart failure is associated with a wide variety of atrial and ventricular arrhythmias, among which atrial fibrillation and nonsustained ventricular tachycardia are the most common.

Multifactorial etiologies and multiple patho-physiologic mechanisms of heart failure suggest the need for a multidimensional approach to the management of patients with heart failure and cardiac arrhythmias.

ACE inhibitors, beta-blockers, and spirono-lactone have been shown to reduce total mortality, decrease the risk of worsening heart failure, and prevent sudden cardiac death in an additive fashion. There is evidence that ACE inhibitors may prevent or delay the development of atrial fibrillation in patients with left ventricular dysfunction.

It is now generally accepted that the use of class I antiarrhythmic drugs and sotalol for the management of arrhythmias should be avoided in patients with heart failure because of increased total mortality, proarrhythmic risk, and worsening heart failure associated with these agents. Presently, amiodarone is considered a safe agent in patients with heart failure who require antiarrhythmic therapy for recurrent atrial fibrillation or symptomatic sustained ventricular arrhythmias. Treatment with amiodarone is not associated with increased mortality and proarrhythmic risk and may reduce the risk of sudden death by about 30%. However, empiric prophylactic use of amiodarone for primary prevention of sudden death has not been shown to confer a noticeable survival benefit.

New agents are being tested that might favorably affect both sudden death and progressive pump failure, such as the new class III antiarrhythmic drugs, dofetilide and azimilide. Their role for primary prevention of sudden death in patients with heart failure or in those with sustained ventricular tachyarrhythmias and cardiac arrest has not yet been established. However, both drugs appear to have neutral effects on total mortality and to be efficacious in the restoration and maintenance of sinus rhythm in patients with atrial fibrillation.

'Ablate and pace' strategy for the management of drug refractory atrial fibrillation has proved to be safe and efficacious in patients with heart failure, often resulting in a noticeable improvement in ventricular function and quality of life. Clinical studies have suggested possible beneficial effects of physiologic pacing over ventricular pacing in terms of prevention of the development of heart failure and atrial fibrillation. However, this benefit has been observed only after a relatively long follow-up, has been limited to patients with sinus node dysfunction, and has not translated into improved survival. Novel pacing algorithms for the prevention and termination of atrial arrhythmias incorporated in implantable ICD and pacemakers are currently under investigation. They may offer a valuable alternative to antiarrhythmic drug therapy in patients with severe left ventricular dysfunction at high risk of proarrhythmias or worsening heart failure.

There is compelling evidence from both primary and secondary prevention trials that an ICD may be the first choice in patients with severe myocardial infarction (left ventricular ejection fraction 35% or less) and the presence of sustained ventricular arrhythmias or nonsustained ventricular tachycardia. These patients should be referred for electrophysiologic assessment and, in the case of inducible ventricular tachycardia should be considered as candidates for ICD implantation. However, whether patients with better-preserved ejection fraction and a noninducible ventricular tachycardia might benefit from ICD implantation is not evident, and the use of amiodarone may be considered in the first instance.

Finally, biventricular pacing appears to be a valuable adjunctive therapy to an ICD in patients with heart failure due to its beneficial effects on left ventricular function and possible prevention of sustained ventricular tachyarrhythmias that may require shock.

References

1. Uretsky BF, Sheahan RG. Primary prevention of sudden cardiac death in heart failure: will the solution be shocking? J Am Coll Cardiol 1997; 30:1589–97.

2. MERIT-HF Study Group. Effect of metoprolol CR/XL in chronic heart failure: Metoprolol CR/XL Randomized Intervention Trial in Congestive Heart Failure (MERIT-HF). Lancet 1999; 353:2001–7.

3. Cohn JN, Archibald DG, Franciosa SA, et al. Effects of vasodilator therapy on mortality in chronic congestive heart failure: a result of a Veterans Affairs Cooperative Study (V-HeFT). N Engl J Med 1986; 314:1547–52.

4. Doval HC, Nul DR, Grancelli HO, et al. Nonsustained ventricular tachycardia in severe heart failure: independent marker of increased mortality due to sudden death: GESICA-GEMA Investigators. Circulation 1996; 94:3198–203.

5. Singh SN, Fisher SG, Carson PE, Fletcher RD. Prevalence and significance of nonsustained ventricular tachycardia in patients with premature ventricular contractions and heart failure treated with vasodilator therapy: Department of Veterans Affairs CHF STAT Investigators. J Am Coll Cardiol 1998; 32:942–7.

6. Teerlink JR, Jalaluddin M, Anderson S, et al., on behalf of the PROMISE (Prospective Randomized Milrinone Survival Evaluation) Investigators. Ambulatory ventricular arrhythmias in patients with heart failure do not specifically predict an increased risk of sudden death. Circulation 2000; 101:40–6.

7. Nolan J, Batin PD, Andrews R, et al. Prospective study of heart rate variability and mortality in chronic heart failure: results of the United Kingdom Heart failure Evaluation and Assessment of Risk Trial (UK-Heart). Circulation 1998; 98:1510–16.

8. Stevenson WG, Stevenson LW, Middlekauff HR, Saxon LA. Sudden death prevention in patients with advanced ventricular dysfunction. Circulation 1993; 88:2953–61.

9. Goldman S, Johnson G, Cohn JN, et al., for the V-HeFT VA Cooperative Studies Group. Mechanism of death in heart failure: the Vasodilator-Heart Failure Trials. Circulation 1993; 87:VI-24–31.

10. Cleland JGF, Thygesen K, Uretsky BF, et al., on behalf of the ATLAS Investigators. Cardiovascular critical event pathways for the progression of heart failure: a report from the ATLAS study. Eur Heart J 2001; 22:1601–12.

11. Luu M, Stevenson WG, Stevenson LW, et al. Diverse mechanisms of unexpected cardiac arrest in advanced heart failure. Circulation 1989; 80:1675–80.

12. Benedict C, Shelton B, Johnstone DE, et al., for the SOLVD Investigators. Prognostic significance of plasma norepinephrine in patients with asymptomatic left ventricular dysfunction. Circulation 1996; 94:690–7.

13. Vantrimpont P, Rouleau JL, Ciampi A, et al., for the SAVE Investigators. Two-year time course and significance of neurohumoral activation in the Survival and Ventricular Enlargement (SAVE) Study. Eur Heart J 1998; 19:1552–63.

14. Sato R, Koumi S. Characterization of the stretch-activated chloride channel in isolated human atrial myocytes. J Membr Biol 1998; 163:67–76.

15. Sadoshima J, Izumo S. The cellular and molecular response of cardiac myocytes to mechanical stress. Ann Rev Physiol 1997; 59:551–71.

16. Rydèn L, Armstrong PW, Cleland JGF, et al., on behalf of the ATLAS Study Group. Efficacy and safety of high-dose lisinopril in chronic heart failure patients at high cardiovascular risk, including those with diabetes mellitus: results from the ATLAS trial. Eur Heart J 2000; 21:1967–78.

17. Swedberg K, Idanpaan Heikkila U, Remes J, and the CONSENSUS Trial Study Group. Effects of enalapril on mortality in severe congestive heart failure: results on the Cooperative North Scandinavia Enalapril Survival Study

(CONSENSUS). N Engl J Med 1987; 316:1429–35.

18. Fonarow GS, Chelimsky-Fallick C, Stevenson LW, et al. Effect of direct vasodilatation with hydralazine versus angiotensin-converting enzyme inhibition with captopril on mortality in advanced heart failure: the Hy-C trial. J Am Coll Cardiol 1992; 19:842–50.

19. The SOLVD Investigators. Effects of enalapril on survival in patients with reduced left ventricular ejection fraction and congestive heart failure. N Engl J Med 1991; 325:303–10.

20. The SOLVD Investigators. Effects of enalapril on mortality and the development of heart failure in asymptomatic patients with reduced left ventricular ejection fraction. N Engl J Med 1992; 327:685–91.

21. Køber L, Torp-Pedersen C, Carlsen JE, et al., for the Trandolapril Cardiac Evaluation (TRACE) Study Group. A clinical trial of the angiotensin converting enzyme inhibitor trandolapril in patients with left ventricular dysfunction after myocardial infarction. N Engl J Med 1995; 333:1670–6.

22. The Acute Infarction Ramipril Efficacy (AIRE) Study Investigators. Effect of ramipril on mortality and morbidity of survivors of acute myocardial infarction with clinical evidence of heart failure. Lancet 1993; 342:821–8.

23. Pfieffer MA, Braunwald E, Moue LA, et al. Effect of captopril on mortality and morbidity in patients with left ventricular dysfunction after myocardial infarction. N Engl J Med 1992; 327:669–77.

24. Domanski MJ, Exner DV, Borkowf CB, et al. Effect of angiotensin converting enzyme inhibition of sudden cardiac death in patients following acute myocardial infarction: a meta-analysis of randomized clinical trials. J Am Coll Cardiol 1999; 33:598–604.

25. Fletcher RD, Cintron GB, Johnson G, et al., for the V-HeFT II VA Cooperative Studies Group. Enalapril decreases prevalence of ventricular tachycardia in patients with chronic congestive heart failure. Circulation 1993; 87:VI-49–55.

26. Priori SG, Aliot E, Blomstrom-Lundqvist C, et al. Task Force on Sudden Cardiac Death of the European Society of Cardiology. Eur Heart J 2001; 22:1374–450.

27. Pratt CM, Gardner M, Pepine C, et al. Lack of long-term ventricular arrhythmia reduction by

enalapril in heart failure. Am J Cardiol 1995; 75:1244–9.

28. Søgaard P, Thygesen K. Potential proischemic effect of early enalapril in hypotension-prone patients with acute myocardial infarction: the CONSENSUS II Holter substudy group. Cardiology 1997; 88:285–91.

29. Billman GE, Castillo LC, Hensley J, et al. Beta$_2$-adrenergic receptor antagonists protect against ventricular fibrillation: in vivo and in vitro evidence for enhanced sensitivity to β$_2$-adrenergic stimulation in animals susceptible for sudden death. Circulation 1997; 96:1914–22.

30. Molina-Viamonte V, Anyukhovsky EP, Rosen MR. An alpha$_1$-adrenergic receptor subtype is responsible for delayed repolarizations and triggered activity during simulated ischemia and reperfusion of isolated canine Purkinje fibers. Circulation 1991; 84:1732–40.

31. Brophy JM, Joseph L, Rouleau JL. β-blockers in congestive heart failure: a Bayesian meta-analysis. Ann Intern Med 2001; 134:550–60.

32. CIBIS Investigators and Committees. A randomized trial of β-blockade in heart failure: the Cardiac Insufficiency Bisoprolol Study (CIBIS). Circulation 1994; 90:1765–73.

33. Bristow NIR, Gilbert EM, Abraham VYT, et al., for the MOCHA Investigators. Carvedilol produces dose-related improvements in left ventricular function and survival in subjects with chronic heart failure. Circulation 1996; 94:2807–16.

34. The Metoprolol in Dilated Cardiomyopathy (MDC) Trial Study Group. 3-year follow-up of patients randomised in the metoprolol in dilated cardiomyopathy trial. Lancet 1998; 351:1180–1.

35. Australia–New Zealand Heart Failure Research Collaborative Group. Randomised, placebo-controlled trial of carvedilol in patients with congestive heart failure due to ischemic heart disease. Lancet 1997; 349:375–80.

36. Packer M, Bristow MR, Cohn JN, et al., for the US Carvedilol Heart Failure Study Group. The effect of carvedilol on morbidity and mortality in patients with chronic heart failure. N Engl J Med 1996; 334:1349–55.

37. Chadda K, Goldstein S, Byington R, Curb D. Effect of propranolol after acute myocardial infarction in patients with congestive heart failure. Circulation 1986; 73:503–10.

38. CIBIS-II Investigators and Committees. The Cardiac Insufficiency Bisoprolol Study II (CIBIS-II): a randomised trial. Lancet 1999; 353:9–13.

39. Parker M, Coats AJS, Fowler MB, et al., for the Carvedilol Prospective Randomized Cumulative Survival Group. Effect of carvedilol on survival in severe chronic heart failure. N Engl J Med 2001; 344:1651–8.

40. The CAPRICORN Investigators. Effect of carvedilol on outcome after myocardial infarction in patients with left-ventricular dysfunction: the CAPRICORN randomised trial. Lancet 2001; 357:1385–90.

41. The Beta-Blocker Evaluation of Survival Trial Investigators. A trial of the beta-blocker bucindolol in patients with advanced chronic heart failure. N Engl J Med 2001; 344:1659–67.

42. Remme WJ, Swedberg K. Guidelines for the Diagnosis and Treatment of Chronic Heart Failure. Task Force of the European Society of Cardiology. Eur Heart J 2001; 22:1527–60.

43. Lichstein E, Morganroth J, Harrist R, Hubble E. Effect of propranolol on ventricular arrhythmia: the Beta-blocker Heart Attack Trial experience. Circulation 1983; 67:I-5–10.

44. Cice G, Tagliamonte E, Ferrara L, Iacono A. Efficacy of carvedilol on complex ventricular arrhythmias in dilated cardiomyopathy: double-blind, randomized, placebo-controlled study. Eur Heart J 2000; 21:1259–64.

45. Navarro-López F, Cosin J, Marrugat J, et al., for the SSSD investigators. Comparison of the effects of amiodarone versus metoprolol on the frequency of ventricular arrhythmias and on mortality after acute myocardial infarction. Am J Cardiol 1993; 72:1243–8.

46. Uretsky BF, Thygesen K, Armstrong PW, et al. Acute coronary findings at autopsy in heart failure patients with sudden death: results from the Assessment of Treatment with Lisinopril And Survival (ATLAS) trial. Circulation 2000; 102:611–16.

47. Leier C, Dei CL, Metra M. Clinical relevance and management of the major electrolyte abnormalities in congestive heart failure: hyponatremia, hypokalemia, and hypomagnesemia. Am Heart J 1994; 128:564–74.

48. Cooper HA, Dries DL, Davis CE, et al. Diuretics and risk of arrhythmic death in patients with left ventricular dysfunction. Circulation 1999; 100:1311–15.

49. Barr CS, Lang CC, Hanson J, et al. Effects of adding spironolactone to an angiotensin-converting enzyme inhibitor in chronic congestive heart failure secondary to coronary artery disease. Am J Cardiol 1995; 76:1259–65.

50. Pitt B, Zannad F, Remme WJ, et al., for the Randomized Aldactone Evaluation Study Investigators. The effect of spironolactone on morbidity and mortality in patients with severe heart failure. N Engl J Med 1999; 341:709–17.

51. Cardiac Arrhythmia Suppression Trial (CAST) Investigators. Preliminary report: effect of encainide and flecainide on mortality in a randomised trial of arrhythmia suppression after myocardial infarction: the Cardiac Arrhythmia Suppression Trial (CAST) Investigators. N Engl J Med 1991; 324:781–8.

52. Hallstrom A, Pratt CM, Greene HL, et al. Relations between heart failure, ejection fraction, arrhythmia suppression and mortality: analysis of the Cardiac Arrhythmia Suppression Trial. J Am Coll Cardiol 1995; 25:1250–7.

53. Flaker GC, Blackshear JL, McBride R, et al. Antiarrhythmic drug therapy and cardiac mortality in atrial fibrillation. J Am Coll Cardiol 1992; 20:527–32.

54. Siebels J, Cappato R, Rüppel R, et al., and the CASH Investigators. ICD versus drugs in cardiac arrest survivors: preliminary results of the Cardiac Arrest Study Hamburg. Pacing Clin Electrophysiol 1993; 16:552–8.

55. Wyse GD, Talajic M, Hafley GE, et al., for the MUSTT Investigators. Antiarrhythmic drug therapy in the Multicenter UnSustained Tachycardia Trial (MUSTT): drug testing and as-treated analysis. J Am Coll Cardiol 2001; 38:344–51.

56. Klein RC, and the ESVEM Investigators. Comparative efficacy of sotalol and class I antiarrhythmic agents in patients with ventricular tachycardia or fibrillation: results of the Electrophysiology Study versus Electrocardiographic Monitoring (ESVEM) trial. Eur Heart J 1993; 14(Suppl H):78–84.

57. Waldo AL, Camm AJ, DeRuyter H, et al. Effect of d-sotalol on mortality in patients with left ventricular dysfunction after recent and remote myocardial infarction. The SWORD Investigators. Survival with Oral d-Solatol. Lancet 1996; 348:7–12.

58. Pratt CM, Camm AJ, Cooper W, et al. Mortality in the Survival With Oral D-sotalol (SWORD)

trial: why did patients die? Am J Cardiol 1998; 81:869–76.

59. Julian DG, Camm AJ, Franglin G, et al., for the European Myocardial Infarct Amiodarone Trial Investigators. Randomised trial of effect of amiodarone on mortality after myocardial infarction in patients with left ventricular dysfunction after recent myocardial infarction: EMIAT. Lancet 1997; 349:667–74.

60. Cairns JA, Connolly SJ, Roberts R, Gent M, for the Canadian Amiodarone Myocardial Infarction Arrhythmia Trial Investigators. Randomised trial of outcome after myocardial infarction in patients with frequent or repetitive ventricular premature depolarisations: CAMIAT. Lancet 1997; 349:675–82.

61. Doval HC, Nul DR, Grancelli HO, et al., for Gruppo de Estudio de la Sobrevida en la Insuficiencia Cardiaca en Argentina (GESICA): randomised trial of low-dose amiodarone in severe congestive heart failure. Lancet 1994; 344:493–8.

62. Singh SN, Fletcher RD, Fisher SG, et al., for the Survival Trial of Antiarrhythmic Therapy in Congestive Heart Failure: amiodarone in patients with congestive heart failure and asymptomatic ventricular arrhythmia. N Engl J Med 1995; 333:77–82.

63. Amiodarone Trials Meta-Analysis Investigators. Effect of prophylactic amiodarone on mortality after acute myocardial infarction and in congestive heart failure: meta-analysis of individual data from 6500 patients in randomised trials. Lancet 1997; 350:1417–24.

64. Connolly SJ, Hallstrom AP, Cappato R, et al., for the Investigators of the AVID, CASH, and CIDS Studies. Meta-analysis of the implantable cardioverter defibrillator secondary prevention trials. Eur Heart J 2000; 21:2071–8.

65. Boutitie F, Boissel JP, Connolly SJ, et al. Amiodarone interaction with beta-blockers: analysis of the merged EMIAT (European Myocardial Infarct Amiodarone Trial) and CAMIAT (Canadian Amiodarone Myocardial Infarction Trial) databases. Circulation 1999; 99:2268–75.

66. Exner DV, Reiffel JA, Epstein AE, et al. Beta-blocker use and survival in patients with ventricular fibrillation or symptomatic ventricular tachycardia: the Antiarrhythmics Versus Implantable Defibrillators (AVID) trial. J Am Coll Cardiol 1999; 34:325–33.

67. Boriani G, Lubinski A, Capucci A, on behalf of Ventricular Arrhythmias Dofetilide Investigators. A multicentre, double-blind randomised crossover comparative study on the efficacy and safety of dofetilide vs sotalol in patients with inducible sustained ventricular tachycardia and ischaemic heart disease. Eur Heart J 2001; 22:1–12.

68. Cardiovascular and Renal Drugs Advisory Committee 87th Meeting. U.S. Food and Drug Administration. January 28, 1999.

69. Torp-Pedersen C, Møller M, Bloch-Thomsen PE, et al., for the Danish Investigations of Arrhythmia and Mortality on Dofetilide Study Group. Dofetilide in patients with congestive heart failure and left ventricular dysfunction. N Engl J Med 1999; 341:857–65.

70. Al-Khalidi H, Brum J, Hislop C, et al. Azimilide reduces the frequency of shocks in patients with an implantable cardioverter defibrillator programmed for pacing and shock: Ansersen–Gill model. Eur Heart J 2000; 21:592 [Abstract].

71. The Antiarrhythmics Versus Implantable Defibrillators (AVID) Investigators. A comparison of antiarrhythmic drug therapy with implantable defibrillators in patients resuscitated from near-fatal ventricular arrhythmias. N Engl J Med 1997; 337:1576–83.

72. Connolly SJ, Gent M, Roberts RS, et al., for the CIDS Investigators. Canadian Implantable Defibrillator Study (CIDS): a randomized trial of the implantable cardioverter defibrillator against amiodarone. Circulation 2000; 101:1297–302.

73. Kuck KH, Cappato R, Siebels J, Rüppel R, for the CASH Investigators. Randomized comparison of antiarrhythmic drug therapy with implantable defibrillators in patients resuscitated from cardiac arrest: the Cardiac Arrest Study Hamburg (CASH). Circulation 2000; 101:748–54.

74. Moss AJ, Hall WJ, Cannom DS, et al. Improved survival with an implanted defibrillator in patients with coronary artery disease at high risk for ventricular arrhythmia: Multicenter Automatic Defibrillator Implantation Trial Investigators. N Engl J Med 1996; 335:1933–40.

75. Buxton AE, Lee KL, Fisher JD, et al., for the Multicenter Unsustained Tachycardia Trial Investigators. A randomized study of the prevention of sudden death in patients with coronary artery disease. N Engl J Med 1999; 341:1882–90.

76. Moss AJ, Zareba W, Hall WJ, et al., for the Multicenter Automatic Defibrillator Implantation Trial II Investigators. Prophylactic implantation of a defibrillator in patients with myocardial infarction and reduced ejection fraction. N Engl J Med 2002; 346:877–83.

77. Bigger JT Jr, Whang W, Rottman JN, et al. Mechanisms of death in the CABG Patch Trial: a randomized trial of implantable cardiac defibrillator prophylaxis in patients at high risk of death after coronary artery bypass graft surgery. Circulation 1999; 99:1416–21.

78. Strickberger SA, for the AMIOVIRT Investigators. Multicenter randomized trial comparing amiodarone to implantable defibrillator in patients with nonischemic cardiomyopathy and asymptomatic nonsustained ventricular tachycardia: AMIOVIRT trial. Circulation 2000; 102:2794.

79. Bänsch D, Antz M, Boczor S, et al., for the CAT Investigators. Primary prevention of sudden cardiac death in idiopathic dilated cardiomyopathy: the Cardiomyopathy Trial (CAT). Circulation 2002; 105:1453–8.

80. Bardy GH, Lee KL, Mark DB, and the SCD-HeFT Pilot Investigators. The Sudden Cardiac Death in Heart Failure Trial: pilot study. Pacing Clin Electrophysiol 1997; 20:1148 [Abstract].

81. Raviele A, Bongiorni MG, Brignole M, et al. Which strategy is 'best' after myocardial infarction? The beta-blocker strategy plus implantable cardioverter defibrillator trial: rationale and study design. Am J Cardiol 1999; 83: 104D–111D.

82. Mathew J, Hunsberger S, Fleg J. et al., for the Digitalis Investigation Group. Incidence, predictive factors, and prognostic significance of supraventricular tachyarrhythmias in congestive heart failure. Chest 2000; 118:914–22.

83. Dries DL, Exner DV, Gersh BJ, et al. Atrial fibrillation is associated with an increased risk for mortality and heart failure progression in patients with asymptomatic and symptomatic left ventricular systolic dysfunction: a retrospective analysis of the SOLVD trials. J Am Coll Cardiol 1998; 32:695–703.

84. Crijns HJGM, Tjeerdsma G, De Kam PJ, et al. Prognostic value of the presence and development of atrial fibrillation in patients with advanced chronic heart failure. Eur Heart J 2000; 21:1238–45.

85. Carson PE, Johnson GR, Dunkman WB, et al., for the V-HeFT VA Cooperative Studies Group. The influence of atrial fibrillation on prognosis in mild to moderate heart failure: the V-HeFT Studies. Circulation 1993; 87:102–10.

86. Pederson OD, Bagger H, Køber L, et al., for the TRACE Study Group. Trandolapril reduces the incidence of atrial fibrillation after acute myocardial infarction in patients with left ventricular dysfunction. Circulation 1999; 100: 376–80.

87. Van Noord T, Van Gelder IC, Van Den Berg M, et al. Pre-treatment with ACE inhibitors enhances cardioversion outcome in patients with persistent atrial fibrillation. Circulation 2001; 104:II-699 [Abstract].

88. Madrid AH, Bueno MG, Rebollo JM, et al. Use of irbesartan to maintain sinus rhythm in patients with long-lasting persistent atrial fibrillation: a prospective and randomized study. Circulation 2002; 331–6.

89. Kühlkamp V, Schirdewan A, Stangl K, et al. Use of metoprolol CR/XL to maintain sinus rhythm after conversion from persistent atrial fibrillation: a randomized, double-blind, placebo-controlled study. J Am Coll Cardiol 2000; 36: 139–46.

90. McMurray JJ, Dargie HJ, Ford I, et al. Carvedilol reduces supraventricular and ventricular arrhythmias after myocardial infarction: evidence from the CAPRICORN study. Circulation 2001; 104:II-700 [Abstract].

91. Lechat P, Hulot JS, Escolano S, et al., on behalf of the CIBIS II Investigators. Heart rate and cardiac rhythm relationships with bisoprolol benefit in chronic heart failure in CIBIS II trial. Circulation 2001; 103:1428–33.

92. The Digitalis in Acute Atrial Fibrillation (DAAF) Trial Group. Results of a randomized, placebo-controlled multicentre trial in 239 patients. Eur Heart J 1997; 18:649–54.

93. Tieleman RG, Blaau Y, Van Gelder IC, et al. Digoxin delays recovery from tachycardia-induced electrical remodeling of the atria. Circulation 1999; 100:1836–42.

94. Pedersen OD, Bagger H, Keller N, et al., for the Danish Investigations of Arrhythmia and Mortality ON Dofetilide Study Group. Efficacy of dofetilide in the treatment of atrial fibrillation–flutter in patients with reduced left ventricular function: a Danish Investigations of Arrhythmia and Mortality on Dofetilide (DIAMOND) Substudy. Circulation 2001; 104:292–6.

95. Van Gelder IC, Crijns HJGM, Van Gilst WH, et al. Prediction of uneventful cardioversion and maintenance of sinus rhythm from direct-current electrical cardioversion of chronic atrial fibrillation and flutter. Am J Cardiol 1991; 68:41–6.

96. Hohnloser SH, Kuck KH, Lilienthal J, for the PIAF Investigators. Rhythm or rate control in atrial fibrillation – Pharmacological Intervention in Atrial Fibrillation (PIAF): a randomised trial. Lancet 2000; 356:1789–94.

97. Carlsson J, Tebbe U. Rhythm control versus rate control in atrial fibrillation: results from the STAF Pilot Study (Strategies of Treatment in Atrial Fibrillation). Pacing Clin Electrophysiol 2001; 24:561 [Abstract].

98. The Atrial Fibrillation Follow-up Investigation of Rhythm Management (AFFIRM) Investigators A Comparison of Rate Control and Rhythm Control in Patients with Atrial Fibrillation. N Engl J Med 2002; 347: 1825–33.

99 Van Gelder IC, Hagens VE, Bosker HA, et al. for the Rate Control versus Electrical Cardioversion for Persistent Atrial Fibrillation Study Group. A Comparison of Rate Control and Rhythm Control in Patients with Recurrent Persistent Atrial Fibrillation. N Engl J Med 2002; 347:1834–40.

100. Vora AM, Goyal VS, Naik AM, et al. Maintenance of sinus rhythm by amiodarone is superior to ventricular rate control in rheumatic atrial fibrillation: a blinded placebo-controlled study. Pacing Clin Electrophysiol 2001; 24:546 [Abstract].

101. Roy D, Talajic M, Dorian P, et al., for the Canadian Trial of Atrial Fibrillation Investigators. Amiodarone to prevent recurrence of atrial fibrillation. N Engl J Med 2000; 342:913–20.

102. Deedwania PC, Singh BN, Ellenbogen K, for the Department of Veterans Affairs CHF-STAT Investigators. Spontaneous conversion and maintenance of sinus rhythm by amiodarone in patients with heart failure and atrial fibrillation: observations from the Veterans Affairs Congestive Heart Failure Survival Trial of Antiarrhythmic Therapy (CHF-STAT). Circulation 1998; 98:2574–9.

103. Singh S, Zoble RG, Yellen L, et al., for the Dofetilide Atrial Fibrillation Investigators. Efficacy and safety of oral dofetilide in converting to and maintaining sinus rhythm in patients with chronic atrial fibrillation or atrial flutter. Circulation 2000; 102:2385–90.

104. Pritchett ELC, Page RL, Connolly SJ, et al. Antiarrhythmic effects of azimilide in atrial fibrillation: efficacy and dose–response. J Am Coll Cardiol 2000; 36:794–802.

105. Connolly SJ, Schnell DJ, Page RL, et al. Dose–response relations of azimilide in the management of symptomatic, recurrent atrial fibrillation. Am J Cardiol 2001; 88:974–9.

106. Camm AJ, Pratt CM, Schwartz PJ, et al. Azimilide Post Infarct Evaluation (ALIVE): azimilide does not affrect mortality in post-myocardial infarction patients. Late-breaking clinical trial abstractsa. Circulation 2001;104:1.

107. Kober L, Bloch-Thompsen PE, Moller M, et al. Effect of dofetilide in patients with recent myocardial infarction and left ventricular dysfunction: a randomized trial. Lancet 2000; 356: 2052–2058.

108. Kay GN, Ellenbogen KA, Giudici M, et al. The Ablate and Pace Trial: a prospective study of catheter ablation of the AV conduction system and permanent pacemaker implantation for treatment of atrial fibrillation. APT Investigators. J Interv Card Electrophysiol 1998; 2:121–35.

109. Twidale N, McDonald T, Nave K, Seal A. Comparison of the effects of AV nodal ablation versus AV nodal modification in patients with congestive heart failure and uncontrolled atrial fibrillation. Pacing Clin Electrophysiol 1998; 21:641–51.

110. Brignole M, Menozzi C, Gianfranchi L, et al. Assessment of atrioventricular junction ablation and VVIR pacemaker versus pharmacological

treatment in patients with heart failure and chronic atrial fibrillation: a randomised controlled study. Circulation 1998; 98:953–60.

111. Becker R, Klinkott R, Bauer A, et al. Multisite pacing for prevention of atrial tachyarrhythmias: potential mechanisms. J Am Coll Cardiol 2000; 35:1939–46.

112. Israel CW, Ehrlich JR, Grönefeld G, et al. Prevalence, characteristics and clinical implications of regular atrial tachyarrhythmias in patients with fibrillation: insights from a study using a new implantable device. J Am Coll Cardiol 2001; 38:355–63.

113. Adler SW, Wolpert C, Warman EN, et al., for the Worldwide Jewel AF Investigators. Efficacy of pacing therapies for treating atrial tachyarrhythmias in patients with ventricular arrhythmias receiving a dual-chamber implantable cardioverter defibrillator. Circulation 2001; 104:887–92.

114. Faggiano P, D'Aloia A, Gualeni A, et al. Mechanisms and immediate outcome of in-hospital cardiac arrest in patients with advanced heart failure secondary to ischemic or idiopathic dilated cardiomyopathy. Am J Cardiol 2001; 87:655–7.

115. Cleland JGF, Erhardt L, Murray G, et al., on behalf of the AIRE Study Investigators. Effect of ramipril on morbidity and mode of death among survivors of acute myocardial infarction with clinical evidence of heart failure: a report from the AIRE Study Investigators. Eur Heart J 1997; 18:41–51.

116. Kjekshus J, Gullestad L. Heart rate as a therapeutic target in heart failure. Eur Heart J 1999; 1(Suppl H):H64–9.

117. Alboni P, Menozzi C, Brignole M, et al. Effects of permanent pacemaker and oral theophylline in sick sinus syndrome. The THEOPACE study: a randomized controlled trial. Circulation 1997; 96:260–6.

118. Alpert MA, Curtis JJ, Sanfelippo JF, et al. Comparative survival following permanent ventricular and dual-chamber pacing for patients with chronic symptomatic sinus node dysfunction with and without congestive heart failure. Am Heart J 1987; 113:958–65.

119. Alpert MA, Curtis JJ, Sanfelippo JF, et al. Comparative survival after permanent ventricular and dual-chamber pacing for patients with chronic high degree atrioventricular block with and without pre-existent congestive heart failure. J Am Coll Cardiol 1986; 7:925–32.

120. Nielsen JC, Andersen HR, Thomsen PE, et al. Heart failure and echocardiographic changes during long-term follow-up of patients with sick sinus syndrome randomised to single-chamber atrial or ventricular pacing. Circulation 1988; 97:987–95.

121. Lamas GA, Orav EJ, Stambler BS, et al., for the Pacemaker Selection in the Elderly Investigators. Quality of life and clinical outcomes in elderly patients treated with ventricular pacing as compared with dual-chamber pacing. N Engl J Med 1998; 338:1097–104.

122. Connolly SJ, Kerr CR, Gent M, et al. Effects of physiologic pacing versus ventricular pacing on the risk of stroke and death due to cardiovascular cause: Canadian Trial of Physiologic Pacing Investigators. N Engl J Med 2000; 342:1385–91.

123. Lamas GA, Lee KL, Sweeney MO, et al., for the Mode Selection Trial in Sinus-Node Dysfunction. Ventricular pacing or dual-chamber pacing for sinus-node dysfunction. N Engl J Med 2002; 346:1854–62.

124. Cazeau S, Leclercq C, Lavergne T, et al., for the Multisite Stimulation in Cardiomyopathies (MUSTIC) Study Investigators. Effects of multisite biventricular pacing in patients with heart failure and intraventricular conduction delay. N Engl J Med 2001; 344:873–80.

125. Abraham VT, Fisher WG, Smith AL, et al., for the MIRACLE Study Group. Cardiac resynchronization in chronic heart failure. N Engl J Med 2001; 346:1845–53.

126. Linde C, Leclercq C, Rex S, et al. Long-term benefits of biventricular pacing in congestive heart failure: results from the MUltisite STimulation In Cardiomyopathy (MUSTIC) study. J Am Coll Cardiol 2002; 40:111–8.

127. Etienne Y, Mansourati J, Gilard M, et al. Evaluation of left ventricular based pacing in patients with congestive heart failure and atrial fibrillation. Am J Cardiol 1999; 83:1138–40.

128. Leon AR, Greenberg JM, Kanuru N, et al. Cardiac resynchronization in patients with congestive heart failure and chronic atrial fibrillation: effect of upgrading to biventricular pacing after chronic right ventricular pacing. J Am Coll Cardiol 2002; 39:1258–63.

129. Higgins SL, Yong P, Scheck D, et al., for the Ventak CHF Investigators. Biventricular pacing diminishes the need for implantable cardioverter defibrillator therapy. J Am Coll Cardiol 2000; 36:824–7.

130. Walker S, Levy TM, Rex S, et al. Usefulness of suppression of ventricular arrhythmia by biventricular pacing in severe congestive heart failure. Am J Cardiol 2000; 86:231–3.

131. Zagrodzky JD, Ramaswamy K, Page RL, et al. Biventricular pacing decreases the inducibility of ventricular tachycardia in patients with ischemic cardiomyopathy. Am J Cardiol 2001; 87: 1208–10.

132. Saxon LA, DeMarco T, Chatterjee K, et al. Chronic biventricular pacing decreases serum norepinephrine in dilated heart failure patients with the greatest sympathetic activation at baseline. Pacing Clin Electrophysiol 1999; 22:830 [Abstract].

133. Hamdan MH, Zagrodzky JD, Joglar JA, et al. Biventricular pacing decreases sympathetic activity compared with right ventricular pacing in patients with depressed ejection fraction. Circulation 2000; 102:1027–32.

13

Heart failure and peripheral vascular disease
Jan Östergren

Introduction

The mortality and morbidity of chronic heart failure has become a major public health issue, as the care of patients with heart failure accounts for a substantial utilization of health care resources.[1] However, the treatment of heart failure patients has improved dramatically during the last decades following the incorporation of the evidence from several large clinical trials in the therapeutic arsenal. Thus, treatment with angiotensin-converting enzyme (ACE) inhibitors,[2] beta-blockers,[3–5] and spironolactone[6] has been shown to be highly beneficial for patients with chronic heart failure. These advances have not been fully implemented in clinical practice, however, as several studies have shown under-treatment of large patient populations. A reason for withholding these effective agents in the treatment of heart failure may be a fear among physicians that certain patient groups may have difficulties in tolerating treatment, or may even have contraindications to treatment, e.g. with beta-blockers or ACE inhibitors. A large example of such a group is most probably patients with peripheral vascular disease, in whom fear of complications from the peripheral vasculature may lead to an unwillingness to use treatments that would otherwise be indicated to relieve symptoms from heart failure and which could considerably improve long-term prognosis. This chapter will discuss the treatment of heart failure in patients with peripheral vascular disease and try to relate the existing evidence of heart failure treatment in this group of patients.

The peripheral circulation in heart failure

A high resistance in the peripheral vasculature is one of the hallmarks of hypertension, which, with or without coexisting ischemic heart disease, is the most common background disease to heart failure in terms of etiology. Consequently, it is evident that there is an important interaction between changes in peripheral vascular resistance and left ventricular function. In more severe stages of heart failure, blood pressure is most often normal or even low, sometimes due to an impaired cardiac output. But, also in such cases, the peripheral vascular resistance is increased due to neurohormonal activation, which attempts to maintain blood pressure at a higher level than would otherwise be possible. A reduced compliance in the peripheral vasculature is also a complicating factor in relation to cardiac performance. Thus, in patients with atherosclerosis the arterial compliance is reduced, which leads to an increased strain on left ventricular systolic performance.

It has been shown that heart failure leads to maladaptive changes in the peripheral circulation and in the skeletal muscle.[7] Impaired peripheral vasodilation occurs in the exercising muscle, which leads to reduced muscle blood flow. A high sympathetic activity due to heart failure may be one of the reasons for this abnormality in vascular tone. Derangements of various types in the skeletal muscle itself are associated with fatigue during exercise; among these are a decrease in capillary-to-muscle fiber ratio and a reduction in aerobic metabolism.[8] Thus, in patients with both peripheral vascular disease and heart failure, several mechanisms contribute to a reduced muscle blood flow and to a poor exercise ability.[9]

Peripheral vascular disease and comorbidity with heart failure

Peripheral vascular disease is common in elderly patients, as is heart failure. It is estimated that 20% of the population in the United States aged over 70 years is afflicted by peripheral vascular disease.[10] Both peripheral vascular disease and heart failure tend to affect the same individuals, as the risk factors are the same: hypertension, hyperlipidemia, smoking, and diabetes are the most important ones.

Although there are no reliable data regarding the prevalence of peripheral vascular disease in patients with heart failure, it is very plausible from the data cited above that considerably more than 20% of heart failure patients also have peripheral vascular disease, either symptomatic or asymptomatic. As indicated previously, the coexistence of peripheral vascular disease and heart failure is an unfortunate combination with regard to exercise ability and may lead to a vicious circle with further deterioration of physical performance and general well-being. Thus, it is important

to try to maintain physical activities in these patients. Structured exercise programs have been evaluated and found to be of benefit.[9]

Pharmacologic treatment of heart failure in patients with peripheral vascular disease

Data on peripheral vascular disease as a background factor in the large heart failure intervention trials are largely lacking. However, peripheral vascular disease has not been an exclusion criterion in these studies. Hence, a substantial proportion of such patients has probably been included in the trials, although separate results in this subset of patients have not been published.

Beta-blockers

The use of beta-blockade in patients with peripheral vascular disease has been questioned due to the potential negative effects on peripheral blood flow. There have been reports of worsening intermittent claudication after institution of beta-blockers. However, conflicting data exist, as some controlled trials have not been able to show a difference between beta-blockers and control treatment with regard to walking distance or symptoms in patients with intermittent claudication. A meta-analysis and a critical review of these studies concluded that beta-blockers are safe in patients with peripheral vascular disease except in the most severely affected patients, in whom the drug should be administered with caution.[11,12]

Thus, intermittent claudication or asymptomatic peripheral vascular disease (i.e. discovered by a low ankle–brachial index) is not a contraindication to beta-blockade in patients with heart failure. It is to be kept in mind that mortality in patients with peripheral vascular disease is not a result of the disease in the peripheral vessels but of complications to the disease in the central vessels, such as myocardial infarction, stroke, and heart failure. Treatment with proven life-saving effects should not be withheld without a very good reason.

Blood pressure lowering drugs in patients with critical limb ischemia

In patients with critical limb ischemia (rest pain or ulcers in combination with an ankle blood pressure below 50 mmHg) the situation is more difficult. In such patients even small changes in blood pressure may result in a detrimental decrease in skin perfusion in the affected area, causing a rapidly evolving gangrene that in some cases may lead to amputation. In patients with critical limb ischemia, beta-blockers as well as other drugs with blood pressure lowering effects should be given only after carefully weighing the potential benefits against the risks. ACE inhibitors should be given as the first-line treatment but with careful surveillance on the effects on systemic and local (ankle) blood pressure as well as on subjective symptoms (pain) and objective signs (local temperature, ulcers).

Trials on beta-blockers

In the MERIT trial there was no excess of withdrawal of metoprolol due to signs of impaired peripheral circulation.[4] However, patients with severe peripheral vascular disease might not have been recruited into the study, as one of the exclusion criteria was 'contraindications for beta-blockers.' In a retrospective analysis of the tolerance to carvedilol in patients with heart failure, the 58 patients with peripheral vascular disease who were included tolerated carvedilol at an equal degree to the rest of the patients.[13] This is thus in accordance with the CIBIS-II[3] and MERIT trials,[4] which were also unable to find baseline predictors of poor tolerance.

In the longer perspective, an improvement of central hemodynamics, due to an optimal pharmacologic treatment of heart failure, for example, may improve the peripheral circulation, leading to a reduced risk for amputation.

Conclusion

In conclusion, patients with intermittent claudication and no signs of severe peripheral ischemia should receive the ordinary evidence-based treatment for heart failure, including ACE inhibitors and beta-blockers. In patients with critical limb ischemia, special attention should be given to the local peripheral circulation when instituting drugs with blood pressure lowering effects. Beta-blockers are generally contraindicated in such patients, but in certain cases the positive effects of beta-blockade in the heart failure situation may be beneficial overall.

References

1. Cowie MR, Mosterd A, Wood DA, et al. The epidemiology of heart failure. Eur Heart J 1997; 18:208–25.

2. Garg R, Yusuf S. Overview of randomized trials of angiotensin-converting enzyme inhibitors on the mortality and morbidity in patients with heart failure. JAMA 1995; 18:1450–5.

3. CIBIS-II Investigators and Committees. The Cardiac Insufficiency Bisoprolol Study II (CIBIS-II). Lancet 1999; 353:9–13.

4. MERIT-HF Study Group. Effect of metoprolol CR/XL in chronic heart failure: Metoprolol CR/XL Randomised Intervention Trial in Congestive Heart Failure (MERIT-HF) Lancet 1999; 353:2001–7.

5. Packer M, Bristow MR, Cohn JN, et al., for the US Carvedilol Heart Failure Study Group. The effect of carvedilol on morbidity and mortality in patients with chronic heart failure. N Engl J Med 1996; 334:1349–55.

6. Pitt B, Zannad F, Remme WJ, et al. Randomized Aldactone Evaluation Study Investigators. The effect of spironolactone on morbidity and mortality in patients with severe heart failure. N Engl J Med 1999; 341:709–17.

7. Schaufelberger M, Eriksson BO, Grimby G, et al. Skeletal muscle fiber composition and capillarization in patients with chronic heart failure: relation to exercise capacity and central hemodynamics. J Card Fail 1995; 1:267–72.

8. Sullivan MJ, Green HJ, Cobb FR. Altered skeletal muscle metabolic response to exercise in chronic heart failure: relation to skeletal muscle aerobic enzyme activity. Circulation 1991; 84:1597–1602.

9. Hiatt WR, Regensteiner JG, Wolfel EE. Special populations in cardiovascular rehabilitation. Peripheral arterial disease, non-insulin dependent diabetes mellitus and heart failure. Card Clin 1993; 11:309–21.

10. Criqui MH, Fronek A, Barret-Connor E, et al. The prevalence of peripheral arterial disease in a defined population. Circulation 1985; 71:510–15.

11. Radack K, Deck C. Beta-adrenergic blocker therapy does not worsen intermittent claudication in subjects with peripheral arterial disease: a meta-analysis of randomized controlled trials. Arch Intern Med 1991; 151:1769–76.

12. Heintzen MP, Strauer BE. Peripheral vascular effects of beta-blockers. Eur Heart J 1994; 15(Suppl C):2–7.

13. Krum H, Ninio D, MacDonald P. Baseline predictors of the tolerability to carvedilol in patients with chronic heart failure. Heart 2000; 84:615–19.

14

Heart failure and depression

Wei Jiang and Christopher M O'Connor

Introduction

Depression, or depressive disorder, is common in patients with heart failure and its presence in such patients is associated with higher risks of mortality and morbidity. Although we await evidence from clinical trials, depression in these patients must be treated without delay. In this chapter, we provide a review of the literature on the relationship between heart failure and depression. Further, we discuss key issues related to diagnosing depression in patients with heart failure and the considerable interventions targeting depressive disorder in this population, based on expert opinion and our own experience.

Prevalence and prognosis of depression in patients with heart failure

Over the past several decades, abundant evidence has emerged to support the adverse impact of depression on ischemic heart disease.[1–5] Recently, several studies have focused on the impact of depression on patients with heart failure. Not surprisingly, depression has been found to be a common occurrence and to be associated with an increased risk of poor prognosis in these patients.

In studies that assessed depression with self-administered questionnaires and standardized

diagnostic psychiatric interviews, the point prevalence of major depressive disorder (*Diagnostic and Statistical Manual* [DSM]-IV criteria) has been reported to be from 14% to 36.5%.[6–8] The variation in rates among those studies likely reflects the different characteristics of patients studied and interpersonal differences in establishing a diagnosis of major depressive disorder. Koenig[8] reported the highest rate (36.5%) in a sample of 107 patients aged 60 or older with heart failure, who were admitted to the general medicine, cardiology, or neurology service of a tertiary-care hospital and stayed on this service for at least 3 days. Patients who were transferred to or from other services or nursing homes were excluded. All 107 patients underwent a standardized diagnostic psychiatric interview by the same psychiatrist. All of these features likely explain the higher rate of major depression in this study compared with others.

In a sample of 357 patients with New York Heart Association (NYHA) class II or greater heart failure, we found the point prevalence of major depression to be 14%.[7] All participants in our study had been screened by a self-administered questionnaire, the Beck Depression Inventory (BDI). Only patients who scored ≥10 on the BDI underwent standardized diagnostic psychiatric interview to diagnose major depressive disorder. Of those patients, 26 patients did not complete the interview, which is probably a major effect on the lower rate of major depression. Ten years ago, Freedland and colleagues reported a 17% incidence of major depression in a sample of 60 patients aged 70 or older with heart failure. In their very recent study of 432 patients aged 40 or older with heart failure, the rate of major depression was estimated at 18%. They noted that the rate of depression was much higher in those under age 65 (24%) than in those age 65 or older (13%) (Freedland, unpublished data). Despite the large variation in incidence in these studies, it is fair to say that the prevalence of major depressive disorder is indeed high in patients with heart failure, probably three to five times higher than its prevalence in the general population.[9]

In addition to major depression, a large proportion of patients with heart failure are considered to have subclinical or minor depression, 16% in our study[7] and 21.5% in Koenig's study,[8] as indicated by self-administered questionnaires, such as the BDI or Center for Epidemiological Studies-Depression (CES-D) scale.

Depression is independently associated with significant adverse prognosis in patients with ischemic heart disease and normal cardiac function.[10-16] Early studies investigating depression in patients with heart failure had failed to show a relationship with outcome, possibly because of inadequate sample sizes or some degree of patient selection bias. In the study by Freedland and colleagues, the 1-year mortality rate was considerably higher for the depressed patients than for the nondepressed patients. That this difference was not statistically significant was thought to reflect too few endpoints, related to the small sample size (total $n = 60$). The study by Koenig showed that although patients with major depression were more likely to have severe medical illness and functional impairment and use more inpatient and outpatient services than the non-

depressed, mortality did not differ significantly between patients with major depression (28.2%) and the nondepressed (20.0%). Again, the lack of significance is likely a result of low power.

In a sample of 357 patients with heart failure, we found that, compared with patients who were not depressed, those with major depression were two to three times more likely to die or be readmitted to the hospital during 1 year of follow-up. This difference had become significant within 3 months after the assessment for depression. More important, the adverse effects of depression on prognosis in patients with heart failure were independent of traditional risk factors such as age, Killip class, and baseline ejection fraction (Table 14.1).[7] Although one easily could conclude that such an adverse association is just an extension of the relationship seen between depression and outcome in ischemic heart disease, the etiology of heart failure (ischemic vs nonischemic) did not alter the results in our study. Clearly, there is another mechanism at work.

Lesperance, Frasure-Smith and colleagues have reported that cardiac patients with a BDI score ≥10, whether they meet the DSM-IV criteria for major depression or not, and whether they have unstable angina or acute myocardial infarction, have significantly higher mortality during an 18-month follow-up compared with patients with a BDI score <10.[13-15,17] In patients with heart failure, we found that mortality among patients with a BDI score ≥10 was almost 2.5 times higher than that among patients with a BDI score <10 at 3 months after depression assessment (Figure 14.1).[7] Morbidity followed a similar pattern. However, such predictive power diminished as time progressed. Murberg et al. followed 119 patients with clinically stable heart failure after assessing the severity of their depressed

Univariate analysis	Odds ratio (95% confidence interval)	P
Mortality at 3 months	2.50 (0.90–6.98)	0.079
Mortality at 1 year	2.23 (1.04–4.77)	0.038
Morbidity at 3 months	1.90 (1.00–3.59)	0.043
Morbidity at 1 year	3.07 (1.41–6.66)	0.005
Multivariate analysis[a]		
Mortality at 3 months	2.74 (0.95–7.87)	0.062
Mortality at 1 year	2.18 (0.97–4.92)	0.059
Morbidity at 3 months	1.86 (0.96–3.63)	0.068
Morbidity at 1 year	2.62 (1.19–5.79)	0.017
Multivariate analysis[b]		
Mortality at 3 months	2.68 (0.93–7.72)	0.068
Mortality at 1 year	2.12 (0.94–4.81)	0.072
Morbidity at 3 months	1.83 (0.93–3.57)	0.079
Morbidity at 1 year	2.57 (1.16–5.68)	0.019

[a] Adjustment for age, Killip class, and baseline ejection fraction.
[b] Adjustment for age, Killip class, baseline ejection fraction, and etiology of heart failure.
Data from Jiang et al.[7]

Table 14.1 Odds of mortality and morbidity in patients with heart failure and major depressive disorder vs no depression

mood by means of the Zung depression scale.[18] They found that for every 1-point increase in the depression scale, the hazard ratio was 1.08 in multivariate modeling, indicating that the severity of depressed mood was linearly related to decreased survival during a 2-year follow-up period.

Many possible mechanisms could explain the poorer outcomes in patients with heart failure and depression. First, depressed patients generally are in a higher NYHA class than are nondepressed patients, which may represent greater deterioration in cardiopulmonary function, increased fluid retention, or both. This finding could explain reports of greater somatic symptoms[19,20] and diminished functional status[21] in depressed patients. Patients with heart failure and depression also have been found to have or perceive reduced social contacts and support networks[18,22–26]

and to have lesser compliance with treatment.[27,28] Furthermore, platelet aggregation may be greater in patients with depression compared with the nondepressed.[29] Finally, heart rate variability is reduced in patients with depression.[30,31] Decreased heart rate variability has been shown to be associated with poorer prognosis in the heart failure population[32] and in patients with ischemic heart disease.[33,34]

Diagnosis of depression in patients with heart failure

According to the DSM-IV criteria, a major depressive episode is diagnosed when five or more symptoms listed in the DSM-IV[9] have been present for at least 2 weeks. If symptoms include either depressed or dysphoric mood or

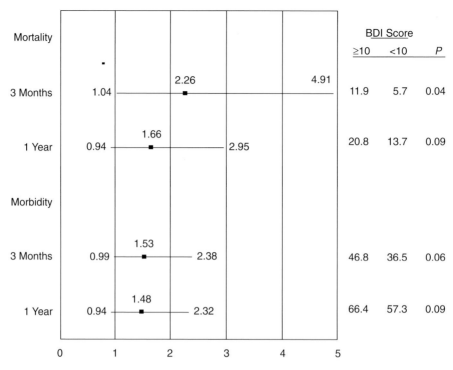

				BDI Score		
				≥10	<10	*P*
Mortality						
3 Months	1.04	2.26	4.91	11.9	5.7	0.04
1 Year	0.94	1.66	2.95	20.8	13.7	0.09
Morbidity						
3 Months	0.99	1.53	2.38	46.8	36.5	0.06
1 Year	0.94	1.48	2.32	66.4	57.3	0.09

Figure 14.1 Mortality and morbidity at 3 months and 1 year after depression assessment, by BDI score. Data from Jiang et al.[7]

pervasive loss of interest or pleasure in daily activities, it is no longer necessary to meet the requirement of having at least five symptoms to establish the diagnosis. If patients have less than five but at least two of the listed symptoms with either depressed mood or loss of interest or symptoms lasting for 2 weeks or longer, a minor depressive disorder is diagnosed.

Although less common, but because of the significantly different treatment approach and prognosis, it is important to exclude the possibility that patients may have bipolar disorder or schizoaffective disorder. In addition, substance-abuse or dependence-related depressive disorder must be differentiated. Premenstrual dysphoric disorder should be considered when interviewing premenopausal female patients. Finally, although suicidal ideation has appeared extremely infrequently in our experience[7] and that

of others, any patient expressing such thoughts requires immediate psychiatric evaluation.

Hypothyroidism is a common medical problem that is related to clinical depression as well as to heart failure. Thyroid function should be tested routinely in all patients with depressive symptoms, and hypothyroidism should be treated with synthetic thyroid hormone. Neurovegetative symptoms of depressive disorder – fatigue, sleep disturbance, weight gain or loss, poor appetite, etc. – that develop in a physically healthy person can assist in identification of depression, but they are not particularly indicative of depression in patients with heart failure. The following symptoms or complaints usually are helpful in identification of patients suffering from depressive disorder: reduced or lack of interest in previously pleasurable activities or hobbies, sadness or grieving without clear reason, passivity, low or diminished spirits, or getting upset easily at minor things that are not typically bothersome.

In practical terms, simply asking patients about their spirit or mood can offer clues. Evidence of noncompliance with medications or risk modifications, frequent visits to the clinic or emergency room, or somatic complaints not well-explained by pathophysiological findings warrants assessment for depression. Because more than one-third of patients with heart failure (who are preoccupied by their heart condition and unaware of their mental illness) suffer from some degree of depression, the nonpsychiatric professionals they often encounter, such as primary care physicians and cardiologists, must be vigilant in the recognition of depression.

Self-administered questionnaires such as the BDI[35] and the CES-D scale[36] can be used as screening tools. Patients should be informed about the purpose for the questionnaires. Patients who score positively on items targeting emotional activities – such as feeling sad, discouraged, impatient or easily irritated, like a failure, as though being punished, worthless, or uninterested or less interested in other people – are likely to have some degree of depression or other mental illness, regardless of the total scores on the scale. Patients are more likely to be depressed if they have had previous depression or if a family member has had depression.

Concomitant medications utilized in heart failure and depression

Soon after the beta-adrenergic receptor-blocking agent propranolol was approved for the treatment of hypertension in the United States, concern arose that it was associated with an increased risk of depression.[37] More cases linking other beta-blockers to depression were then reported,[38–44] which resulted in hesitation in prescribing beta-blockers for patients with signs of depression who otherwise would have been benefited from such treatment. Other researchers have found no such association between the use of beta-blockers and increased depression.[45–48]

The most convincing data are likely tobe that of Gerstman et al., who followed new users of beta-blockers (propranolol users, $n = 704$; other beta-blockers, $n = 587$) for 6 months for the occurrence of depression, as well as patients taking calcium channel blockers ($n = 742$), diuretics ($n = 773$), and angiotensin-converting enzyme (ACE) inhibitors ($n = 976$).[49] The rates of major depression in the users of beta-blockers and users of other drugs were 5.8/1000 and 9.6/1000 person-years, respectively, whereas the estimated annual incidence of major depression is 15.9 per 1000 persons according to the population-based Epidemiologic Catchment Area Study of the National Institute of Mental Health.[50] The relative risk of major depression associated with the use of beta-blockers was 0.5 (95% confidence interval, 0.0–2.5) compared with no beta-blocker.

Although depression also was reported to be associated with the use of some ACE inhibitors, Gerstman's study revealed a rate of major depression much lower than the estimated annual incidence (7.9 vs 15.9/1000 person-years). The rate of depression in this study was highest among patients taking calcium channel blockers, but even this rate (12.7/1000 person-years) was lower than the estimated annual incidence. Patients taking diuretics (hydrochlorothiazide or combined triamterene/hydrochlorothiazide) had a rate of major depression of 9.3/1000 person-years.

Spironolactone and digitalis, both commonly prescribed for patients with heart failure, were not included in the Gerstman study. In a sample of 190 patients who had had myocardial infarction, Schleifer et al. found that digitalis treatment was associated with increased depression during 3–4 months of follow-up ($P < 0.05$).[46] Duplication of this finding in larger samples and in heart failure populations will be needed. The recommendation at present is to monitor for depressive symptoms if patients are taking digitalis. Discontinuation of digitalis, psychiatric care, or both may be needed with new or worsening depression. Spironolactone has not been reported to be associated with depression.

There is some evidence that pindolol, the beta-adrenoceptor/5-hydroxytryptamine-1A receptor antagonist, can augment the action of certain antidepressant drugs, especially the selective serotonin-reuptake inhibitors (SSRIs),[51,52] and of electroconvulsive therapy.[53] It may be considered a better choice for beta-blockade in depressed patients with heart failure, although its prognostic effects must be further investigated in these patients.

Interventions for depression in patients with heart failure

Despite its high prevalence and poor prognostic outcome, depressive disorder as a comorbid illness in patients with heart diseases is underdiagnosed and undertreated.[54] In a recent survey study of depression,[7] we noted that only about one in five in patients with heart failure who met DSM-IV criteria for major depression were prescribed an antidepressant at discharge. This phenomenon could be attributed to underrecognition of depression and its impact, concern about the side effects of antidepressants, or a lack of supporting evidence for treatment of depression in this population.

Current approaches for treatment of depression include antidepressant drugs, psychotherapy, and electroconvulsive therapy, or some combination of these. The major goals of treatment are to reduce the intensity of depressive symptoms, improve the level of daily functioning, and prevent suicide. Antidepressants have been broadly chosen as the first approach for comorbid depression in patients with medical illnesses. Besides being the treatment of choice for major depressive episodes, antidepressants also are indicated for chronic mild depression or dysthymia and may be helpful in minor or subclinical depression, which puts patients at higher risk of chronic or recurrent major depression. The anxiolytic properties of antidepressants can also substantially reduce the irritability or hostility of many patients.

All clinically useful antidepressants potentiate, either directly or indirectly, the action of norepinephrine (noradrenaline), dopamine, or serotonin in the brain through interaction with receptors or alteration of the level(s) of particular neurotransmitter(s). These actions provide the pharmacologic foundation for the current classifications of various antidepressants: the classic antidepressants, monoamine oxidase (MAO) inhibitors and tricyclic antidepressants; the SSRIs; and the noradrenergic- and dopamine-reuptake blockers. Newer agents include the dual serotonin- and noradrenergic-reuptake inhibitors, alpha-2 antagonists, which affect both serotonin and noradrenergic action, and dual serotonin 2A antagonists/serotonin-reuptake inhibitors.

Similar efficacy for depression among the various antidepressants (about 65%) has been supported by many well-controlled studies against placebo (35%).[55] However, side-effect profiles of each class and each agent within a class differ considerably, presumably because of their interaction with neurotransmitters and their metabolic mechanisms, making them the basis for antidepressant selection for targeted populations. The famous Cardiac Arrhythmia Suppression Trials (CAST)[56–58] taught clinicians that the safety profile of an agent is no less important than its efficacy when applying it to a patient. Further, the deleterious effects of class I antiarrhythmic agents in patients with ischemic heart disease shown in the CAST studies call into doubt the presumed relative safety of tricyclic antidepressants in these patients, given that they are, in fact, type IA antiarrhythmics.

The relative safety of short-term use of SSRIs and other newer antidepressants, such as bupropion and mirtazapine, has been assessed through changes in heart rate, blood pressure, and electrocardiographic characteristics in depressed patients with and without heart disease. These agents have been reported to have no cardiotoxic effects compared with tricyclic antidepressants.[59–66] Bupropion was not found to have the cardiotoxicity of tricyclic antidepressants, but Kiev et al. showed that it was associated with mean increases in supine diastolic blood pressure, ranging from 5.6 mmHg on day 7 to 7.5 mmHg on day 28 in patients with major depression and no underlying heart disease.[63] Venlafaxine, another newer antidepressant, has not been associated with clinically significant conduction abnormalities or arrhythmia, but its potential to elevate blood pressure cautions against its use in patients with concomitant cardiovascular disease.[67,68] Trazodone appears to have no anticholinergic or quinidine-like properties compared with amitriptyline in depressed non-cardiac patients, but it did show minor effects on systolic time intervals.[69] The orthostatic hypotension related to trazodone use makes it less favorable for cardiac patients. Whether nefazodone may be relatively safer in patients with heart disease and depression is unknown. Despite their high efficacy, MAO inhibitors generally are reserved for patients who are unresponsive or unable to tolerate other antidepressants, because of the restrictions in diet required with MAO use. They are not recommended for patients with heart diseases because of the potential for hypertensive crisis and its sympathomimetic effects, which interfere with other medications commonly used in these patients. Mirtazapine, one of the newest tricyclic antidepressants, has been found to relieve not only depressive symptoms but also anxiety and insomnia. The major concern with its use in patients with heart diseases is the potential for weight gain.

Among the available antidepressants, the SSRIs have been considered the better choice for patients with heart diseases, given their limited cardiotoxicity, lack of increase in seizure risk, and lesser associated weight gain. Recently, the Sertraline AntiDepressant HeaRt Attack Trial (SADHART) compared the efficacy and safety of sertraline, an SSRI, vs placebo in a multicenter, randomized, double-blind trial of inpatients with recent (≤30 days) myocardial infarction or unstable angina and comorbid major depression. In this study, sertraline significantly improved depression during 24 weeks of treatment. There also were trends toward reduced mortality and morbidity in the sertraline arm, but, possibly because of the relatively small sample size, the differences did not reach statistical significance.[70]

The SSRIs alter the activity of the cytochrome-P450 metabolic pathway. This pathway is also involved in the breakdown of many drugs taken by patients with heart disease, including beta-blockers, warfarin, type I antiarrhythmics, and calcium channel blockers. As a result, significant adverse drug interactions can occur with the use of SSRIs in these patients. On the other hand, each SSRI interacts differently with the cytochrome-P450 enzymes, and careful selection of an SSRI may reduce the risk of adverse effects from drug interactions. Results from clinical trials in this regard are lacking. Table 14.2 lists the commonly encountered cytochrome-P450 enzymes and the cardiovascular and psychiatric medications that they metabolize.

The other important question in the treatment of comorbid depression in heart failure is whether it can modify or aggravate the poor prognosis of these patients. To date, all investigations have targeted patients with normal cardiac function. Patients with unstable angina or recent myocardial infarction who showed clinical signs of heart failure or a left ventricular ejection fraction <35% were excluded from the SADHART study. The pathophysiological features and biochemical alterations of heart failure uniquely affect drug absorption, metabolism, and excretion in patients with heart disease and compensated or normal range of cardiac function. Although evidence is lacking, these factors must be considered when using antidepressants in patients with heart failure. The full results of the SADHART trial, and a large randomized, controlled clinical trial (ENhancing Recovery In Coronary Heart Disease [ENRICHD]) of the safety and efficacy of cognitive behavioral therapy in patients with recent myocardial infarction and comorbid major depression or social isolation, should be available soon. The results

	Substrate	Inducer	Inhibitor
CYP2C9	Irbesartan, losartan, torsemide, warfarin (s-warfarin)	Fluoxetine	Amiodarone, fluvastatin, warfarin (r-warfarin) Fluoxetine > fluvoxamine > paroxetine > sertraline > citalopram
CYP2D6	Captopril Labetalol, carvedilol, metoprolol, penbutolol, pindolol, propranolol, timolol Encainide, flecainide, mexiletine, propafenone		Amiodarone, propafenone, quinidine Diltiazem, labetalol, paroxetine > fluoxetine = fluvoxamine > sertraline > citalopram
CYP3A3/4	Amiodarone, digoxin, quinidine, lidocaine, atorvastatin, cerivastatin, lovastatin, simvastatin, bepridil, diltiazem, felodipine, nifedipine, nicardipine, nimodipine, verapamil, enalapril, losartan, warfarin (r-warfarin) Fluvoxamine, fluoxetine, sertraline		Amiodarone, quinidine, diltiazem, verapamil Fluvoxamine > sertraline > fluoxetine > paroxetine > citalopram

Table 14.2 Commonly encountered cytochrome P-450 enzymes and cardiovascular and psychiatric medications that they metabolize

of these two trials may assist in the selection of antidepressive treatment in patients with heart failure.

For patients whose depression is severe, intractable, or life-threatening, requiring immediate relief, electroconvulsive therapy is recommended for its high efficacy and relative safety. Evidence suggests that most patients with an underlying cardiac condition can undergo electroconvulsion, if appropriate precautions are taken before the procedure.[71]

In summary, patients with heart failure are more likely than the general population to suffer from depression. Patients with heart failure and comorbid depression are at higher risk of death or rehospitalization than their nondepressed counterparts. Nonpsychiatric clinicians must be vigilant about recognition of and proper intervention for depression. Although antidepressants, particularly the SSRIs, are recommended as first-line treatment for depression in patients with heart failure, evidence from randomized trials is lacking. Drug safety requires particular attention when antidepressants are used, especially the potential for drug interactions. Clinical trials of the efficacy and safety of different interventions for depression are critical to improve outcomes in these patients.

References

1. Hallstrom T, Lapidus L, Bengtsson C, et al. Psychosocial factors and risk of ischaemic heart disease and death in women: a twelve-year follow-up of participants in the population study of women in Gothenburg, Sweden. J Psychosom Res 1986; 30:451–9.
2. Anda R, Williamson D, Jones D, et al. Depressed affect, hopelessness, and the risk of ischemic heart disease in a cohort of U.S. adults. Epidemiology 1993; 4:285–94.
3. Barefoot JC, Helms MJ, Mark DB, et al. Depression and long-term mortality risk in patients with coronary artery disease. Am J Cardiol 1996; 78:613–17.
4. Pratt LA, Ford DE, Crum RM, et al. Depression, psychotropic medication, and risk of myocardial infarction: prospective data from the Baltimore ECA follow-up. Circulation 1996; 94:3123–9.
5. Ford DE, Mead LA, Chang PP, et al. Depression is a risk factor for coronary artery disease in men: the precursors study. Arch Intern Med 1998; 158:1422–6.
6. Freedland KE, Carney RM, Krone RJ, et al. Psychological factors in silent myocardial ischemia. Psychosom Med 1991; 53:13–24.
7. Jiang W, Alexander J, Christopher E, et al. Relationship of depression to increased risk of mortality and rehospitalization in patients with congestive heart failure. Arch Intern Med 2001; 161:1849–56.
8. Koenig HG. Depression in hospitalized older patients with congestive heart failure. Gen Hosp Psychiatry 1998; 20:29–43.
9. American Psychiatric Association. Diagnostic and Statistical Manual of Mental Disorders, 4. Washington, DC: American Psychiatric Association, 1994.
10. Schleifer SJ, Macari-Hinson MM, Coyle DA, et al. The nature and course of depression following myocardial infarction. Arch Intern Med 1989; 149:1785–9.
11. Ahern DK, Gorkin L, Anderson JL, et al. Biobehavioral variables and mortality or cardiac arrest in the Cardiac Arrhythmia Pilot Study (CAPS). Am J Cardiol 1990; 66:59–62.

12. Ladwig KH, Kieser M, Konig J, et al. Affective disorders and survival after acute myocardial infarction. Eur Heart J 1991; 12:959–64.

13. Frasure-Smith N, Lesperance F, Talajic M. Depression following myocardial infarction. Impact on 6-month survival. JAMA 1993; 270:1819–25.

14. Frasure-Smith N, Lesperance F, Talajic M. Depression and 18-month prognosis after myocardial infarction. Circulation 1995; 91:999–1005.

15. Frasure-Smith N, Lesperance F, Juneau M, et al. Gender, depression, and one-year prognosis after myocardial infarction. Psychosom Med 1999; 61:26–37.

16. Kaufmann MW, Fitzgibbons JP, Sussman EJ, et al. Relation between myocardial infarction, depression, hostility, and death. Am Heart J 1999; 138:549–54.

17. Lesperance F, Frasure-Smith N, Juneau M, et al. Depression and 1-year prognosis in unstable angina. Arch Intern Med 2000; 160:1354–60.

18. Murberg TA, Bru E, Svebak S, et al. Depressed mood and subjective health symptoms as predictors of mortality in patients with congestive heart failure: a two-years follow-up study. Int J Psychiatry Med 1999; 29:311–26.

19. Waxman HM, McCreary G, Weinrit RM, et al. A comparison of somatic complaints among depressed and non-depressed older persons. Gerontologist 1985; 25:501–7.

20. Lesperance F, Frasure-Smith N, Talajic M. Major depression before and after myocardial infarction: its nature and consequences. Psychosom Med 1996; 58:99–110.

21. Sullivan MD, LaCroix AZ, Baum C, et al. Functional status in coronary artery disease: a one-year prospective study of the role of anxiety and depression. Am J Med 1997; 103:348–56.

22. Myers JK, Weissman MM, Tischler GL, et al. Six-month prevalence of psychiatric disorders in three communities 1980 to 1982. Arch Gen Psychiatry 1984; 41:959–67.

23. Krishnan KR, George LK, Pieper CF, et al. Depression and social support in elderly patients with cardiac disease. Am Heart J 1998; 136:491–5.

24. Zipfel S, Lowe B, Paschke T, et al. Psychological distress in patients awaiting heart transplantation. J Psychosom Res 1998; 45:465–70.

25. Steffens DC, O'Connor CM, Jiang WJ, et al. The effect of major depression on functional status in patients with coronary artery disease. J Am Geriatr Soc 1999; 47:319–22.

26. Dracup K, Walden JA, Stevenson LW, et al. Quality of life in patients with advanced heart failure. J Heart Lung Transplant 1992; 11:273–9.

27. Blumenthal JA, Williams RS, Wallace AG, et al. Physiological and psychological variables predict compliance to prescribed exercise therapy in patients recovering from myocardial infarction. Psychosom Med 1982; 44:519–27.

28. Richardson JL, Marks G, Johnson CA, et al. Path model of multidimensional compliance with cancer therapy. Health Psychol 1987; 6:183–207.

29. Musselman DL, Tomer A, Manatunga AK, et al. Exaggerated platelet reactivity in major depression. Am J Psychiatry 1996; 153:1313–17.

30. Krittayaphong R, Cascio WE, Light KC, et al. Heart rate variability in patients with coronary artery disease: differences in patients with higher and lower depression scores. Psychosom Med 1997; 59:231–5.

31. Watkins LL, Grossman P. Association of depressive symptoms with reduced baroreflex cardiac control in coronary artery disease. Am Heart J 1999; 137:453–7.

32. Jiang W, Hathaway WR, McNulty S, et al. Ability of heart rate variability to predict prognosis in patients with advanced congestive heart failure. Am J Cardiol 1997; 80:808–11.

33. Kleiger RE, Miller JP, Bigger JT Jr, et al. Decreased heart rate variability and its association with increased mortality after acute myocardial infarction. Am J Cardiol 1987; 59:256–62.

34. Carney RM, Saunders RD, Freedland KE, et al. Association of depression with reduced heart rate variability in coronary artery disease. Am J Cardiol 1995; 76:562–4.

35. Beck AT, Ward CH, Mendelson M, et al. An inventory for measuring depression. Arch Gen Psychiatry 1961; 4:561–71.

36. Radloff LS. The CES-D scale: a self-report depression scale for research in the general population. Appl Psychol Measure 1977; 1:385–401.

37. Waal HJ. Propranolol-induced depression. Br Med J 1967; 2:50.

38. Petrie WM, Maffucci RJ, Woosley RL. Propranolol and depression. Am J Psychiatry 1982; 139:92–4.

39. Nolan BT. Acute suicidal depression associated with use of timolol. JAMA 1982; 247:1567.

40. Kalayam B, Shamoian CA. Propranolol, psychoneuroendocrine changes, and depression. Am J Psychiatry 1982; 139:1374–5.

41. Faber R. Nadolol and antidepressant response. Biol Psychiatry 1983; 18:1338–9.

42. Pollack MH, Rosenbaum JF, Cassem NH. Propranolol and depression revisited: three cases and a review. J Nerv Mental Dis 1985; 173: 118–19.

43. Avorn J, Everitt DE, Weiss S. Increased antidepressant use in patients prescribed beta-blockers. JAMA 1986; 255:357–60.

44. Thiessen BQ, Wallace SM, Blackburn JL, et al. Increased prescribing of antidepressant subsequent to beta-blocker therapy. Arch Intern Med 1990; 150:2286–90.

45. Carney RM, Rich MW, teVelde A, et al. Prevalence of major depressive disorder in patients receiving beta-blocker therapy versus other medications. Am J Med 1987; 83:223–9.

46. Schleifer SJ, Slater WR, Macari-Hinson MM, et al. Digitalis and beta-blocking agents: effects on depression following myocardial infarction. Am Heart J 1991; 121:1397–402.

47. Bright RA, Everitt DE. B-blockers and depression. Evidence against an association. JAMA 1992; 267:1783–7.

48. Sorgi P, Patey J, Knoedler D, et al. Depression during treatment with beta-blockers: results from a double-blind placebo-controlled study. J Neuropsychiatry Clin Neurosci 1998; 4:187–9.

49. Gerstman BB, Jolson HM, Bauer M, et al. The incidence of depression in new users of beta-blockers and selected antihypertensives. J Clin Epidemiol 1996; 49:809–15.

50. Eaton WW, Dryman A, Sorenson A, McCutcheon A. DSM-III major depressive disorder in the community. A latent class analysis of data from the NIMH epidemiologic catchment area programme. Br J Psychiatry 1989; 155:48–54.

51. Rasanen P, Hakko H, Tiihonen J, Mitchell B. Balter Award – 1998. Pindolol and major affective disorders: a three-year follow-up study of 30,485 patients. J Clin Psychopharmacol 1999; 19:297–302.

52. Perez V, Puiigdemont D, Gilaberte I, et al., for the Grup de Recerca en Trastorns Afectius. Augmentation of fluoxetine's antidepressant action by pindolol: analysis of clinical, pharmacokinetic, and methodologic factors. J Clin Psychopharmacol 2001; 21:36–45.

53. Shiah IS, Yatham LN, Srisurapanont M, et al. Does the addition of pindolol accelerate the response to electroconvulsive therapy in patients with major depression? A double-blind, placebo-controlled pilot study. J Clin Psychopharmacol 2000; 20:373–8.

54. Sheline YI, Freedland KE, Carney RM. How safe are serotonin reuptake inhibitors for depression in patients with coronary heart disease. Am J Med 1997; 102:54–9.

55. Frank E, Kupfer DJ, Perel JM, et al. Three-year outcomes for maintenance therapies in recurrent depression. Arch Gen Psychiatry 1990; 47:1093–9.

56. The Cardiac Arrhythmia Suppression Trial (CAST) Investigators. Preliminary report: effect of encainide and flecainide on mortality in a randomized trial of arrhythmia suppression after myocardial infarction. N Engl J Med 1989; 321: 406–12.

57. Greene HL, Roden DM, Katz RJ, et al. The Cardiac Arrhythmia Suppression Trial: first CAST . . . then CAST-II. J Am Coll Cardiol 1992; 19:894–8.

58. Epstein AE, Hallstrom AP, Rogers WJ, et al. Mortality following ventricular arrhythmia suppression by encainide, flecainide, and moricizine after myocardial infarction. JAMA 1993; 270: 2451–5.

59. Roose SP, Glassman AH, Giardina EG, et al. Cardiovascular effects of imipramine and bupropion in depressed patients with congestive heart failure. J Clin Psychopharmacol 1987; 7:247–51.

60. Roose SP, Dalack GW, Glassman AH, et al. Cardiovascular effects of bupropion in depressed patients with heart disease. Am J Psychiatry 1991; 148:512–16.

61. Upward JW, Edwards JG, Goldie A, et al. Comparative effects of fluoxetine and amitriptyline on cardiac function. Br J Clin Pharmacol 1988; 26:399–402.

62. Laird LK, Lydiard RB, Morton WA, et al. Cardiovascular effects of imipramine, fluvoxamine, and placebo in depressed outpatients, J Clin Psychiatry 1993; 54:224–8.

63. Kiev A, Masco HL, Wenger TL, et al. The cardiovascular effects of bupropion and nortriptyline in depressed outpatients. Ann Clin Psychiatry 1994; 6:107–15.

64. Hewer W, Rost W, Gattaz WF. Cardiovascular effects of fluvoxamine and maprotiline in depressed patients. Eur Arch Psychiatry Clin Neurosci 1995; 246:1–6.

65. Tulen JH, Bruijin JA, de Man KJ, et al. Cardiovascular variability in major depressive disorder and effects of imipramine or mirtazapine (Org 3770). J Clin Psychopharmacol 1996; 16: 135–45.

66. Baker B, Dorian P, Sandor P, et al. Electrocardiographic effects of fluoxetine and doxepin in patients with major depressive disorder. J Clin Psychopharmacol 1997; 17: 15–21.

67. Feighner JP. Cardiovascular safety in depressed patients: focus on venlafaxine. J Clin Psychiatry 1995; 56:574–9.

68. Thase ME. Effects of venlafaxine on blood pressure: a meta-analysis of original data from 3744 depressed patients. J Clin Psychiatry 1998; 59:502–8.

69. van de Merwe TJ, Silverstone T, Ankier SI, et al. A double-blind non-crossover placebo-controlled study between group comparison of trazodone and amitriptyline on cardiovascular function in major depressive disorder. Psychopathology 1984; 17:64–76.

70. Glassman AH. SADHART preliminary results. Presented at the 2001 American Psychiatric Association Annual Meeting, New Orleans, May 2001.

71. Rayburn BK. Electroconvulsive therapy in patients with heart failure or valvular heart disease. Convulsive Ther 1997; 13:145–56.

Index

Note: References to figures are indicated by 'f' and references to tables are indicated by 't' when they fall on a page not covered by the text reference.